THE POLITICS OF MENTAL HEALTH

THE POLITICS OF
MENTAL HEALTH

Organizing Community Mental Health

in Metropolitan Areas

Robert H. Connery

Charles H. Backstrom · David R. Deener

Julian R. Friedman · Morton Kroll · Robert H. Marden

Clifton McCleskey · Peter Meekison

John A. Morgan, Jr.

1968

COLUMBIA UNIVERSITY PRESS

New York and London

The authors' research was supported by a grant
from the National Institute of Mental Health.

PREFACE

IN AN AGE of rapid advances in the care of the mentally ill and emotionally disturbed, one should not forget the importance of the political framework in which public programs must operate. For the first time in history the federal government is becoming heavily involved in mental health programs, an area long thought to be the exclusive domain of the states. But the new approach relies quite as much on local communities as on the federal government, and the states have by no means withdrawn from the field. Thus, in the future, government mental health programs will involve federal, state, and local political agencies as well as voluntary ones. Sound intergovernmental relations in planning and operating programs consequently become a major objective.

The goal of local participation, however, presents difficulties. The majority of the American people today live in some 200 metropolitan communities varying in population from 50,000 to several million. The modern metropolis, however, is not a legal political entity but rather a miscellaneous collection of cities, counties, villages, and independent districts. As mental health programs develop they will depend more and more upon coordination with other community services which bear upon the individual's normal growth and development, such as schools, recreation facilities, housing, mass transportation, and special public health and welfare services. At the local level, in a single metropolitan community, these may be provided by hundreds of different school districts, townships, counties, boroughs, and municipalities.

The purpose of this study is to demonstrate the effect of fragmented government in metropolitan urban areas on mental health programing; to indicate ways to overcome obstacles that fragmentation presents in developing new mental health programs; and to indicate the range of political and administrative accommodations which might be made to assure full utilization of community resources in mental health programing. The study suggests patterns of action to cope with the confusion which divided responsibilities introduce into the planning and operation of mental health programs. Thus, it should be of value both to mental health administrators and to political leaders who must deal with mental health problems in their communities.

Recent studies concerned with health have emphasized the impact of metropolitan living on mental health and the consequent need for counteraction. The Joint Commission on Mental Illness and Health report emphasized again and again the importance of mobilizing community agencies at the local level to promote mental health more effectively. But can effective community action be brought about in rapidly growing urban areas whose government is as fragmented as that of most American metropolitan areas?

The problem of fragmentation is not limited, of course, to mental health services. The report of the Committee on Environmental Health Problems sponsored by the Public Health Service noted that "most threats to environmental health cover geographic areas which are larger than the traditional political boundaries which constitute the basic state and local governmental system of this country. The problem of fragmented government is particularly acute in metropolitan areas, and it is in these areas that the problems of environmental health are most serious. Further, these health problems are no respecters of the boundaries which divide these areas into literally hundreds of semi-independent principalities."

If there were any hope that the problems of government fragmentation would be met by political action in the near future and if government in metropolitan communities were to be reorganized on some more rational basis, the matter could be safely left to political means. But there is no evidence that the situation will change materially in the foreseeable future. Thus, the development of a comprehensive program of mental health centers must be accommodated to the existing structure of government. Political fragmentation, therefore, becomes a problem with which mental health planners and administrators will have to cope.

Political scientists have not been much concerned with the area of policy programs in recent years, although there have been a few exceptions. The analysis of the field of public health in general is of unusual value in considering the total American governmental system. Mental health offers the additional advantage of being currently in a state of dynamic expansion. Insights about program formulation, intergovernmental relations, and community dynamics in mental health may be useful for the political scientist interested in the broad implications of political action.

This study developed from discussions over a period of years in the National Institute of Mental Health (NIMH) Committee on Social and Environmental Variables as Determinants of Mental Health, better known in Washington as "The Space Cadets" because of the wide-ranging nature of the topics discussed. The committee, made up of psychiatrists, psychologists, biologists, economists, and political scientists, was the brainchild of its chairman, Dr. Leonard Duhl, who early recognized the impact of social conditions as a factor in mental health. Dr. Duhl played a leading role in expanding research to include appropriate community action to assist in preventing mental illness. I am greatly indebted to him for encouraging this study.

The dimensions of mental health and public health programs have always been ambiguous. Sometimes they have been combined, and sometimes they have been separated under different government agencies. In an endeavor to understand this relationship I undertook a study of mental health activities in Philadelphia, New Orleans, and the North Carolina crescent in 1961, which was later published in mimeograph form by NIMH under the title *Mental Health in Metropolitan Areas: A Pilot Study*. The Institute of Public Administration in New York City acted as housekeeper for the project. Professor David Deener of Tulane University and Professor Bert Swanson of Sarah Lawrence were co-authors of the study.

The impending passage of the Kennedy Mental Health Act in 1963 led to the present study, which was also supported by a grant from NIMH. Duke University in North Carolina was the original home of the project, but in 1966 it was transferred to Columbia University in New York City. Six field studies in widely separated but representative metropolitan areas were the bases for the project.

The original staff consisted of Professor John A. Morgan, Jr., now of George Washington University; Professor Peter Meekison, now at the University of Alberta; and Professor David R. Deener, now Provost of Tulane University. As the six field studies got under way, the staff was expanded to include Professors Charles H. Backstrom of the University of Minnesota; Morton Kroll of the University of Washington; Julian R.

Friedman of Syracuse University; Clifton McCleskey of the University of Texas; and Dr. Robert H. Marden of Harvard University.

This study is the product of the joint endeavors of the whole group. Each field director was responsible for his own study, but the manuscript as a whole was subject to general discussion of all the participants. While we aimed at consensus, there were times when I had to assume responsibility for a decision. Given the interplay of ideas among the group, it is difficult to assign authorship to parts of the study. Morgan did the research and the original drafts for Chapters III and IV, with assistance from Deener on Chapter III. Meekison did the research and the draft of Chapter II as well as sections of Part Three. In addition, Morgan and Deener acted as associate editors for all of Part Three as well as for many of the field studies. Deener, of course, made the New Orleans field study. All of the field directors contributed substantially to sections of Part Three.

The field studies were made in 1963–1964. Important events since that time have been noted, but the basic statistical data are from that period, or in some instances earlier if that was the only information available. Printed reports and written records were, of course, widely used in the field studies, but there were also interviews with a great many individuals familiar with mental health and community activities in general. These persons numbered too many to list here by name. Nevertheless, I wish to express our thanks for their cooperation.

From the beginning the project was fortunate in having the advice of some of the country's leading authorities in the area of mental health. We are particularly indebted to the project consultants who included the following: Dr. Ray E. Brown, Director, Hospital Administration Program, Medical Center, Duke University; Dr. H. Elaine Cumming, Department of Mental Hygiene, State of New York; Dr. Howard P. Rome, Chief of Psychiatry, Mayo Clinic, and Past President of the American Psychiatric Association; Dr. Jack R. Ewalt, Past President, American Psychiatric Association, Bullard Professor of Psychiatry in Harvard University, and Superintendent, Massachusetts Mental Health Center; Dr. Charles M. Strother, Chairman, Department of Psychology, University of Washington; Dr. Robert H. Felix, Director, National Institute of Mental Health; Dr. John Connorton, Executive Vice President, Greater New York Hospital Association; Dr. Gerald Caplan, Director, Department of Psychiatry, School of Public Health, Harvard University; and

Dr. Paul M. Gross, Chairman, U.S. Public Health Service Special Committee on Environmental Health Problems, and former Provost, Duke University.

Some of the consultants advised on the general plan of the study; others read and commented on particular portions of the manuscript of which they had some special knowledge. The authors alone, of course, are responsible for the final manuscript, since they decided not only on the final form but set forth the study's conclusions.

I am indebted to a number of my political science colleagues, Wallace Sayre, Eaton Professor of Public Administration in Columbia University; Luther Gulick, President Emeritus, Institute of Public Administration, and former City Administrator of New York City; and Lindsay Rogers, Burgess Professor Emeritus of Public Law in Columbia University, who read the manuscript and consulted on the project at various stages.

Finally, I would like to express appreciation on behalf of all the authors for the research and clerical assistance of a score of people. William V. Farr of The Academy of Political Science was particularly helpful in editing the final manuscript, and to Susan Bass particular thanks go for typing the whole manuscript twice.

ROBERT H. CONNERY

Columbia University
March 28, 1968

CONTENTS

CONTENTS

ONE: THE BOLD NEW PROGRAM

I: ACTION FOR MENTAL HEALTH

SOCIETIES HAVE REACTED to mental illness in strange ways. Some prehistoric cavemen punched holes in the skull to release demons supposedly causing mental aberrations. Other societies put unfortunate victims to the stake or drowned them in attempts to loosen the diabolic grip. At the other extreme, in some ancient lands and others not so ancient, mental affliction was regarded as a supernatural gift and those touched by it were elevated to the role of priest or witch doctor.

Countless prescriptions for mental illness developed through the ages. Some were psychic, such as hypnotism and incantations. Others were mechanical, such as Rush's tranquilizer chair. And still others were medicinal, including weird potions concocted of ewes' bladders or lizards' eyes or gantweed and cropleek, perhaps steeped in ale or holy water. One prescription required a potion to be drunk on nine successive mornings out of a church bell. Some communities left madmen to shift for themselves. Roaming about, begging, they were often stoned if they came too near normal people. In other places, the mentally ill were incarcerated in asylums and hospitals, out of society's reach and society out of theirs.

Even in more recent times, both in Europe and the United States, incarceration, or custodial care, of the mentally ill has been the approach most generally adopted. Institutions supported by churches, private charities, and various governments have served as depositories for an increasing number of mentally disturbed persons for whom private or family arrangements could not be made.

The first state asylum for the mentally ill in the United States was opened in 1773, and from that time the public came to accept isolation of mentally ill persons in large hospitals as the proper way of dealing with mental illness. And despite the ever-increasing number of people afflicted and the steady advance of potentially useful medical knowledge, the public reliance on custodial isolation endured well into the twentieth century. In 1963 the average daily number of resident patients in mental hospitals and institutions for the mentally retarded was 800,000, and the number of people receiving treatment each year had reached a million and a half. Small wonder, then, that Senator Lister Hill observed in 1963: "Our present programs for the treatment of the mentally ill have changed very little since the first public mental hospital opened at Williamsburg."

Yet, by the mid-twentieth century, portents of major change were clearly apparent. During World War I the rejection of large numbers of men by the armed services on grounds of mental defects and the large number of cases of mental illness among the troops attracted wide attention but did not lead to significant reforms. The experience of World War II, however, revealing even larger numbers of mentally disturbed men, led to the intervention of a new participant in mental health activities, and later to new and radically different efforts to deal with the problem.

The new participant was the federal government. World War II was hardly over when the National Mental Health Act of 1946 propelled the federal government into a position of prominence in mental health. The National Institute of Mental Health was created in 1949 and funds began to be made available for research, training, and grants-in-aid to stimulate state and local efforts. A decade later the report of the Joint Commission on Mental Illness and Health of 1960 led to the "bold new national mental health program" proposed by President John F. Kennedy in a message to Congress in 1963.

The President's message had the revolutionary aim of shifting "the locus of treatment of the mentally ill from State mental hospitals into community mental health centers." Accepting in principle the objectives of the President's program, Congress passed the Mental Retardation Facilities and Community Mental Health Centers Construction Act of 1963. Thus the means were provided, in the words of a proponent of the legislation, for a "dramatic start" toward a shift from the "warehousing" of patients in "houses of horror" to treatment in the patient's own community.

Not all state hospitals deserved this lurid description, of course. But far too many had failed to make needed advances in the kind of service offered or the physical facilities necessary to provide even adequate custodial care for their resident populations. As more people moved

from rural areas into cities, many state hospitals found themselves increasingly isolated from the centers of population and consequently less
able to provide services and recruit a qualified staff. The 1963 legislation,
however, was not aimed primarily at improving state mental hospitals
but at providing an alternative. Indeed, as one supporter said, "the
basic premise" underlying the President's program was "the disappear-
ance of the state mental hospital as it is known today."

This assumption involved a commitment to a kind of analysis and
theory about which there were strong differences of opinion. Neither
the 1963 legislation nor the official pronouncements regarding the new
community mental health program provided a clear definition of "mental
health." Standard texts on psychiatry define certain types of mental
illness but seldom attempt to say when an individual enjoys mental
health. For some people the term "mental health" means the absence
of any specific mental illness; for others it means a broad, tolerant, well-
adjusted person operating effectively in his social and political environment. Even among psychiatrists the definition of the line between mental
health and mental illness is not "a sharp impenetrable barrier, but rather
a hazy area, now distinct, and then again barely discernible." To be
sure, the recent works of a number of psychiatrists are helpful, but
fundamental differences in approach make consensus difficult. Political
scientists can take a sympathetic view toward this problem in the light
of their own difficulties with concepts and methodology. Nevertheless,
it is virtually impossible to define mental health in a way that satisfies
all professionals in medicine, psychiatry, psychology, and sociology.

Even the term "community mental health center" might be mis-
understood by laymen. One might assume that it means a single physical
structure somewhat like a community hospital. Actually, the regulations issued pursuant to the Act require that a center provide a wide
range of services but permit them to be physically separated so long as
the program is administratively integrated. Thus a center is not necessarily
a complex of resources housed in a fine new building.

The political problems arising from the new program are labyrinthine.
Caring for the mentally ill in the United States, like most other public
health activities, has traditionally been a function of state governments.
With the national government joining in the esablishment of community
mental health centers, questions of intergovernmental relations become
vital. If the federal government intervenes with massive amounts of

money, will this action produce new funds for mental health or will states simply shift funds from one segment of their program to another? Will federal grants effectively equalize present inequalities between the states? Or will the opposite be true—will states with the most resources receive the most federal matching funds? Will restrictive federal regulations inhibit state and local action or will federal permissiveness provide so much latitude as to prevent the goals of the new program from being reached? In other words, what will be the impact of the "bold new program" on existing practices?

Great variations prevail from one state to another, both in the types of mental health services available and in the kinds of organizations that administer the programs. The most common organizational pattern is the dispersion of mental health functions among public agencies within the same state. Although in every state there is a designated "mental health authority," rarely does that authority administer all state mental health services. These are dispersed among departments of hospitals, health, education, welfare, and perhaps others. Nor is the pattern of splintering any less at the local level, where a myriad of private agencies, each with its own program, commonly adds to the confusion.

In an administrative structure where assigned functions overlap, internecine warfare and empire building are to be expected. To what extent will the dispersion of mental health activities present an obstacle to the implementation of the new program? Will mental hospital officials attempt to overcome criticism of their institutions and improve their image by trying to make the hospital rather than the new centers the focal point of mental health programs? Moreover, to be successful, a high degree of cooperation between the mental health center and workers in welfare, education, probation, public health, and recreation is essential. Can such coordination of programs be attained?

The most revolutionary aspect of the new program is its emphasis upon services provided by numerous small community centers. Assigning a precise meaning to the word "community" as used in the Act is difficult, but the importance attached to some kind of local involvement is unmistakable. Does "community" refer to a geographic area? Or does it describe a group of people having some identifiable social unity, which might be residential, occupational, or organizational? If community is simply a geographic area it could be taken as synonymous with "catchment area." Would such a concept serve the purposes envisioned by the mental health professionals who advocate community involvement? If a social unit of some therapeutic significance can be identified, is such a "community" likely to consist of enough people to justify committing the resources necessary to provide a full range of services? Or, contrarily, will these communities be small enough geographically so that the provision of services through community centers will offer significant advantages over what can be done through outpatient clinics of mental hospitals?

There are still other aspects of the problem of community. As one Administration spokesman put it, "It is vital to bear in mind that the entire concept of a comprehensive community mental health center is new. Therefore, community acceptance and support is essential." Must the community as a whole express support, or if not, what is sufficient? What kind of local participation is envisaged? Does community acceptance and support mean local recognition and utilization of the services provided by a state-supported center, or does it require the assumption by the community of a major responsibility for financing and operating the new facility? One thing is clear. Even in states where local mental health clinics have become significant, their support in the past has come principally from the state government. Will the new program change this pattern?

Answers to these question are complicated by certain basic facts of population location and governmental organization. In the 1960s, any attempt to locate comprehensive mental health centers close to the individual involves placing most of those centers in a relatively small number of very densely populated areas. The bulk of the nation's population has become urban. In fact, approximately two-thirds now live in some 200 metropolitan areas ranging in population from 50,000 to more than 10,000,000. Moreover, these areas accounted for four-fifths of the nation's population growth between 1950 and 1960. Consequently, implementing the mental health legislation of 1963 means primarily successful mental health programing in densely populated urban areas.

These metropolitan areas vary greatly, not merely in population, but in countless other ways. One area depends mainly on manufacturing, another on trading and transportation, and still another on government payrolls. Some are great seaports; others are landlocked. Some areas are predominantly Protestant, others are Catholic. Racial minorities abound

in many cities, North and South. Some cities are old; others burst with
the growing pains of youth. But one characteristic is common to all larger
metropolitan areas—governmental fragmentation.

Metropolitan areas in the United States are not single governmental
units, but a patchwork of political jurisdictions. The boundaries of counties, cities, townships, and school districts crisscross the metropolitan
map. Frequently they are all but lost in a maze of other jurisdictional
lines marking special health districts, park districts, sewage districts,
water districts, and so on. A multiplicity of quasi-independent authorities
with a variety of functions, powers, and purposes, and ruled by as many
types of councils, boards, and commissions completes the picture of
metropolitan government in the United States. Moreover, some metropolitan communities spill over state or national boundaries.

The federal program calls for mental health centers designed to serve
a population of 75,000 to 200,000. Whatever the likelihood of identifying social or economic or ethnic communities of the size contemplated by
the 1963 Act, as governmental entities they are largely nonexistent.
Nonetheless, if there are to be such localized centers, some government
must assume responsibility for them if public action is to be taken.

To be sure, the number of jurisdictions says nothing about the number
of people who are governed. The mere existence of a number of governments within an area does not preclude the possibility that most people
might reside within the boundaries of a single local authority. Given such
a situation, the problem presented by a multiplicity of jurisdictions within
a metropolis might well be more apparent than real. Nor does the presence of a host of governments preclude the possibility of creating a new
areawide mental health district.

Still, the governmental tangle of urban America has crucial significance
for the successful implementation of the new federal program. It is out
of this milieu that a community response must be evoked if the concept of
the community mental health center is to have any reality. And it is
within this political environment that the necessary coordination of activities must be achieved if the range of services available in the centers is
to be "comprehensive." Implementation of the 1963 Act involves, then,
not only programing mental health in urban areas; it requires programing
mental health in fragmented metropolitan areas.

Recent studies have emphasized the impact of urban living on mental
health and the consequent need for counteraction. The report of the Joint

Commission on Mental Illness and Health emphasized again and again the importance of total mobilization of community resources at the local level to promote mental health more effectively. But can effective community action be brought about in rapidly growing urban areas whose government is as fragmented as that of most metropolitan areas? Larger community goals can rarely be achieved when local governments independently pursue their separate ends.

Given the approach of the 1963 Act, what is already a serious problem of poor coordination may become an even worse one. The development of comprehensive community mental health programs emphasizing early diagnosis, prevention, and continuity of care will lead to greater and greater necessity for coordination with other community services bearing upon the individual's normal growth and development, such as schools, recreation facilities, housing, mass transportation, and other public health and welfare activities. Yet in a single metropolitan community these may be provided by hundreds of different school districts, townships, counties, special purpose governments, and municipalities.

There is no reason to believe that the problem of fragmentation will be met by political action leading to governmental reorganization on a more rational basis. Consequently, the comprehensive program envisioned by the 1963 Act will require the community centers to be accommodated to the existing pattern of government organization. How to satisfy the diverse interests found in a fragmented metropolitan community is a basic and crucial question.

Local in impact, federal in structure, broad in scope, and revolutionary in concept, the very dimensions of President Kennedy's "bold new national mental health program" indicate that its implementation will be vastly difficult and its realization far from instantaneous. It has received congressional approval, but many obstacles lie in the way of achieving its goals. Fitting the new program into the highly complex administrative network of a modern social welfare state will be difficult. The federal structure complicates an already formidable task.

It would be a serious mistake to look at mental health problems solely in terms of medicine, psychiatry, and social reform. The budgets of state mental health agencies have been among the largest of all state programs. With hundreds of thousands of inmates, state mental institutions have had bigger budgets and more employees than most other state programs. The location of a mental hospital in a community brings jobs and money to the area in which it is located. Consequently, the location of state hospitals was frequently influenced by political log rolling at the state capitals. On the surface the concern might have seemed to be solely with programs, but real battles were often fought over power, dollars, and jobs.

So long as federal appropriations for mental health were small relative to the total federal budget, decisions could be made by a small group of professionals in the National Institute of Mental Health and in universities, a few congressmen, and some state mental health directors. To be sure, there were disputes even among these individuals; but it was a relatively closed system. A very few people made the most important decisions and for the most part determined the future course of mental health programs.

The 1963 Act will propel new actors into the decision-making process because the payoff is greater. The financial rewards of vastly larger federal appropriations will make the political stakes more attractive. Thus the question of who will make decisions in mental health becomes more important. Some answers can be found in diagnosing the present influence patterns—national, state, and local. What part have political leaders, congressmen, state governors, and mayors had in mental health? What has been the role of the American Medical Association, the American Psychiatric Association, United Funds, and community health organizations? Who has made decisions about mental health in metropolitan areas? To gauge the probable interaction of decision makers in the future, it is necessary to identify the actors in the current political drama and the methods they use. The same stakes of power will be present in the future. Political prestige, the rewards of public office, the control of public funds, profits from construction contracts, and indirect economic advantages—all will be involved in the new mental health center program.

Even if financial resources to support "a great society" are at hand, mental health will have to compete with other social programs. How financial resources will be allocated among these programs is a problem which by its very nature in a democratic society is a political one. After the decision is made to commit the necessary resources to the achievement of a given program, the problems that remain are administrative, but obviously of concern to many groups and therefore likely subjects for political action.

Certainly one problem which the new program will face involves competing for already scarce medical and welfare manpower to staff the new centers. Expanded mental health services presumably will require more trained personnel. How extensive is the deficiency in metropolitan areas and what are the possibilities of meeting this need?

Any new program requires popular backing, and one that presupposes extensive community action demands widespread and continuing support. If lacking, popular support must be generated and then sustained. The necessary money must be found and committed, and qualified personnel must be recruited and trained. All of these activities must be carried on in areas where governmental authority is splintered among many units. This fragmentation of power is the universal condition under which the new mental health program must operate.

To examine the effect that these conditions will have on mental health programing is the prime objective of this study. The first step is to examine in some detail the development of the new federal program and the milieu in which it must be implemented. The second step is to identify through field studies the problems arising from fragmentation, splintering, and dispersal of governmental power. The third step is to suggest the range of political and administrative accommodations necessary for adequate utilization of community resources in implementing the national mental health program.

Intergovernmental relations in the United States appear to be in the process of important alteration. One may suggest that the mix is changing. The input proportions at the local, state, and federal levels of governmental activity seem to be shifting radically, not only financially, but also in respect to initiative, leadership, and administrative organization. The development of new patterns of regional organization, like Appalachia, appears well underway. Complaints are already being heard that the federal government is undermining the traditional system. By-passing state governments, it is dealing directly with local jurisdictions in efforts to cope with the pressing problems of the burgeoning metropolis. It may be that "cooperative federalism" has become as inadequate a description of federal-state relations today as "dual federalism" was a generation ago. Perhaps a new descriptive term such as "creative federalism" will answer the need. Hopefully, this study of the politics of mental health will serve the more general purpose of shedding some light on the realities of policy development and implementation in the complex political atmosphere of a modern federal state committed to extensive social welfare services.

II: MENTAL HEALTH ORGANIZATION

THE NEW PROGRAM called for by the 1963 Act requires fitting new and expanded efforts into a maze of ongoing mental health activities involving an already extensive and intricate administrative apparatus. Currently, each level of government in the United States is involved to some extent in providing mental health services, and coordinating public programs becomes a complex affair of intergovernmental relations. In some areas, particularly at the local level, the importance of the private sector exceeds that of the public. The historical development of mental health activities explains, in large part, the present system.

THE EARLY PERIOD

For a long while the mentally ill were confined in jail cells and often chained to walls or floors.[1] Indeed, one popular amusement was to visit "bedlam" to taunt the "crazy people." Sometimes famous men in their dotage were exhibited like wild animals in a zoo for a penny a head.

The Pennsylvania General Hospital of Philadelphia, established in 1756 by the Society of Friends, was the first institution in the United States that attempted to emphasize treatment and care as contrasted to confinement. Steps were taken to discourage abusive practices common elsewhere, and the care provided was quite humane.

The first public asylum for the mentally ill was erected by Virginia in 1773 at Williamsburg. Five decades elapsed before another was opened in 1824, when Kentucky established a state hospital in Lexington, followed by South Carolina in 1828. In the mid-nineteenth century several additional state institutions were opened, but these were insufficient to meet the demand. The dependent insane usually were incarcerated in poorhouses or were auctioned off to the person who agreed to maintain

[1] Albert Deutsch, *The Mentally Ill in America* (2d ed.; New York: Doubleday, Doran, 1949). This standard work on the history of the treatment and care of the mentally ill has been drawn upon extensively for this section.

them at the lowest cost to the community. The unfortunate victims of this custom usually were bought to be used as laborers.

Revolutionary theories calling for a minimum of restraint and a maximum of intelligent understanding and sympathy, first expressed by Philippe Pinel in France during the closing decade of the eighteenth century, spread to other European countries and finally across the Atlantic to America. As early as 1811 Dr. T. R. Beck, in a little book published in New York, summarized the new approach as "moral management." It involved

removing patients from their residence to some proper asylum; and for this purpose a calm retreat in the country is to be preferred. . . . Coercion by blows, stripes and chains . . . is now justly laid aside. . . . Have humane attendants . . . strictly exclude visitors. . . . The diet ought to be light . . . introduce entertaining books, . . . exhilarating music; . . . and admit friends under proper restrictions.[2]

But "moral management" found little acceptance in the United States for several decades.

Probably the most militant crusader for improved care of the mentally ill in America during the nineteenth century was Dorothea Lynde Dix, a retired Boston school teacher. Her crusade was to have an important effect on which level of government should bear responsibility for the care of the mentally ill. Asked to teach a Sunday school class among the women inmates of the East Cambridge jail in the winter of 1841, she was shocked to find insane persons locked up in unheated cells, unheated because of the widely held belief that the insane were insensible to cold. The East Cambridge Court granted a petition brought by Miss Dix to provide heat. For the next forty years she traveled around the country advocating humane treatment for the mentally ill. Get the insane out of local jails and county poorhouses into hospitals built and operated by the state—this was her constant theme. Over the years some twenty states responded to her appeal by establishing or enlarging mental hospitals.

Despite the increase in hospital facilities the number of beds available in these institutions fell far short of the number required. "Hardly were hospitals opened than their capacities became overtaxed by the never-ceasing flow of patients. Overcrowding soon forced upon authorities the

[2] T. Romeyn Beck, *An Inaugural Dissertation on Insanity* (New York, 1811), pp. 27–28, quoted in Deutsch, pp. 91–92.

problem of selection." [3] The basis of selection was a diagnosis of acute (potentially curable) versus chronic (incurable) as doctors of that time defined those terms. Acute cases were admitted to the hospitals while the chronically ill were still confined in jails or poorhouses.

After the Civil War the number and variety of state hospitals increased rapidly. The first major step taken to develop centralized state control was the formation of a single board to supervise all state institutions, including prisons, orphanages, insane asylums, and sometimes the state university. While the primary purpose of this centralization was the more economical administration of these institutions, the care provided under the new system was considerably better. In 1890 the passage of the New York Care Act, by which the state assumed financial responsibility for the treatment and care of the mentally ill, marked the end of one era and the beginning of another. This act and similar statutes passed by other states broadened the base for financing institutional care.

Later, state mental hospitals were sometimes combined for administrative purposes with welfare or public health activities in a single department. In more recent years further refinement and the expansion of public services has resulted in the emergence of separate departments of mental health. This is not to suggest, of course, that every state followed the same pattern or the same order of development.

Centralization of control at the state level was accompanied by the construction of new state facilities, which helped in relieving overcrowded conditions and allowed the gradual transfer of mental patients from local jails and county poorhouses. Nevertheless, treatment of patients was slow to change. Partly as a result of interest created by Clifford W. Beers's revolutionary book, *A Mind That Found Itself,* the National Committee for Mental Hygiene was founded in 1909 with Beers as its secretary. Many of the reforms urged by the mental hygiene movement had a distinctively modern flavor. The national committee emphasized research into the causes of mental illness, treatment leading to cure, the development of preventive measures, and even the enlistment of federal aid.

Despite these efforts progress was slow. A study launched by the Public Health Service and the National Committee for Mental Hygiene in 1937 demonstrated that conditions in many mental hospitals were abominable. [4]

[3] Deutsch, *The Mentally Ill in America,* p. 231.
[4] Samuel W. Hamilton *et al., A Study of the Public Mental Hospitals of the United States, 1937–39,* U.S., Public Health Service, Supplement No. 164 to the Public Health Reports (Washington: U.S. Government Printing Office, 1941).

Ten years later Albert Deutsch, reporting on a survey of mental hospitals, stated that "in some of the wards there were scenes that rivalled the horrors of the Nazi concentration camps—hundreds of naked mental patients herded into huge barn-like, filth-infested wards, in all degrees of deterioration, untended and untreated, stripped of every vestige of human decency, many in stages of semi-starvation." The plight of the mental patient of this period received further dramatization in Mary J. Ward's highly personalized account, *The Snake Pit,* which together with its movie adaptation did much to focus public attention on the conditions inside many of the mental hospitals.

Efforts of the national government in public health date back to 1789, when Congress provided for federal hospitals to care for merchant seamen. Federal activity regarding mental health, however, is of much more recent origin. To be sure, Dorothea Lynde Dix had prevailed on Congress to pass an act as early as 1854 granting federal lands to finance the erection of state hospitals for the insane, but President Franklin Pierce vetoed it on grounds that the federal government had no business in mental health.

With the passage of the Selective Service Act of 1917 the Army became concerned about the mental fitness of inductees and a Division of Neurology and Psychiatry was created under the War Department's Surgeon General to screen recruits and to bar from enlistment all men suffering from psychiatric disorders. The division also was charged with the treatment of mentally ill service personnel. While this work involved a larger number of people, it was limited to members of the armed forces. These activities were continued after the war, but long-term treatment of veterans was given to the newly created Veterans Administration.

Federal activity in the mental health field was increased somewhat in 1930, when a Division of Mental Hygiene in the Public Health Service was established. While continuing to study drug addiction and operating limited facilities for addicts, the new division also undertook to provide psychiatric care for federal prisoners, to extend psychiatric diagnostic services to federal courts, and to carry on some research. This agency continued its activities until the National Institute of Mental Health began operation in 1949. But it is important to recognize that federal activity was primarily for a restricted clientele consisting of military veterans, merchant seamen, residents of the District of Columbia, and other special groups. It was not until the National Mental Health Act of 1946 that the federal government began to treat mental health as a general public health problem.

THE NATIONAL MENTAL HEALTH ACT OF 1946

The recruitment of forces in World War II was a major factor in bringing about a great expansion in the federal government's mental health activities and the direction of those efforts toward the general public rather than solely to special clienteles. Almost two million men were rejected by the Army and Navy because of mental problems. This aroused widespread concern about the problem of mental illness. Ultimately it led to the passage of the National Mental Health Act of 1946, which authorized extensive research, demonstration projects, training programs, and grants-in-aid to the states for mental health purposes. Testifying during the hearings on the 1946 bill, General Lewis B. Hershey, director of the Selective Service System, described the staggering dimensions of the problem:

As of August 1 [1945] we show somewhere around 4,800,000 men ages 18 to 37 have been rejected for the armed forces, and of this number 856,000 have been rejected for mental diseases and an additional 235,000 have been rejected for what we tabulate as neurological cases. In addition to that there are 676,000 that have been turned down for mental deficiency. . . . [Mental illness] is the greatest single cause by a very, very large percentage, that is, we haven't any other single cause probably that runs above 400,000.[5]

Other witnesses not only stressed the alarming proportions of mental illness, but also emphasized the need for a new approach to the whole problem. As Dr. George S. Stevenson, medical director of the National Foundation of Mental Hygiene, put it, "Mental health functions as they have been conducted to date are based upon requirements and facilities conceived in the middle of the last century."

All witnesses who appeared before the Senate and House committees supported increased federal activity. Dr. Stevenson said, "For a problem of the size indicated, the research aspects have been sorely neglected. . . . For the most part psychiatric training has been left to chance." Dr. Robert Felix, then chief of the Division of Mental Hygiene in the Public Health Service and later the first director of the National Institute of

[5] U.S., Congress, House, Committee on Interstate and Foreign Commerce, *Hearings on H.R. 2550, National Neuropsychiatric Institute Act,* 79th Cong., 1st Sess., 1945, p. 36.

Mental Health, described his conception of the role of the national government as follows:

While the primary responsibility for operating and financing services of public health belongs to the State and local communities to the limit of their resources, it is the responsibility of the Public Health Service . . . to mobilize the collective knowledge of the nation in matters pertaining to the prevention, diagnosis, and treatment of illness; . . . to equalize the opportunities of the several States to provide comparable service to their citizens by technical aid and grants.

"The institutional care of psychotics," said Albert Deutsch, "has been traditionally mainly a State responsibility. It should remain so. But the job of getting preventive devices and using them is a national responsibility." [6] Dr. Stevenson added: "This bill does not wait for such complete breakdown as is found in the patients in our mental hospitals in order to begin its usefulness. It speaks of prevention; it can help the communities to begin treatment when treatment is most promising at the first sign of illness."

Arguing for grants-in-aid, Dr. Felix stressed the importance of outpatient psychiatric clinics as "an effective means for the provision of early diagnosis and [saving] the states money by permitting earlier release of patients from their mental hospitals." The economics of the existing situation was summarized by Dr. C. C. Burlingame's comment that "we just can't keep on building bigger and better mental hospitals."

All of the witnesses who testified during the hearings were favorably disposed toward the bill, and the committees heard few criticisms. To be sure, one member of the House subcommittee, Representative Clarence J. Brown of Ohio, continually questioned witnesses as to how extensive federal aid should be, intimating that he believed some limit should be placed on the federal invasion of state and local government prerogatives. In a similar vein Senator Robert Taft was concerned over the expansion of federally supported research. Some administrative provisions also were questioned. For example, Sanford Bates, commissioner of the New Jersey Department of Institutions and Agencies, criticized the bill's designation of the state health department as the agency to administer the federal grants. Mr. Bates argued that this would confuse administration in those states which had separate departments of mental health, and his objection was met by making an exception for those states. The only di-

[6] U.S., Congress, Senate, Committee on Education and Labor, *Hearings on S. 1160, National Neuropsychiatric Institute Act*, 79th Cong., 2d Sess., 1946, p. 107.

rect criticism of the principles behind the legislation came from the Citizens Medical Reference Bureau. In a letter to the House subcommittee, this group stated its opposition to the bill on the grounds that it interfered with state functions and "would regiment the individual in matters pertaining to the mind."

The reports of the House and Senate subcommittees made plain the rationale underlying the extensive federal support for training and research which the bill authorized. Both emphasized the retarded state of mental health activity, highlighting the twin problems of inadequate manpower and knowledge. The House subcommittee reported that:

research on the causes, prevention, diagnosis, and treatment of psychiatric disorders has not kept pace with research in the other branches of the medical sciences, nor has the training of specialists in this field kept pace with the growing demands for psychiatrists. . . . Finally, services for prevention and early diagnosis of psychiatric disorders, such as those which have been developed and made available in other fields of medicine during the past decade, have not been available to the public to a sufficient extent.[7]

The Senate report commented on the amount spent for mental health services as compared to other areas of public health by pointing out that:

all public and private Government agencies together are spending not more than 25 cents per year for each estimated case of mental illness and only $1.00 for each known case of total disability because of mental ill health, as compared, for example, with $100.00 per case of poliomyelitis, a disease which is far less widespread.[8]

Commenting on the inadequacy of research, the Senate subcommittee observed that:

not more than $2,500,000 is spent annually on research in psychiatry and related fields, as compared to an expenditure of at least $250,000,000 or 100 times as much for the maintenance of mental institutions. This is an extremely inefficient way of attacking the mental health problem.

The subcommittees estimated the number of additional people needed to staff an adequate mental health program would be 2,000 psychiatrists, 1,700 psychologists, 15,000 psychiatric nurses, 4,500 psychiatric social workers, 1,000 occupational therapists, 15,000 attendants, and 3,000 other technical personnel. It was this situation which the bill was de-

---

[7] U.S., Congress, House, Committee on Interstate and Foreign Commerce, *National Mental Health Act*, 79th Cong., 1st Sess., 1945, H. Rep't. No. 1445 to accompany H.R. 4512, p. 3.

[8] U.S., Congress, Senate, Committee on Education and Labor, *National Mental Health Act*, 79th Cong., 2d Sess., 1946, S. Rep't. No. 1353 to accompany H.R. 4512, p. 6.

signed to remedy, and both houses passed it with few dissenting voices. There was, however, no evidence as to how these figures were arrived at and they were little more than "guesstimates."

The National Mental Health Act of 1946 [9] created the National Institute of Mental Health (NIMH) and the National Advisory Mental Health Council. NIMH was to be the unit within the Public Health Service responsible for the research, training, and service activities authorized by the Act. The advisory council was composed of six members appointed for three-year terms with the Surgeon General as ex officio chairman. It was to advise and make recommendations to the Surgeon General on matters relating to mental health activities of the Public Health Service, to review research and training applications, and to collect and disseminate information on mental health.

Under the Act research grants could be made to universities, hospitals, laboratories, and other public or private institutions, and in some instances to private individuals. Grants for training, instruction, and demonstrations could also be made to public and other nonprofit institutions.

Perhaps most significantly, the 1946 Act included two sections that gave direct aid to states for the development of their mental health services. One form of assistance was grants-in-aid, which were to be apportioned among the states according to a formula based on population size, extent of the mental health problem, and financial need. The second form of direct federal aid was the assignment of Public Health Service personnel to states or localities to provide technical assistance.

It is important to recognize that the federal aid authorized by the Act was not intended to subsidize the operating costs of mental hospitals. Instead, the objective of the legislation was to stimulate a new form of community mental health activity. The desirability of treating mental illness in the patient's normal environment rather than in a mental hospital had been recognized in the case of children.[10] The 1946 Act sought to provide similar services for adults through a network of outpatient psychiatric clinics.

At the time the Act was passed the problem was that "less than 20 per cent of the number of outpatient clinics required . . . are now avail-

[9] 60 Stat. 421.
[10] See George S. Stevenson and Geddes Smith, *Child Guidance Clinics* (New York: The Commonwealth Fund, 1934).

able, and these are concentrated largely in cities having more than 150,000 population and are devoted almost exclusively to child care." [11] The House subcommittee reported that supporters of the bill had suggested that "the nation should have as a minimum one all-purpose psychiatric out-patient clinic for each 100,000 of the population." [12] The Senate subcommittee report stated that "mental out-patient clinics, conveniently located and offering facilities for early diagnosis and treatment, give every promise of being the most effective means at our disposal for combating mental disease." Testifying before the Senate subcommittee, Dr. Felix said: "The initial goal is the establishment of 100 clinics during the first full year of the operation of the program proposed in this bill. These would be set up in the areas of the greatest need, based on one clinic for 500,000 population." Congress recognized that most mental hospitals were equipped to provide treatment only for the chronically ill, and even that treatment primarily consisted of custodial care. For that reason, the funds authorized under the Act were not intended to "be used to finance routine bed care in mental hospitals but should be devoted in large measure to further development of existing and new techniques of preventive and treatment methods as well as to training of much-needed personnel." In short, the proponents of the Act sought to stimulate program developments centered in the community and in particular the establishment of outpatient psychiatric clinics.

Each state was required to designate a "mental health authority" to receive the grant-in-aid funds and to plan for and govern their disbursement within the state. This state mental health authority was to be "the state health authority, except that, in the case of any State in which there is a single agency, other than the state health authority, charged with responsibility for administering the mental health program of the State, it means such other state agency." In reporting the bill the House committee spelled out very clearly that the mental health authority was not to be a state agency "whose activities in the mental health field are restricted to jurisdiction over mental institutions and their patients." Thus it was clearly the purpose of the Act to expand as well as to improve the mental health services available.

[11] Senate Report No. 1353, 79th Cong., p. 5.
[12] House Report No. 1445, 79th Cong., p. 4.

FEDERAL MENTAL HEALTH PROGRAMS

The National Institute of Mental Health became one of several bureaus in the Public Health Service of the Department of Health, Education, and Welfare. From a modest beginning in the 1948 fiscal year with a budget of $4.5 million, federal mental health programs have blossomed into a major health activity with a budget of over $230 million in the 1966 fiscal year and a staff of approximately 1,280.

From its beginning until late 1964, NIMH was directed by Dr. Robert H. Felix. Announcing Dr. Felix's retirement after a long and distinguished career in the Public Health Service, Dr. Luther L. Terry, Surgeon General of the United States, commented on his importance to the development of the Institute and its work:

The entire program of the Institute reflects his foresight, administrative skills, professional knowledge and his ability to articulate its technical, scientific, and humanitarian needs and achievements. . . . His qualities of leadership and persuasion have helped to rally thousands of professional persons and interested citizens to his belief that the mentally ill can best be served by a community-based program of treatment providing a continuity of care, available to everyone at the time of need.

NIMH activities fell into two broad categories, intramural research and extramural programs, each under the supervision of an associate director. Although the Institute's external programs were larger in terms of expenditures as well as the number of projects supported, its internal research program was far from unimportant.

Intramural research activities were conducted primarily in NIMH's extensive laboratories at its Bethesda, Maryland, headquarters, where an interdisciplinary approach to the elimination of mental disorders was emphasized. In addition to the Bethesda operations other intramural centers were maintained. In these the Institute studied a wide range of community mental health problems, clinical techniques, and the pharmacological, neurophysiological, biochemical, psychological, and socioeconomic aspects of drug addiction.

NIMH's external programs could be divided into three broad categories—research, training, and community services. All three of these programs when first formulated were quite modest. However, they have been expanded to support a great variety of mental health services.

As Table 1 shows, total program expenditures have risen steadily and, in recent years, rapidly. In fiscal 1948, research and training grant expenditures were $374,000 and $1,140,000 respectively, while in fiscal 1966 expenditures for these two programs had reached an estimated $85,230,000 and $86,081,000. Although expenditures for grants-in-aid have quadrupled since fiscal 1948, they have remained fairly constant in recent years, averaging about $6,600,000. In short, while all three categories of extramural activity have expanded significantly over the years, support for training and research programs has been increasingly emphasized.

Table 1: Annual Expenditures of the National Institute of Mental Health for Fiscal Years 1948–1966; Total and by Grant Program
(Thousands of Dollars)

		Grant Program			
Year	Total Expenditures[a]	Research Grants	Fellowship Grants	Training Grants	State Grants-in-Aid
1948	$ 4,500	$ 374	$ 64	$ 1,140	$ 1,653
1950	8,258	798	103	2,882	3,294
1952	10,639	1,637	255	3,958	3,009
1954	11,759	2,587	187	4,174	2,308
1956	18,052	3,937	299	5,884	2,981
1958	38,423	12,402	562	13,288	3,955
1960	67,409	23,288	1,996	26,197	4,911
1962	106,220	42,634	3,786	38,608	6,622
1964	170,978	63,510	7,501	67,023	10,858[b]
1965	186,068	75,162	8,053	72,542	6,675
1966[c]	232,650[d]	85,230	8,364	86,081	6,750

[a] Includes direct operating costs of the Institute.
[b] Included an estimated $4.2 million for state mental health planning grants.
[c] Estimates.
[d] Includes $18,899,000 for staffing grants for Community Mental Health Centers constructed under the 1963 Act.
Source: Compiled from U.S., Congress, Senate and House, Appropriations Committees, Hearings, for each year except 1948. Data for that year were taken from Federal Security Agency, Annual Report (Washington: U.S. Government Printing Office, 1948), pp. 49, 349, 352.

Research grants have been made primarily in the medical sciences, but in recent years awards have been made in the physical, biological, and social sciences. In fiscal 1948 NIMH funded 38 projects at a cost of $373,226, while in fiscal 1966 it awarded 1,596 grants at an estimated cost of $58,926,000. Special programs in areas in which NIMH has had a particular interest took another $26,304,000 in research funds, bringing total expenditures for research in fiscal 1966 to an estimated $85,230,000. One activity, hospital improvement grants, accounted for $18,000,000 of the special grant funds. The increasing importance of NIMH's extramural research activities in terms of expenditures can be seen in Table 1.

The Institute's training program has the general objective of increasing manpower available in every phase of mental health activity including clinical services, teaching, research, consultation, and administration. Training grants are awarded to educational institutions and research fellowships are made available to individuals.

At first the preparation of clinical specialists in the core fields of psychiatry, psychology, psychiatric social work, and psychiatric nursing was the major focus. But gradually the training program expanded to include support for training in the social and biological sciences, the teaching and study of mental health, public health, and human behavior. In recent years approximately 10 per cent of the total funds has been used to support undergraduate training, particularly in nursing and psychiatry. A distinctive feature of this extensive federal program is that trainees have not been obligated to work, even for a limited time, in the public arena. Thus the program differs from similar state programs and federal training efforts in most other fields.

A recent extension of the training grant program was the General Practitioner Program, initiated in 1959 at the suggestion of the congressional appropriations committees. Under this program general practitioners can take short courses in psychiatry and then return to their practice or they may receive awards to specialize in psychiatry. During the six-year period 1959–1964 an estimated 14,400 physicians took advantage of the postgraduate short course.

Not surprisingly, there has been wide variation among the states in the amount of federal training funds awarded to institutions within their boundaries. States with great medical centers such as Harvard, Columbia, and the Universities of California, Pennsylvania, and Illinois received a disproportionately large amount of money. Indeed, five states —New York, Massachusetts, California, Pennsylvania, and Illinois—

with a third of the nation's population, received 47 per cent of the training grant funds during the first fourteen years of the program's operation. Nine states plus the District of Columbia, with 47 per cent of the population, received almost two-thirds of the total funds awarded during the same period; and four states—Alaska, Nevada, Idaho, and Wyoming—received nothing. On the basis of population, the Northeast received a disproportionately large share of the training funds while the South received considerably less than its share.

The variation among the states in the amount of federal training funds received was in itself not necessarily important, unless the trainees tended to locate in the area where they received their training. But areas with the most training facilities were not necessarily those which had the greatest need for mental health personnel. A statistical study by NIMH based on a 25 per cent sample of former trainees suggested that the place where one was trained was related to the place where one practiced.[13] The five states that had received 47 per cent of the training grant funds through fiscal 1961 also employed 47 per cent of the former trainees. Moreover, of the eighteen states employing the largest numbers of former trainees in 1962, sixteen also ranked in the top eighteen in the amount of federal training funds received through 1961.

The third type of NIMH extramural activity, community services, consisted of a series of grant and technical assistance programs designed to stimulate a greater interest in community mental health services. Grants-in-aid states were authorized by the National Mental Health Act of 1946. Over the years there has been a great increase in state and local expenditures for community mental health purposes, a development attributable in large part to the availability of federal funds. While federal grant-in-aid expenditures rose from $1,653,000 in fiscal 1948 to $6,675,000 in fiscal 1965, state and local expenditures during the same period increased from $2,398,000 to an estimated $119,950,000 in fiscal 1965.

Demonstration projects were also employed by NIMH to assist states and localities in the development of their mental health programs. The

[13] U.S., Public Health Service, National Institute of Mental Health, *Current Professional Status of Mental Health Personnel Supported Under National Institute of Mental Health Training Grants,* Public Health Service Publication No. 1088 (Washington: U.S. Government Printing Office, 1963).

federal government paid the cost of certain mental health services for a limited time as a means of evaluating the effectiveness of new forms of treatment. Projects were directed at a variety of mental health concerns, including alcoholism, community psychiatry, mental retardation, and mental health aspects of public health and manpower utilization.

In addition, a technical assistance program included the loan of federal personnel to states and localities and the sponsoring of conferences for mental health professionals in various states. The program was designed to help state and local officials to improve their services by keeping them informed of the latest developments in treatment techniques and concepts of care.

One of the most significant expansions of NIMH programs in recent years resulted from a 1956 amendment to the Public Health Service Act. Title V of that amendment authorized grants to states or local governments and nonprofit agencies for research on improving methods of diagnosis and treatment of mental illness.

The areas studied have included mental health planning, mental hospital administration, diagnosis and treatment, attitudes toward mental illness, mental health education, delinquency, mental retardation, alcoholism, and rehabilitation. From some sixty-eight grants totalling slightly less than two million dollars in 1958, the Title V program has expanded to an estimated $18,235,000 in fiscal 1966.

One of the principal purposes of the research grants authorized under the 1956 amendment was the improvement of conditions in state mental hospitals. Funds were not, however, to be used to subsidize routine bed care, but for research and experiments in techniques and management. Few grants were made until fiscal 1964 when NIMH initiated the Hospital Improvement Program under Title V. Expenditures were expected to approximate $18,000,000 a year.

One of the most recently initiated NIMH community service programs was planning grants to states. Testifying before the Senate Appropriations Committee in 1962, Mike Gorman of the National Committee Against Mental Illness urged the committee to grant NIMH "$4 to $5 million in the coming year for the purpose of providing matching grants to the states for the development of comprehensive mental health plans." Mr. Gorman warned the committee that "we are losing precious time in implementing the Joint Commission report. We can make up

for some of this lag by developing a system of planning grants." [14]
His plea was heeded and Congress provided $4.2 million for fiscal 1963
and 1964 to help states develop long- and short-range comprehensive
community mental health plans. Grants were to be on a dollar for
dollar matching basis, but no state was to receive less than $50,000.
To qualify for federal aid each state had to submit a "plan for planning" indicating specific areas of study and the staff it proposed to
employ. The plans had to consider facilities and services, legislation and
finance, research and training, as well as many other matters. The long-
range objective was to mobilize the state's total resources for the prevention, diagnosis, and treatment of mental illness. All fifty states accepted planning grants.

Despite the extensive activities of NIMH, not all federal mental health
services are under its jurisdiction. The Department of Defense and
U.S. Bureau of Prisons care for their own clientele; of even greater
significance is the Veterans Administration, which operates a chain of
mental hospitals and clinics.

While a large part of the $600,000,000 annual mental health expendi-
tures of the Veterans Administration has been for disability pensions,
approximately half has been for the operation of mental hospitals and
outpatient clinics. Thirty-eight of the 168 VA hospitals were, in 1965,
classified as psychiatric;[15] and of a total 118,896 operating beds, 58,746
were for psychiatric patients. The Veterans Administration also under-
takes extensive research on various aspects of mental illness. It is generally conceded that the Veterans Administration program is among the
best in the nation. It spends considerably more per patient per day than
do most states. However, it competes for scarce manpower with other
federal and state programs.

The Hill-Burton hospital construction program, initiated in 1946, has
also resulted in some minor splintering of federal efforts relating to
mental health. Administered by the PHS Bureau of State Services, the
program has included psychiatric facilities as well as others. By mid-
1965, some $72 million had been expended to add 19,295 beds to

[14] U.S., Congress, Senate, Committee on Appropriations, *Hearings, Departments
of Labor, and Health, Education, and Welfare Appropriations for 1963, Part II,*
87th Cong., 2d Sess., 1962, p. 1585.

[15] U.S., Veterans Administration, *Annual Report, Administration of Veterans'
Affairs, 1965* (Washington: U.S. Government Printing Office, 1965).

mental hospitals; and another 10,020 beds for psychiatric patients had been added to general hospitals. While indirectly involved in mental health activity, the role of the Bureau of State Services in the Hill-Burton program has been *solely* that of construction supervisor.

Mental retardation activities represent another area related to mental health and are divided among a number of federal agencies. While the assistant secretary of HEW for legislation is charged with overall staff coordination of mental retardation activities, operational responsibility is scattered throughout the entire department. Within the Public Health Service itself, responsibility for various aspects of the mental retardation program is spread among the Bureau of State Services and the various National Institutes of Health. This division raises questions as to precise program responsibilities and the jurisdiction of each agency, as well as problems of coordination.

It is all very well to say, as did the Secretary's (HEW) Committee for Mental Retardation, that "mental retardation and mental illness are in most instances separate health problems" [16] and to conclude therefore that mental health and mental retardation programs should be separately administered. The problem is illustrated by the operations of the National Institute of Child Health and Human Development (NICHD), established in 1962. During its first year, NICHD activities were financed with funds transferred from other institutes, including NIMH. Dr. R. A. Aldrich, director of NICHD, commenting on the responsibilities of his institute as compared with NIMH, told the House Appropriations Committee: "We are very much interested in and consider ourselves as having a primary interest in normal intellectual development and the normal learning process. Now, we feel that the National Institute of Mental Health should place its primary emphasis on disorders of learning rather than on normal learning." Dr. Felix indicated his agreement with this division of labor but pointed out that overlapping was possible "because two people sometimes look at the same thing differently." He might well have added that, for the same reason, disagreement between the two institutes could be expected, particularly as their programs continued to expand.

[16] U.S., Department of Health, Education, and Welfare, Secretary's Committee for Mental Retardation, *Mental Retardation* (Washington: U.S. Government Printing Office, 1963), p. 95.

STATE PROGRAMS AND ORGANIZATION

Today, confinement in a mental hospital continues to be the principal method of state care for the mentally ill, both in terms of the number of patients treated and the extent of financial support. In 1963 there were 284 mental hospitals in operation. Admissions to these hospitals increased from 130,872 in 1947 to 297,139 in 1963.[17] While admissions have risen, so have separations. Despite the increase in the number of admissions, the average daily resident population from 1955 to 1963 decreased by 46,692, showing a decline in total hospital population. In other words, the duration of hospitalization has become shorter, and with the increase in local facilities many patients can now be treated on an outpatient basis in their communities.

Hospital personnel have more than doubled since 1947. In 1963 there were 195,356 on hospital payrolls, thus indicating a far more favorable patient-staff ratio. During the same period operating costs of mental hospitals rose from $256,231,000 to $1,142,841,000.[18] Since President Kennedy reported that all public expenditures for mental health in the United States totaled only $1,800,000,000 it is evident that state mental hospitals remain by far the most important facet of mental health programs.

With the use of new drugs and techniques, state hospitals have begun to place greater emphasis on treatment leading to eventual cure as opposed to custodial care. Many hospitals have been increasing the range of their activities by supporting research and training as well as establishing and expanding outpatient facilities. As a result, the once isolated mental hospital in some states is becoming involved in community mental health services. The growth of local mental health programs, the increased patient turnover in mental hospitals, the development in a few states of mental health regions, and the adoption by a number of state hospitals of the unit system are all indications of the necessity of coordinating hospital and community mental health programs.

Unfortunately the expansion of state mental health activities that was

[17] For more complete statistical data on mental hospitals for the years 1952–1963, see U.S., Public Health Service, National Institute of Mental Health, *Patients in Mental Institutions, Part II, State and County Mental Hospitals* (Washington: U.S. Government Printing Office, 1964).

[18] The last year for which complete data are available.

stimulated by the National Mental Health Act of 1946 tended to divorce mental hospitals and community mental health programs. The Act prohibited states from naming agencies solely responsible for mental hospitals as their mental health authority since state hospitals had shown little interest in community services. Consequently, a variety of state agencies was named to handle community services, with public health departments predominating.

As of 1966 the agencies designated as mental health authorities in the fifty states were as follows:[19]

Departments of health	13
Departments of mental health	16
Departments of institutions or state mental hospitals	5
Departments of welfare	5
Departments of health and welfare	6
Departments of mental health and corrections	2
Others	3

The most notable change since the Act was passed has been the trend to shift the location of the mental health authority from state health departments to more recently established departments of mental health.

Since the mental health authority is the custodian of federal aid and is also the principal agency responsible for the development of community mental health programs, its administrative location is of considerable significance. The emphasis placed on mental health depends in large measure on the primary function of a department responsible for it. Thus, if the principal function of a department is public health or welfare, improved health and welfare programs are likely to be given priority over community mental health services, or if the primary func-

[19] The source for this breakdown is the third U.S., Public Health Service *Directory of State and Territorial Health Authorities*, 1966 revised edition. States in each category are as follows: Public Health (13)—Arizona, Arkansas, Georgia, Hawaii, Idaho, Mississippi, Nebraska, New Mexico, North Dakota, Oklahoma, Utah, Washington, and Wyoming; Mental Health (16)—Alabama, Connecticut, Delaware, Illinois, Indiana, Massachusetts, Michigan, New York, North Carolina, South Carolina, South Dakota, Tennessee, Texas, Vermont, Virginia, and West Virginia; Institutions (5)—Colorado, Florida, Montana, New Jersey, and Oregon; Welfare (5)—Kansas, Minnesota, Pennsylvania, Rhode Island, and Wisconsin; Health and Welfare (6)—Alaska, California, Kentucky, Missouri, Nevada, and New Hampshire; Mental Health and Corrections (2)—Maine and Ohio; Other (3)—Iowa (psychopathic hospital of the state university), Louisiana (Department of Hospitals), Maryland (Board of Health and Mental Hygiene). While California, Kentucky, and Maryland have departments of mental health, they were under the jurisdiction of the state health and welfare agency or, as in the case of Maryland, the Board of Health and Mental Hygiene.

tion is administering state institutions, better mental hospitals and prisons are likely to be considered more important. Such program favoritism may well be reflected in both budget and staffing patterns.

Regardless of which administrative unit is designated the mental health authority, however, the provision of services is complicated in many, if not most, states by a splintering of functions among several agencies. Some states deal with alcoholism as part of their public health program, others place it under the jurisdiction of a separate agency. Law enforcement authorities, welfare departments, public health or mental health units—any or all of these agencies may bear responsibility for the problem of narcotics addiction. Some states have separate youth commissions, separate boards for the care of the aging, and may operate extensive mental health facilities under the department of corrections. Partly the result of the historical development of various kinds of services, the tendency toward splintering has been given additional impetus by confusion over the proper definition of mental health. But, whatever the cause, a number of different state agencies are usually concerned to some extent with diagnosing, treating, rehabilitating, or otherwise dealing with the mentally ill.

Locating community mental health services in one department and the administration of state mental hospitals in another can lead to serious conflicts. The division in state programs caused by the 1946 Act had created certain administrative problems by the mid-fifties. One study group reported:

The events of recent years . . . have tended to draw a sharp line of demarcation between mental-health programs and mental-hospital programs, with mental health on one side and mental illness on the other, quite separate. . . . The mental health programs of health departments . . . devote their special attention to what are called "educational and preventive services," and with few exceptions shy away from having much, if anything, to do with the treatment of mental illness.[20]

However, there seems to be a trend toward overcoming this kind of splintering. While in 1950 only seventeen states combined community mental health activities and mental hospitals within the same department, by 1965 the number had risen to thirty-nine. Of the eleven states which have not combined these two activities, ten have maintained the public health department as the mental health authority.

[20] Raymond G. Fuller, "A Study of Administration of State Psychiatric Services," *Mental Hygiene,* XXXVIII (April 1954), 227.

There have been two forces at work in determining the administrative location of mental health activities. One argument has been that community mental health activities should be most closely related organizationally with other community health programs and consequently should be the responsibility of the state health department. The usual result was the administrative separation of community programs and hospitals, even though both were crucial segments of the overall mental health effort. The other argument has been that the prevention and cure of mental illness is a single function and therefore state mental hospitals and community mental health programs should be administered by the same agency. This often led to the unification of those two aspects of mental health activity but also the separation of community mental health services from other community health programs. What effect the 1963 Act's emphasis on the importance of integrated mental health services in community centers will have on the pattern of state organization remains to be seen.

LOCAL PROGRAMS AND ORGANIZATION

With the gradual assumption by the states of responsibility for the care and treatment of the mentally ill in the closing decades of the nineteenth century, what little local governmental activity there had been was largely supplanted. Apart from a few states where county mental hospitals continued to operate, local governmental efforts all but disappeared.

Some aspects of the mental health problem continued to receive local attention, of course, but only because of their relation to some other governmental concern. Law enforcement agencies were necessarily concerned with some of the results of drug addiction and alcoholism. Domestic relations courts, juvenile courts, and welfare agencies continued to be obliquely concerned with mental illness as a contributor to broken homes, delinquency, and other social problems. But, as was the case with federal activity prior to 1945, local government efforts in regard to mental health were directed toward a limited clientele posing specific problems.

Private efforts in this field, however, were and still are primarily local. To be sure, national philanthropic organizations such as the Rockefeller and Hogg Foundations and the Milbank Memorial Fund contribute to research and training programs as well as to the provision of services,

But child guidance clinics, pastoral counseling, nursing homes, and private hospitals are usually local undertakings. Even the funds raised by local chapters of the National Association for Mental Health are expended for local projects. Most mental health activities at the local level are uncoordinated and frequently unrelated.

Increasing emphasis on the importance of treating the mentally ill in their own communities has led to a renewed interest in locally based services and the growth of outpatient psychiatric clinics. The first outpatient clinic was opened in 1885 as a service of the Pennsylvania Hospital. An experiment, the clinic was opened "under a conviction that in a city of one million inhabitants, a large number were suffering from premonitory symptoms of insanity such as nervous prostration and depression, who might receive kindly advice and treatment, and that a further development of mental disorder might thus be arrested." [21]

As late as 1920 there were only 60 clinics in the whole country.[22] But by 1930, largely as a result of subsidies from the Commonwealth Fund, the number of outpatient psychiatric clinics had increased to 217. Many of these, however, operated only as child guidance centers. The number continued to grow slowly and in 1945 there were approximately 450 clinics in operation. But in that year 15 states still had no facilities of this kind and the outpatient services available in the others were far less than adequate.

After the passage of the National Mental Health Act of 1946, the increase in the number of outpatient psychiatric clinics was remarkable. Indeed, the growth was so rapid that of the 1,234 clinics in operation at the end of 1954 nearly two-thirds were opened in 1946 or later. As of April 1965 there were 2,007 such facilities in the United States, providing more than 406,000 professional man-hours per week, an increase of more than 200 per cent over 1954. Moreover, every state had at least 3 clinics in operation.

In recent years a major new development has given increased impetus to local government provision of mental health services. In 1954 New York became the first state to enact a community mental health law

---

[21] Franklin G. Ebaugh and Charles A. Rymer, *Psychiatry in Medical Education* (New York: The Commonwealth Fund, 1942), p. 5.

[22] Anita K. Bahn and Vivian B. Norman, *Outpatient Psychiatric Clinics in the United States, 1954–1955: Characteristics and Professional Staff*, U.S., Public Health Service, Public Health Monograph No. 49 (Washington: U.S. Government Printing Office, 1957), p. 3.

that permitted counties or groups of counties, municipalities of specific size, and in some instances other governmental jurisdictions to operate mental health clinics. As of 1965 twenty-four states had provided for sharing the operating costs of these mental health clinics with local governments. In general, state funds were used for salaries, maintenance, and travel. These acts vary considerably in both the extent of their support and the manner in which it is given. Some of them, such as Colorado, Minnesota, and New Jersey, match local expenditures up to a specified maximum contribution per capita, while others, such as Maine and Wyoming, match all local contributions. The states of Michigan, Oregon, California, and Louisiana are the most generous. Under the Short-Doyle Act, California provides up to 75 per cent state support. Louisiana provides 75 per cent state support in all instances. The existence of these acts illustrates the increasing tendency to decentralize responsibility for mental health services from the state level to the local community.

As a consequence of the community mental health acts and varied programs of local assistance in other states, the rapid growth of outpatient psychiatric clinics in recent years has been accompanied by a growing involvement of local government in the provision of mental health services. While the increase in the number of locally based facilities during recent years has been considerable, the range of community services still leaves much to be desired. While there were 2,007 outpatient psychiatric clinics in operation in 1965, many clinics served only children. Some were directed toward special groups such as college students, veterans, court cases, and alcoholics. Many clinics offered services only on a part-time basis and many spent little time on community-oriented activities.

Consultation and conferences with other agencies, in-service training for professional groups, informational and educational services for the general public, participation in community planning—all of these were important community services which an outpatient psychiatric clinic could provide. But according to a NIMH survey conducted in 1958, "Outpatient psychiatric clinics, regardless of hours open, groups served, or agency operating the clinic, typically devote a relatively small proportion of time to community oriented services." [23] The continued lack of

[23] Vivian B. Norman, Beatrice M. Rosen, and Anita K. Bahn, "Community Oriented Services of Psychiatric Clinics, 1958," *Public Health Reports*, LXXVI (1961), 231–32.

emphasis on these programs was undoubtedly a major factor in causing Dr. Felix to say in 1961, "There probably is no ideal community mental health program in the United States today. The integration of mental health services into community health and welfare programs is a task for the decade ahead." [24]

If community-oriented functions are to receive increased emphasis in the future, a case can be made for accentuating the trend toward greater local government participation. But the decentralization of treatment facilities and the localization of responsibility that have occurred to date are already sufficient to point up a number of organizational problems. There is the problem of how to divide responsibility between state and local governments. In the past, by providing hospitals for the mentally ill, state governments have borne the major financial burden. The decentralization of mental health services raises the question of the extent to which financial responsibility can be shifted downward. And even if this can be answered satisfactorily, there remains the difficulty of delineating the administrative authority of state mental health agencies on the one hand and local units on the other. Speaking to this problem, Dr. Jack Ewalt said:

The local clinic should be responsible for determining matters of local policy, such as eligibility for clinic treatment in terms of finances, sources of referral, location of the clinic's office, and hours of operation. The Central Department of Mental Health should determine the basic organization of the offices, the competence of employees, and should take primary responsibility for recruiting the staff, subject to the approval of the local committee.[25]

But will political realities within the various states permit such a division of responsibility?

The question of which agencies should be assigned administrative responsibility is as pertinent at the local level as it is at the state. Should the local mental health agency be part of the public health department or should it be separate? The dispute has both theoretical and practical overtones. As a recent study put it:

The Public Health Program is significant for mental health in three special ways. First is the leadership role played by public health officers in planning, research, financial support, and provision of certain mental health services.

[24] Robert H. Felix, "A Comprehensive Community Mental Health Program," in *Mental Health and Social Welfare* (New York: Columbia University Press, 1961), p. 13.
[25] Jack R. Ewalt, *Mental Health Administration* (Springfield, Ill.: Charles C. Thomas, 1956), p. 22.

Secondly, the general level of health in a community is significant for maintaining and supporting the level of mental health. . . .

Thirdly, the more adequate the public health services, the more likely they are to provide a supply of public health nurses under high-grade supervision and with mental health consultation.[26]

But the easy conclusion that mental health activities should be administratively united with the public health program ignores the long-standing dispute over whether clinical or preventive measures should receive primary emphasis.

Numerous local agencies other than health departments perform mental health functions. Welfare departments, school boards, law enforcement authorities, and planning boards are the most obvious. Indeed, activities closely related to mental health so pervade the local administrative structure that interagency cooperation is necessary if diagnosis and treatment services are to be fully effective. Furthermore, with the existence of a large number of voluntary organizations involved in various types of mental health activities, the coordination of public and private efforts, as well as interagency cooperation, is important to the success of local mental health programs.

In summary, the extent of governmental efforts on behalf of mental health by 1963 was a far cry from what it was a hundred years ago. Governmental involvement had become so great that it reached all levels of the federal structure and concerned directly or tangentially a number of different agencies at each level. State governments continued to bear the principal burden of caring for the mentally ill, and the mental hospital remained the essential core of their operations. But treatment leading to cure, as opposed to mere custodial care, was receiving ever-growing emphasis; and despite the rapidly growing population and an accompanying increase in admissions, the mental hospital resident population was declining. Growing emphasis on community mental health in the wake of increased public awareness of the problems of mental illness and mounting interest in the potential of new approaches had led to a resurgence of local involvement in the provision of services. In many places psychiatric clinics and mental health centers operated by local government agencies alone or in cooperation with state authorities were

[26] Reginald Robinson, David F. De Marche, and Mildred K. Wagle, *Community Resources in Mental Health* (New York: Basic Books, 1960), p. 16.

becoming highly important links in the chain of available services. Part of the credit for the upsurge of public activities on behalf of mental health must go to the increased efforts on the part of the federal government since 1946. In 1963 the federal government enacted the Mental Retardation Facilities and Community Mental Health Centers Construction Act, designed to direct state and local efforts toward a more comprehensive approach. If this attempt is to be more than simply bold words and lofty ideals, it must be fitted into a complex system of ongoing federal, state, and local programs.

III: THE NEW FEDERAL APPROACH

PRESIDENT KENNEDY'S MESSAGE to Congress of February 5, 1963, announced a new federal approach to mental illness and mental retardation. Foundations had been laid several years earlier, however, in the work of the Joint Commission on Mental Illness and Health. In a larger sense, the new mental health approach evolved out of the experience of the National Institute of Mental Health, which had existed for a decade and a half. From the establishment of a professional group to study the problem of mental illness, through the drafting of the President's message, to action by Congress, the story of these efforts provides an excellent example of the workings of the American political process. The train of events leading to the passage of the Act actually began ten years earlier with what might be termed the "Appel appeal," which was as important in its way as the famed Flexner Report of a previous day.

The publication in 1910 of Abraham Flexner's findings on medical education heralded the development of a rapid and radical improvement in the teaching, and thus the practice, of medicine in the United States. Based on a survey Flexner made for the Carnegie Foundation for the Advancement of Teaching, his report was entitled *Medical Education in the United States and Canada*. Written by a layman, this highly literate essay became a landmark development in the history of American medicine. The Flexner Report exposed abuses in medical education and proposed reforms, thereby hastening much-needed improvements in teaching, curricula, and standards of American medical schools. As Dr. Jack R. Ewalt has put it, "The Flexner Report is credited with bringing about the Class A Standardization and AMA approval of all our modern medical schools. As a consequence, something like half of the then existing medical schools—proprietary diploma mills, most of them—were forced to close." [1]

[1] Bullard Professor of Psychiatry, Harvard University; past president of the American Psychiatric Association; formerly superintendent, Massachusetts Mental

Forty-three years later, the public statement of another concerned individual reflected important stirrings of interest, sometimes indignation, in the field of psychiatric medicine. In the fall of 1953 at a conference on mental health held in Washington under the auspices of the American Medical Association (AMA) and the American Psychiatric Association (APA), Dr. Kenneth Appel, then president of the APA, appealed for a survey that would produce for mental health the kind of results that came out of the Flexner Report. Dr. Appel's continued exertions and the vigorous efforts of many of his medical colleagues in cooperation with an ever-growing number of other interested individuals and groups bore significant fruit. Out of their work grew the Joint Commission on Mental Illness and Health and its important report, and thus, indirectly, the renewed, redoubled, and redirected efforts now developing under the Mental Retardation Facilities and Community Mental Health Centers Construction Act of 1963.

THE MENTAL HEALTH STUDY ACT OF 1955

Following his appeal in late 1953, Dr. Appel continued to point out the need for a nationwide survey of the problem of mental illness. Other members of the American Psychiatric Association (APA) together with members of the Council on Mental Health of the American Medical Association (AMA) joined in discussions of how to undertake a nationwide study of the problems of mental and emotional illness. In the meantime, during 1953 and 1954, the need to do something constructive with regard to mental illness was urged at the Mental Hospital Institute, at the Governors' Conference, and in the APA presidential addresses. Then in the fall of 1954, following a symposium on "current directions in psychiatry," the Field Foundation provided funds for the APA and the AMA Council on Mental Health to join forces for a joint attack on the problem of mental illness. This grant of $5,000 served as the initial mobilizing contribution to what was to become the Joint Commission on Mental Illness and Health.

With the assistance of Dr. Daniel Blain, then medical director of the American Psychiatric Association, Senator Lister Hill (Democrat, Ala-

---

Health Center. Paper presented at Summer Research Training Institute in Survey Methods in Research on Health Programs, National Opinion Research Center, Chicago, Ill., Aug. 9, 1956.

bama) drafted a resolution for a study of mental illness, which he introduced in the Senate on February 18, 1955.[2] A short time later, Congressman J. Percy Priest (Democrat, Tennessee) introduced a similar resolution in the House of Representatives.[3] In committee hearings held during March, representatives of the APA, Dr. Leo Bartemeier for the AMA, and Dr. Fillmore Sanford for the American Psychological Association strongly supported the measures. The Mental Health Study Act of 1955,[4] providing for "an objective, thorough, and nationwide analysis and reevaluation of the human and economic problems of mental illness," became law without a dissenting vote. The Surgeon General was authorized to make grants in the amount of $1,250,000 over a three-year period to one or more organizations for the carrying out of a coordinated "program of research into and study of our resources, methods, and practices for diagnosing, treating, caring for, and rehabilitating the mentally ill, such programs to be on a scale commensurate with the problem."

Meantime, the planning begun by the American Psychiatric Association and the AMA's Council on Mental Health under the Field Foundation grant continued. An organizational meeting of what was to be the Joint Commission was held in April of 1955 and was attended by representatives of some twenty organizations in addition to the APA and AMA. A sustaining contribution of $10,000 from the Smith-Klineand-French Company, a pharmaceutical manufacturer, enabled the planning to be carried to completion. In August 1955 the Joint Commission on Mental Illness and Health was incorporated in the District of Columbia. Thus, only one month after the passage of the Mental Health Study Act, there was formally in existence an organization expressly and carefully designed to undertake the nongovernmental, multidisciplinary research which that Act sought to encourage.

In September 1955 the Commission's board of trustees[5] met in

---

[2] U.S., Congress, Senate, *Joint Resolution 46,* 84th Cong., 1st Sess., 1955.
[3] U.S., Congress, House, *Joint Resolution 256,* 84th Cong., 1st Sess.; introduced March 17, 1955.
[4] Public Law 182, 84th Cong., 1st Sess.; approved July 28, 1955. 69 Stat. 381.
[5] The trustees, as named in the incorporation papers, were: For the American Psychiatric Association—Kenneth E. Appel, M.D.; Walter Barton, M.D.; Francis Braceland, M.D.; Jack Ewalt, M.D.; Harvey Tomkins, M.D. For the American Medical Association—Walter Baer, M.D.; Leo H. Bartemeier, M.D.; Hugh Carmichael, M.D.; M. Ralph Kaufman, M.D.; Lauren H. Smith, M.D. For the American Psychological Association—Nicholas Hobbs, Ph.D. For the American Association of Psychiatric Social Workers—Miss Madeline Lay. For the American Hospital

Chicago, elected officers, adopted by-laws, appointed a nominating committee to suggest officers of the Commission as distinguished from the trustees, and called for the first meeting of the whole Commission to be held October 8, 1955, in Washington, D.C. From the beginning, organizational participation was emphasized. Some eighteen organizations originally appointed representatives to the Joint Commission. The American Psychiatric Association and the American Medical Association were allotted five representatives apiece while all other organizations had one spokesman each.[6] Most of these organizations continued as members, and others were added later so that at the time of its final report the Joint Commission could list thirty-six participating agencies and forty-five individual members who served as their representatives.

The Joint Commission held its first formal meeting, as scheduled, in October 1955 in Washington, D.C. Dr. Kenneth Appel, appropriately, was elected president. Necessary decisions regarding responsibilities and procedure were reached, and finance and membership committees were appointed. More significantly, the groundwork was laid for the important study which the Commission was about to make. It was agreed that its task was not to undertake or support basic research but to assess the current situation and to make recommendations concerning the most promising lines of attack on mental illness.

Thus, the Commission's proposed undertaking was brought in line with the statement of purpose of the Mental Health Study Act of 1955. A preview of the direction the Commission's study would take was furnished by the reception given the report of the committee on objectives and methods. The committee, under the chairmanship of Dr. Jack Ewalt, named solution-seeking as the main goal, emphasizing the importance of maximum freedom in this search. It stressed the desirability of discovering and developing new approaches, of taking a new look at the whole problem of mental illness. New perspectives were to be sought, new departures developed and examined, perhaps even radical reconstructions of the present system recommended. Merely an evaluation

---

Association—Russell Nelson, M.D. For the American Nursing Association and the National League of Nursing—Miss Kathleen Black. For the National Education Association—Miss Elizabeth Avery.

[6] For a complete listing of participating agencies and individual members as well as a roster of officers, advisory committee members, and consultants, see Joint Commission on Mental Illness and Health, *Action for Mental Health* (New York: Basic Books, 1961), Appendix II, pp. 306–15.

of the conventional social, legal, and medical approaches would not suffice. Apparently impressed by this report, the Commission asked that the committee carry on as its scientific study and planning committee. Later, Dr. Ewalt accepted the responsibility for directing the Commission's study.

Also at this first meeting, plans were made for the preparation of an application to the Surgeon General of the United States for a grant of $250,000 for the first year of a three-year project as set forth in the provisions of the Mental Health Study Act. The application was submitted, it was approved, and the Joint Commission on Mental Illness and Health, which had been instrumental in bringing to fruition the Mental Health Study Act, became the official designee to conduct the study which that Act authorized. In January of 1956 the Commission received its initial grant of $250,000 and shortly thereafter established headquarters at Cambridge, Massachusetts, assembled a staff, and the study was underway.

During the following five years the Commission, assisted by a highly able staff and an impressive assembly of advisory committee members and consultants, conducted the extensive study contemplated by its organizers and by the congressional Act.[7] Given a study of such breadth, it is hardly surprising that it was costly; and, had more funds been available, the Commission most certainly would have further expanded its effort.[8] The full authorization of the Mental Health Study Act of 1955 was received and expended, as were additional grants totaling $160,000 from the National Institute of Mental Health, bringing the total governmental funds utilized by the Commission to $1,410,600.

[7] The scope of the task it set itself is indicated by the titles included in the Monograph Series which the Commission produced: Marie Jahoda, Current Concepts of Positive Mental Health (1958); Rashi Fein, Economics of Mental Illness (1958); George W. Albee, Mental Health Manpower Trends (1959); Gerald Gurin, Joseph Verhoff, and Sheila Field, Americans View Their Mental Health, A National Interview Survey (1960); Reginald Robinson, David F. De Marche, and Mildred K. Wagle, Community Resources in Mental Health (1960); Richard J. Plunkett and John E. Gordon, Epidemiology and Mental Illness (1960); Wesley Allinsmith and George W. Goethals, The Role of Schools in Mental Health; Richard V. McCann, The Churches and Mental Health (1962); Morris S. Schwartz et al., Social Approaches to Mental Patient Care (1964); and William F. Soskin, Research Resources in Mental Health (unpublished).

[8] See Director Ewalt's comment in the Introduction to the Commission's final report, Action for Mental Health (New York: Basic Books, 1961), p. xxx. It also contains a complete listing of the sources and amounts of financial support for the Commission's endeavors.

While early expectations called for extensive additional support from private sources, and while there were some generous contributions from nongovernmental agencies, the total received in this way came to only $137,427. Even though some concerns may have had to be curtailed, the million and a half dollars available proved sufficient to produce a significant study. On the last day of 1960 the final report of the Joint Commission on Mental Illness and Health, *Action for Mental Health,* was submitted as directed by the Act to Congress, to the Surgeon General, and to the governors of the fifty states.

THE JOINT COMMISSION'S RECOMMENDATIONS

Apart from its proposal of an extensive public information program on mental illness in order to facilitate greater public awareness and understanding of the problem, the Joint Commission's recommendations were summarized under three main headings: (1) "Pursuit of New Knowledge," (2) "Better Use of Present Knowledge and Experience," and (3) "The Cost." Under the first heading, the Commission's general recommendation was "an extension and expansion, combined with certain shifts of emphasis, in the research grant program ably administered at present by the National Institute of Mental Health." Among the shifts of emphasis urged were the investment of a much larger proportion of total funds for mental health research in basic, as contrasted with applied, research and in long-term projects as opposed to short-term research. New efforts by NIMH to "invest in, provide for, and hold the young scientist in his career choice," as well as more salary support for mental health career investigators and the establishment of more full-time positions by the federal government were called for. And in addition to urging that federal support of program research in established scientific and educational institutions be continued and considerably expanded, the Commission proposed that the federal government support the establishment of new mental health research centers or research institutes.

The Commission's recommendations under "Better Use of Present Knowledge and Experience" were even more extensive. The report called for better utilization of available manpower by the adoption and practice by the mental health professions of "a broad, liberal philosophy of what constitutes and who can do treatment within the framework of their hospitals, clinics, or other professional service agencies." To that end the Commission set forth some general guidelines for proper division of responsibilities among professionals and between professionals and subprofessionals, and called for the encouragement and extension of volunteer work with mental hospital patients. The report also stressed the need for launching "a national manpower recruitment and training program, expanding on and extending present efforts and seeking to stimulate the interest of American youth in mental health work as a career," the program to "include all categories of mental health personnel" and to "emphasize not only professional training but also short courses and on-the-job training for partially trained persons." Further, the Commission recommended that the federal government not only support a student scholarship and loan program, but also amend the income tax laws to allow deductions of direct expenses for education.

Under the same general heading, the Commission also called for expansion of secondary prevention efforts by supporting training and consultative programs designed to capitalize on the potential community resources available in the persons and services of such people as pediatricians, clergymen, family physicians, teachers, law enforcement officers, public health nurses, public welfare workers, and others. It asserted that aftercare, intermediate care, and rehabilitation were essential and integral parts of a comprehensive program of patient services and urged expanded efforts toward development and improvement in these areas. And it proposed

expanding treatment of the acutely ill mental patient in all directions, via community mental health clinics, general hospitals, and mental hospitals, as rapidly as psychiatrists, clinical psychologists, psychiatric nurses, psychiatric social workers, and occupational, physical, and other nonmedical therapists become available in the community.[9]

The Commission set as an objective the establishment of one fully staffed, full-time mental health clinic available to each 50,000 of population. It urged that every general hospital of 100 beds or more should accept mental patients for short-term hospitalization and therefore should provide a psychiatric unit or psychiatric beds. It proposed that smaller state hospitals, "of 1000 beds or less and suitably located . . . be converted as rapidly as possible into intensive treatment centers" for the acutely ill. Further, it urged that all new state hospital construction be

[9] *Ibid.*, p. xiv.

devoted to these smaller intensive treatment centers, that not one patient be added to any existing mental hospital already housing 1,000 or more patients. Existing large state hospitals should "be gradually and progressively converted into centers for the long-term and combined care of chronic diseases, including mental illness."

The significant financial recommendations were spelled out under "The Cost." Expenditures for public mental health services should be doubled in the next five years and tripled in the next ten. Only by this magnitude of expenditure could the typical state institutions be made in fact what currently they were in name only—hospitals for mental patients. And only by this magnitude of expenditure could outpatient and expatient programs be sufficiently extended outside the mental hospitals into the community.

Recognizing that the states were an unlikely source for the kind of money needed, the Commission called for extensive financial participation by the federal government. In the words of the report:

We recommend that the States and the Federal government work toward a time when a share of the cost of State and local mental patient services will be borne by the Federal government, over and above the present and future program of Federal grants in aid for research and training. . . . under the present tax structure only the Federal government has the financial resources needed to overcome the lag and to achieve a minimum standard of adequacy. The Federal government should be prepared to assume a major part of the responsibility for the mentally ill insofar as the States are agreeable to surrendering it.[10]

More specifically, pointing to the Veterans Administration mental hospitals as financial models of what could be done in the operation of public mental hospitals, the Commission recommended that Congress and the National Institute of Mental Health should develop a federal subsidy program that would encourage states and local governments to follow the example set by VA mental hospitals.

In order to achieve its ends, the Commission recommended that certain principles be followed in a federal program of matching grants to states for the care of the mentally ill. These were: first, "that the Federal government on the one side and State and local governments on the other should *share in the costs* of services to the mentally ill"; second, "that the total Federal share should be arrived at in a *series of graduated steps* over a period of years, the share being determined each

---

[10] *Ibid.*, p. xx; emphasis in original.

year on the basis of State funds spent in a previous year"; and, third, "that the grants should be awarded according to *criteria of merit and incentive* to be formulated by an expert advisory committee appointed by the National Institute of Mental Health." [11]

In short, the Joint Commission had outlined two major new roles for the federal government. It had proposed substantial financial participation by the federal government in the care of patients who heretofore had been considered the responsibility of the states. And it had made the novel recommendation, having the most far-reaching policy implications, that the federal government establish and maintain standards for the quality of care of the mentally ill.

PRELUDE TO ACTION

Perhaps the heavy emphasis placed on inpatient care explains why the Joint Commission's report produced no immediate governmental response. A number of people, most significantly those in charge of the National Institute of Mental Health, charged that "considerably more attention could have been placed upon steps aimed at prevention of mental illness and upon maintenance of mental health." [12] Nonetheless, after a ten-month lapse, a special Governors' Conference on Mental Health was convened in Chicago on November 9, 1961, followed three weeks later by the appointment of a "cabinet-level" committee by the President. The chain of events which followed augured that the era of exploration of the 1950s would now be followed in the decade of the 1960s with an era of action in the mental health field.

That the Commission's report had made a profound impression on the governors is evident in the policy statement adopted by the conference. Noting that *Action for Mental Health* was the first survey in the nation's history that related the problem of mental illness to the various responsibilities of federal, state, and local governments, the governors commended the Joint Commission for "an excellent study." And the policy statement continued with the assertion that "we accept

[11] *Ibid.*, emphasis in original. The reports of the Joint Commission were reviewed at some length in various periodicals. See especially Elaine Cumming, "A Review Article—The Reports of the Joint Commission on Mental Illness and Health," *Social Problems*, Vol. 9, No. 4 (Spring 1962), pp. 391–400.

[12] Robert H. Felix, *Mental Illness: Progress and Prospects* (New York: Columbia University Press, 1967).

the findings that much remains to be done; and we endorse the concept that Federal, State, and local governments as well as private and voluntary efforts must be combined to achieve the goals we seek."

Perhaps most significantly, the governors indicated at least partial acceptance of the Joint Commission's call for new and substantial financial participation by the federal government in combating mental illness. The conference adopted a resolution noting specifically the importance of one kind of federal financial participation. The Social Security Act specifically precluded patients in public and private institutions for mental disease and in community nursing and foster homes from receiving federal public assistance. This policy should be changed, the governors thought.

On November 30, 1961, President John F. Kennedy asked the Secretary of Health, Education, and Welfare, Abraham Ribicoff, to analyze the Joint Commission report "with a view to developing courses of action which might be appropriate for the Federal Government." The President informed the Secretary that he was asking the Secretary of Labor, the administrator of Veterans Affairs, and representatives of the Council of Economic Advisers and the Bureau of the Budget to join in the consideration of the report and the formulation of possible courses of action. In developing proposals, the Secretary was asked to give careful attention to:

1. What should be the federal role in the mental health field and what responsibility should remain with the states, localities, and private groups?

2. If broadened federal activity is warranted, through what channels should it be directed?

3. What emphasis should be given to federal activity in the mental health field in relation to support for more general health programs?

4. What rate of expansion in public programs for mental health services and research is consistent with the present and prospective supply of trained manpower?

5. In the mental health field, should relatively greater encouragement be given to strengthening institutional services or noninstitutional programs, including means for bringing the cost of noninstitutional services within the financial means of a larger number of people?

During the following year, the cabinet-level committee which the President had called for worked at its task of reviewing the Joint Commission's report. Representatives of the agencies named by the President met and deliberated under the leadership of Mr. Boisfeuillet Jones, Special Assistant for Health and Medical Affairs to the Secretary of Health, Education, and Welfare. The "Bo Jones" committee held many sessions and considered not only the Joint Commission's report but also numerous position papers and other advisory materials prepared by the National Institute of Mental Health. During this period state mental health commissioners and other representatives of state agencies responsible for mental health were frequently brought to Washington and consulted as to what kind of program they could live with and were capable of administering. The committee's internal report to the President was never publicly released, but the committee's deliberations culminated in a special message to Congress from the President.

THE PRESIDENT'S MESSAGE

On February 5, 1963, President Kennedy sent to Congress his "Message on Mental Illness and Mental Retardation." [13] An entire message was devoted to these two health problems because, in Mr. Kennedy's words, "they are of such critical size and tragic impact, and because their susceptibility to public action is so much greater than the attention they have received." The President's treatment of these problems made it clear that his cabinet-level committee had developed proposals for action which accepted most of the Joint Commission's findings and many of its recommendations, including its urgent plea for extensive federal financial participation in combating mental illness. But it was also clear that there had been a shift of emphasis regarding the means for implementing the program of improved mental health services which the Commission envisioned.

The message contrasted the magnitude of the problem with the inadequacy of public activity. The President pointed out that at any one time there were approximately 600,000 patients in the country's institutions for the mentally ill and 200,000 in those for the mentally retarded, with a total of 1,500,000 persons receiving treatment at some time during the year. The cost to the taxpayers came to $1.8 billion for

[13] U.S., *Congressional Record,* 88th Cong., 1st Sess., 1963, CIX, Part 2, 1744–49, and as H.R. Doc. 58.

mental illness and $1.6 billion for mental retardation. Yet the average daily expenditure per patient was only about $4 per day, and in some states it was less than $2 a day.

"Governments at every level—Federal, State, and local—private foundations and individual citizens," the President concluded, "must all face up to their responsibilities in this area." Following the Joint Commission's lead, he asked for a broad attack focused on three major objectives: (1) finding and eradicating the causes of mental illness and mental retardation, (2) strengthening the underlying resources of knowledge and necessary skilled manpower, and (3) strengthening and improving the programs and facilities for the mentally ill and mentally retarded. The President called for a new approach to mental illness and mental retardation, an approach "designed, in large measure, to use Federal resources to stimulate State, local, and private action."

In one very important way the program for mental health which the President proposed involved a significant shift in emphasis from the Joint Commission's report. The Commission had stressed, among many other things, the need for improved treatment facilities, and in this connection had recommended the widespread establishment of community mental health clinics along with the gradual elimination of mental hospitals of more than one thousand beds. Rather than community *clinics,* the President's message emphasized community *centers,* which appeared to be far more broadly conceived than the typical clinic.

Relying heavily on new knowledge and new drugs making it possible for the mentally ill to be successfully and quickly treated in their own communities and returned to a useful place in society, the President asked Congress to authorize grants to the states for construction of "comprehensive community mental health centers," short-term grants for their initial staffing, and a relatively small sum for planning grants. These proposed comprehensive community mental health centers were to focus on both treatment and prevention. They were to provide a continuum of treatment, from diagnosis, to cure, to rehabilitation, without need to transfer to different institutions located in different communities. The message emphasized that private practitioners would be able to participate in the program envisioned, and that private funds as well as public would support it. "Long-range federal subsidies for operating costs are neither necessary nor desirable" was a particular point.

Apparently, the community concept was to be emphasized, in the long run, in financing as well.

The proposed mental retardation program emphasized prevention, particularly the need for better prenatal care among the "medically indigent," though this point did not enter into the Mental Health Act of 1963 as passed. The message also proposed "community-centered agencies" including inpatient clinics as part of university associated hospitals; outpatient diagnostic, evaluation, and treatment clinics also associated with such hospitals; and satellite clinics in outlying cities and counties. The need for expanding special education, training, and rehabilitation services, including supporting research and the training of teachers for mentally retarded and other handicapped children was also stressed. In short, a full-scale national attack on the problems of mental illness and mental retardation was called for, with the federal government leading the way, but primarily in a catalytic role insisting on the crucial significance of the local community.

CONGRESSIONAL ACTION

Following the President's message, the Secretary of the Department of Health, Education, and Welfare transmitted draft legislation to Congress. In the Senate, two bills introduced by Senator Lister Hill (Democrat, Alabama), S.755 and S.756 were referred to the Committee on Labor and Public Welfare. They became the subject of hearings conducted by the Subcommittee on Health on March 5, 6, and 7, 1963.[14]

Under the chairmanship of Senator Hill, the subcommittee received testimony—either direct, written, or both—from Administration witnesses, representative of various organizations and associations, and numerous individuals as well. The Administration delegation was headed by Secretary of Health, Education, and Welfare Anthony J. Celebrezze and included Dr. Luther L. Terry, Surgeon General; Mr. Boisfeuillet Jones, Special Assistant for Health and Medical Affairs; Dr. Robert H. Felix, director, National Institute of Mental Health; Dr.

---

[14] U.S., Congress, Senate, Subcommittee on Health of the Committee on Labor and Public Welfare, *Hearings on S. 755 and 756*, 88th Cong., 1st Sess., 1963; and U.S., Congress, House, Subcommittee of the Committee on Interstate Commerce, *Hearings on H.R. 3688, 3689, and 2567*, 88th Cong., 1st Sess., 1963.

Robert A. Aldrich, director, National Institute of Child Health and Human Development; Dr. Jack C. Haldemann, chief, Division of Hospital and Medical Facilities, Public Health Service; and Mr. Wilbur J. Cohen, Assistant Secretary for Legislation. Representatives of sixteen national organizations testified before the subcommittee. Other organizations submitted prepared statements. All of them supported the proposed mental health legislation.

An impressive array of support came from the states themselves. All in all, thirty-nine states through their governors or high administrative officials concerned with mental health or retardation presented evidence of support to the subcommittee. Of the remaining eleven, Massachusetts might also be considered as represented, for Dr. Jack R. Ewalt, appearing primarily in his capacity as president-elect of the American Psychiatric Association, was at the time superintendent of the Massachusetts Mental Health Center.[15]

Questioning by the Senate subcommittee was friendly and virtually no hostile testimony was given. However, one should not confuse appearance with reality. This was a well-managed production, and most of the testimony came from the "in-group." The fact that there was little hostile testimony did not indicate that hostility was nonexistent, but merely that it had not yet coalesced.

The closest approach to opposition that was heard came from a spokesman from the AMA who pointed out that there were two views within the association on whether the federal government should provide funds to assist in the initial staffing of the proposed mental health centers. He indicated that the association had not come to a firm position on the point. Also, Dr. Robert Felix, director of NIMH, suggested that the subcommittee might give serious consideration to whether the mental health and mental retardation programs should be quite so divorced at the local level as called for by some of the witnesses.

The general tone of the proceedings was reflected in the excellent rapport between Dr. Robert Felix and the members of the subcommittee. When Dr. Felix was called by Chairman Hill to testify, it was in

---

[15] The ten states not included did not represent any regional pattern. Three (Florida, Mississippi, and Texas) were from the South; four (Ohio, Michigan, Oklahoma, and South Dakota) from the Midwest and prairies; and three (Idaho, Montana, and Nevada) from the West. See résumé given during Senate debate, *Congressional Record*, 88th Cong., 1st Sess., 1963, CIX, Part 71, 8970, 8973, 8976.

these words: "Doctor, we are going to ask you to give us the doxology." Among the points made by Dr. Felix was the hoped-for effect of the proposed legislation on the traditional state mental hospital system. "I wish to God I could live and be active for 25 more years," he said, "because I believe if I could, I would see the day when the State mental hospitals as we know them today would no longer exist."

The Senate subcommittee and its parent committee eventually combined the two separate bills before them into one measure (S.1576) and reported this bill to the Senate in late May. Before then, however, House committee proceedings occurred on similar bills (H.R.3688 and 3689), introduced by Representative Oren Harris (Democrat, Arkansas).

Much of the testimony heard by the House body was similar to that presented to the Senate committee. The Administration dispatched virtually the same phalanx of witnesses, although Dr. Felix did not play much of a role this time. Almost all of the associations and organizations which had supported the bills before the Senate subcommittee submitted evidence of support this time as well. Many state governors and mental health administrators endorsing the legislation in the earlier hearings did likewise before the House subcommittee.

The House hearings were, nevertheless, by no means a carbon copy of the Senate proceedings. For one thing, the tone of the House subcommittee hearings was different; questioning seemed sharper, more detailed. Chairman Harris of the parent Committee on Interstate and Foreign Commerce attended the hearings and took particular pains to get into the record the need for the new legislation in view of the already existing body of law and appropriation authorizations.[16] He was also concerned over a possible jurisdictional conflict with the House Committee on Education and Labor. There was considerable probing as to exact costs, the nature of the proposed mental health centers, and research conducted and to be conducted. Under this probing, NIMH submitted estimates indicating that the cost of constructing a community mental health center would be $1,300,000. The number of centers contemplated was 422, each requiring a staff of 108. Each center would serve an area with 100,000 population and cost over $1 million per year to operate. The program called for federal matching

[16] See, for example, his questioning in the House subcommittee hearings on H.R. 3688, 3689, and 2567, pp. 70–74.

funds of 45 to 75 per cent of the construction costs. When asked why this percentage was proposed instead of a 50–50 formula, the Administration witness, Mr. Boisfeuillet Jones, replied that a 50–50 program would not provide sufficient stimulation to communities "that have been reluctant through the years to give special recognition to mental health," and that an additional impetus was necessary.

The House hearings also brought out the difference of opinion within the American Medical Association regarding federal assistance for initial staffing of the mental health centers. A spokesman for the AMA, Dr. Lindsay E. Beaton, said that the association's Council on Mental Health had recommended approval of federal aid for initial staffing, but that the AMA had not been able to reconcile within itself opposing views on the matter. One view favored federal financial assistance provided it was strictly limited to the four-year period proposed in the bill. It was felt that this would ensure that the centers could undertake a properly staffed program from the start and that before long the influx of patients and the transfer of state funds from other institutional facilities would make continued federal financing unnecessary. The other point of view opposed any federal staffing assistance, arguing that once the centers were constructed they should be the communities' responsibility. It was felt that once reliance was placed on a federal subsidy for staffing, the role of the federal government as a provider of funds would not easily be terminated. Apparently opposition within the AMA to federal funds for initial staffing was founded on the twin bases of professional concern over the medical importance of the program's community emphasis and political concern over governmental centralization.[17]

In contrast to the smooth sailing which the bills enjoyed in the Senate hearings, a measure of hostility toward the mental health legislation began to appear in the House proceedings. A representative of one small group, the National Health Federation, objected to failure of the bills to define precisely the terms "mental health, mental illness, and mental retardation." The federation wanted to make it a felony for any person administering the proposed law to attempt to change a person's belief in God. It feared a loss of parental control, and—on the positive side—stressed the relation of diet to physical and mental health. The American

---

[17] For further comment on the AMA position on health legislation see Richard Harris, "Annals of Legislation and Medicare," *New Yorker,* June and July 1966; and Robert Dahl, "American Oppositions: Affirmation and Denial," in *Political Oppositions in Western Democracies* (New Haven: Yale University Press, 1966).

Mental Health Foundation through its director of research, Dr. Stefan DeSchill, submitted written objections, evaluating the final report of the Joint Commission on Mental Illness and Health as "obsolete." The foundation argued that what was needed most, and first, were better methods of treatment and better psychotherapists, rather than billions of dollars from federal funds. A mild statement was submitted by a group of Organizations of Parents and Relatives of Mental Patients in New York; they felt that some attention should be given to the patients already in state mental hospitals. A few individuals sent letters to the subcommittee voicing opposition; one of these evoked the specter of "brain washing."

Senate bill 1576 came up for debate on May 27, 1963, and evoked almost no opposition. The only controversy occurred on a motion by Senator Jacob Javits (Republican, New York) to amend the bill to forbid payments to states in aid of any segregated facilities of a state program. The Senate Democratic leadership took the position that the adoption of Javits' proposed amendment would only defeat the measure itself, and it was laid on the table by a vote of 43 to 27. The bill then passed by a vote of 72 to 1.[18]

Title I of the Senate bill authorized $30 million over a five-year period for grants to pay up to 75 per cent of the construction of research centers by public or nonprofit institutions; $42.5 million over a five-year period for similar grants for college or university associated facilities; and $67.5 million for grants to the states over a four-year period to pay 45 to 75 per cent of construction costs of facilities for the mentally retarded. Title II dealt with construction and staffing of mental health centers. It authorized $230 million for grants to states over a four-year period to pay 45 to 75 per cent of the costs of constructing community mental health centers, and $427 million over an eight-year period to pay part of the costs of staffing the centers. Staffing assistance was to be limited to the first four and one-half years of operation, and to be decreased periodically from a maximum of 75 per cent of cost during the first 18 months of operation to a maximum of 30 per cent during the last year.

Title III, which had not been included in the original bills submitted

[18] Sen. Carl T. Curtis of Nebraska was the lone "nay." There were twenty-seven senators absent. The party leaders stated that twenty-five of these would have voted for the bill if they had been present. The two not included were Harry Byrd of Virginia and John Tower of Texas.

to either the Senate or House committees, dealt with the training of
teachers of mentally retarded and other handicapped children. It authorized $45.5 million over a three-year period for training teachers and
$6 million over the same period for research or demonstration projects
relating to education of the handicapped. Title IV contained general
provisions and definitions, including a definition of "federal share" of
grants.

After S.1576 was passed by the Senate, it went to the House and
was referred to the Committee on Interstate and Foreign Commerce.
The House committee requested the Subcommittee on Public Health
and Safety to hold further hearings, even though the subcommittee on
the basis of the earlier hearings had apparently reported a bill to the
committee. Chairman Harris indicated two major reasons for sending
the measure back to the subcommittee in spite of the "extensive hearings" already held and the "good record" already produced. First, Title
III had not been included in the original bills, and "one of the primary
purposes for going back to hearings . . . was to develop information
in connection with this part of the bill."

Secondly, Chairman Harris commented that it was the feeling of
some members of the committee "that the Senate-passed bill had not
been given the tedious consideration that it should have been given"
and that this led them to request further study of the composite new
bill. Another reason, not stated but apparent from the conduct of the
proceedings, was the "controversial" nature of the provisions of the
proposed bill relating to initial staffing of the community mental health
centers. Increasing AMA opposition to this part of the program was
no doubt a major factor in the decision to hold further public hearings.

The supplemental hearings before the subcommittee took place on
July 10 and 11, 1963.[19] As might be expected, a great deal of attention
was focused on the training of teachers of the retarded and handicapped.
Other questioning focused on mental health research and the relation of
the proposed program to the Hill-Burton Act. Hostility to granting more
money for research purposes was apparent in the complaint by one
subcommittee member that HEW had "money running out of its ears
for research" and his scoffing reference to experiments "to determine

[19] U.S., Congress, House, Subcommittee of the Committee on Interstate and
Foreign Commerce, *Hearings on S. 1576* (*Mental Health, Supplemental*), 88th
Cong., 1st Sess., 1963.

whether a baby monkey can be adjusted to the limb of a tree as well as he can to the arm of his mother." Regarding the relationship of the proposed program to Hill-Burton efforts, leading questions by Representative Harris evoked the response by Mr. Boisfeuillet Jones that placing the mental health proposal under Hill-Burton would require revising the "administrative process all the way up and down." It was further suggested by a member of the subcommittee that the "Hill-Burton people" as well as HEW and the state agencies had hitherto not given "due recognition to mental hospitals."

But again and again, the supplemental hearings were directed at the question of providing funds for initial staffing. Opening testimony by Boisfeuillet Jones, the principal Administration witness, argued (1) that without adequate staffing, the proposed centers would "degenerate into miniature custodial hospitals," (2) that the initial staffing grants were to be "one-time" grants, (3) that no construction project would be approved unless it spelled out sources of support for the first year *after* federal assistance had ceased, (4) that the initial staffing grants would be "stimulatory" and "seed money," (5) that the ultimate financial support would be a "combination of State, local, and/or private funds," and (6) that the states could divert a goodly portion of one billion dollars now being spent on state mental hospitals to the mental health centers. Moreover, state mental health officials were asked again and again about the necessity for assistance in initial staffing of the proposed centers. It was abundantly clear that the staffing provisions were a major concern permeating the later hearings.

The House Committee on Interstate and Foreign Commerce, reporting on August 21, 1963, recommended less funds than the Senate bill, and for shorter periods. But the principal difference was the deletion from the Senate bill of the provision for initial staffing.[20] The subcommittee had recommended a reduced amount for this purpose, but the full committee cut out all authorization for staffing. Nevertheless, Chairman Harris and the chairman of the subcommittee, Mr. Roberts, indicated in House debate that they personally had favored federal support for initial staffing.[21] Another member of the committee revealed

[20] It should also be noted that the House version changed the 75–45 per cent grant range of the Senate bill to 66 2/3 - 33 1/3 per cent.
[21] U.S., *Congressional Record,* 88th Cong., 1st Sess., 1963, CIX, Part 12, 15788 (Harris), 15798 (Roberts).

that the full committee had struck the initial staffing provisions by a vote of 15 to 12. In commenting on this action, he pointed out that the "overwhelming weight of professional opinion" given in congressional hearings, including that of the Council on Mental Health of the AMA, supported initial staffing funds. However, as he put it:

A political decision later resulted in the AMA's opposition to this provision. This body [the House of Representatives] should not fail to note that the competent professionals, the experts on mental health, within the AMA recommended otherwise.

It is unfortunate that the majority of the Committee on Interstate and Foreign Commerce chose to follow the political views of the AMA leadership, rather than the professional views of the AMA's own expert body in this field.

No attempt was made in the House to restore the initial staffing funds. The House passed its version of the mental health and mental retardation legislation by a vote of 335 to 18 on September 10, 1963.[22]

The House insisted on its changes and asked for a conference. The conference committee issued its report on October 21, 1963. On the extent of federal funds a compromise had been struck; in general the conference report provided for more than the House bill but less than the Senate. But the initial staffing provisions were not restored. The conference report was accepted in both the House and Senate, and the legislation went to the President, who signed it October 31, 1963.

REGULATIONS RELATING TO MENTAL HEALTH CENTERS

The Act required that within six months of its enactment the Secretary of Health, Education, and Welfare, after consulting with the Federal Hospital Council and the National Advisory Mental Health Council, should issue regulations "applicable uniformly to all States" regarding the construction of community mental health centers. On May 6, 1964, the regulations governing the construction of the centers were published in the *Federal Register*.[23]

Though Senator Javits had failed in an attempt to prohibit segregated facilities during passage of the legislation, the regulations required that

[22] *Ibid.*, p. 15830. Of the 18 in the negative, 13 were from the South (Virginia -3, Mississippi-3, Texas-5, Louisiana-2); 2 were from California and 1 each from Ohio, Nebraska, and New York.
[23] U.S., *Federal Register*, 1964, pp. 5951–56; 54.201–215.

all portions and services of a grant-aided facility be made available without discrimination on account of race, creed, or color. No professionally qualified person could be discriminated against on account of race, creed, or color with respect to the privilege of professional practice in the facility.

Staffing plans were required for the centers as well as a merit system of personnel. Private practitioners were to be allowed to use the centers and a "reasonable volume" of extensive services had to be provided for those unable to pay. The "essential elements" of a comprehensive mental health center's program were declared to be: inpatient, outpatient, emergency, and partial hospitalization services in addition to consultative educational services for the community.

Each state had to prepare a plan that would divide the state into geographic areas and then rank these areas according to their relative need for mental health services. Each mental health center was to serve a population of not less than 75,000 nor more than 200,000. It had to be readily accessible to the community to be served, "taking into account both political and geographic boundaries." Planning was to take cognizance of other health planning efforts, urban redevelopment, and welfare facilities. For interstate metropolitan areas, there had to be consultation with the states involved. And maximum coordination with city, metropolitan area, and interstate planning agencies was stipulated. Finally, there was the specific provision that services would not be denied "to any person residing within the area served" solely on the grounds that he did not meet a minimum residence requirement.

FROM EXPLORATION TO ACTION— AND ADDITIONAL LEGISLATION

Dr. Appel's appeal had evoked its response. Within eight years of his call for a Flexner-type study of mental illness in the United States, the Joint Commission had produced its report. Only two years later a move for improvement in the mental health field rivaling the advance stemming from the Flexner Report was well underway. During fiscal 1963 and 1964 a total of $8.4 million in federal matching funds was appropriated to assist the states in the development of comprehensive plans, and by March 1965 interim progress reports on their planning activities had been submitted to NIMH by all fifty states. Moreover, a new move to obtain funds for initial staffing of the centers was formally begun on January 7, 1965.

Only three days after his January 4th State of the Union Address, President Lyndon Johnson sent a special health message to Congress. While the most newsworthy of the President's recommendations was the hospital insurance plan for the aged—popularly dubbed "medicare" —among the variety of other health proposals was a five-year program of grants to the states for staffing community mental health centers. Federal aid for constructing community mental health centers authorized by the Eighty-eighth Congress was, according to President Johnson, "an important beginning toward community preparation." However, he went on, "facilities alone cannot assure services." Few communities had funds to support adequate programs and communities with the greatest needs hesitated to build centers without being able to identify the source of operating funds. Accordingly, the President proposed "legislation to authorize a five-year program of grants for the initial cost of personnel to man community mental health centers which offer comprehensive services."

A few days later, Senator Lister Hill and Representative Oren Harris introduced bills embodying the Administration's proposal to authorize assistance in meeting the initial cost of professional and technical personnel for comprehensive community mental health centers.[24] This time the House acted first. On March 2 the Interstate and Foreign Commerce Committee began hearings on the staffing grants measure. The line-up of witnesses and the organizations submitting prepared statements at these hearings did not differ significantly from two years previously when the committee was considering the Kennedy proposal. But there was a striking difference in the general tone of the proceedings. With few exceptions the questioning revealed widespread sympathy among the committee members for the proposal to amend the Act to include grants for staffing purposes.

The most searching, and the most frequently repeated, questioning was directed at the problem of the staffing grants' duration. The American Medical Association took the position that

there does not appear to be any justification for Federal participation in financing this type of expense, nor is it likely to phase out, as stated in the

[24] U.S., Congress, Senate, S. 513, 89th Cong., 1st Sess., Jan. 15, 1965, and House, H.R. 2985, 89th Cong., 1st Sess., Jan. 18, 1965.

bill, once the Federal Government has assumed the responsibility. If the community cannot, or will not, support the program from its beginning years, it is not likely to do so later.[25]

Apparently, the possibility that this might indeed prove to be the case and that federal financing might, as a consequence, become permanent bothered a number of committee members. Over and over witnesses were queried as to the desirability and possibility of phasing out federal staffing assistance.

While the committee shared the AMA's concern over the problem of phasing out the staffing grants, it indicated its general agreement with the Administration as to the need for them. Noting that at the time the 1963 Act was passed, "it was not clear that the problem of funds for initial staffing would represent a critical factor in getting centers underway" and that provisions authorizing federal staffing funds had therefore been deleted, the report declared that federal funds were necessary to enable communities to provide desperately needed services.[26]

The committee reported an amended version of the original proposal. By far the most significant changes were those reflecting the concern over limiting the duration of federal staffing assistance.

The bill authorized grants "not exceeding 75 per cent of eligible staff costs in the first 15 months of operation, 60 per cent in the first subsequent year, 45 per cent in the second, and 30 per cent in the third and final year." [27] In this respect, there was no change from the Administration's proposal. But the committee version made an important change in the period during which such grants could be initiated. Whereas the original bill had provided a June 30, 1970, deadline on new staffing grant awards, the committee version moved that date up two full years to June 30, 1968. Moreover, the committee inserted a new appropriations provision with much more precise language. The bill as reported authorized appropriations in the amount of $19.5 million for fiscal 1966, $24 million for fiscal 1967, and $30 million for fiscal 1968 to be used for initial staffing grants to community mental health centers. The bill provided money for con-

---

[25] U.S., Congress, House, Committee on Interstate and Foreign Commerce, *Hearings on H.R. 2984, 2985, 2986, and 2987,* 89th Cong., 1st Sess., 1965, H. Rep't. 248, p. 218.

[26] *Ibid.,* pp. 4–5.

[27] *Ibid.,* p. 3, summarizing Sec. 220 (b).

tinuation grants only for fiscal 1967, 1968, and 1969. Thus, reflecting its concern that the staffing assistance be strictly limited in duration, the committee had foreshortened the period during which federal seed money should be initially available from five years to three. And the Department of Health, Education, and Welfare would have to seek additional authorization four years hence in order to complete the staffing grants program.

But while it had made changes, the committee had given its blessing to the essentials of the staffing grants proposal. Perhaps the committee could be taken at its word as to the reason for the change in its attitude since 1963. It may well be that the experience of two years' planning efforts had convinced the committee that construction grants were not enough, and that money for initial staffing purposes was equally essential to any realistic move to stimulate the expansion of community mental health services. However, the different fate of the staffing grants proposal this time might be explained simply in political terms. What seemed politically dubious in 1963 may have appeared in a different light in early 1965, so soon after the Democratic Party's sweeping victory at the polls and President Johnson's unrivaled personal triumph. Perhaps some of the committee members favored the staffing grants all along, but adopted a "foot in the door" strategy in 1963, believing that support for that part of the measure would be more easily obtained when the importance of staffing assistance to the success of the program had been more clearly demonstrated. But whatever the explanation, the result in committee was different this time, and the bill as amended was passed by the House by a vote of 389–0.[28]

The staffing grants in 1963 had clear sailing in the upper house. No action had been taken by the Senate committee on S.513 when the House passed its bill. Senator Hill's Committee on Labor and Public Welfare held no formal hearings on H.R.2985. On June 24 the committee reported favorably an amended version which contained one important change in regard to the staffing grants. While the bill retained the House's three-year limitation in initial grants and the amounts authorized for those grants, the Administration's proposal that funds be authorized for the entire period of the program had been restored. On June 28, with only Senators Hill of Alabama, Kennedy

[28] U.S., *Congressional Record,* 89th Cong., 1st Sess., 1965, III, Part 79, 9077.

of Massachusetts, and Yarborough of Texas speaking in favor of the bill and no one on the other side, the Senate passed the bill by a voice vote.[29]

In the conference committee the House managers agreed to the Senate's amendment concerning the authorization of appropriations for continuation grants. Thus the bill now provided for initial staffing grants for three years and continuation funds in the necessary amounts for the succeeding four years. On July 26 the Senate passed the measure by voice vote and the House passed it the following day by a 414–0 roll call vote. On August 4 President Johnson signed into law the staffing grants program that had been stricken from the 1963 community mental health centers legislation.

THE POLITICS OF PASSAGE

Less than two and a half years elapsed between President Kennedy's message of 1963 and enactment of the mental health staffing legislation of 1965. This was a short time for Congress to adopt a program whose aim was to revolutionize the centuries-old mental health system of the United States. It was, moreover, a revolution in which only one hostile shot was fired. As a revolution, then, passage of the mental health legislation of 1963 and 1965 had all the earmarks of a coup d'état, carefully staged and managed, with the full implications for the country at large to come later, after the changing of the palace guard.

Who set the stage for the revolution? In one sense the 1963 Act was but another episode in the continuing story of the expanding activities and influence of the National Institute of Mental Health. From its beginnings in 1949, partly the result of bureaucratic instinct, partly the result of professional dedication, NIMH's aggressiveness in pursuing its own expansion was exceeded only by its success. Strategically placed congressmen, notably Senator Lister Hill and Representative John Fogarty (Democrat, Rhode Island), who chaired the relevant appropriations subcommittees, were carefully cultivated by Dr. Felix, aided and abetted by interested private groups and individuals. Among the more important of these surrogates were the American Psychiatric Association, the National Association for Mental Health and its state affiliates, and—through the good offices of Mike Gorman, executive

[29] *Ibid.*, III, Part 116, 14419.

director of the National Committee Against Mental Illness—Mrs. Mary Lasker, long known for her efforts, both personal and through the Albert and Mary Lasker Foundation, on behalf of medical advances.

The push for the broad-gauged study conducted by the Joint Commission during the late fifties was in large measure inspired by this same group of NIMH supporters. The effectiveness of the interlocking directorate is illustrated by the initiation of the study. While Congress was considering legislation authorizing funds for an extensive study of mental illness, legislation drafted with the assistance of the APA, the groups lobbying for the Mental Health Study Act were at the same time organizing to conduct the study. The Act was passed and the Joint Commission was incorporated almost simultaneously; and since NIMH was in fact to select the investigatory agency, the Commission's application to the Surgeon General for the study funds was immediately successful.

While the Joint Commission's study was itself largely the work of these same people who had vigorously supported NIMH activities in the past, the formal organization of the Commission was calculated to minimize potential opposition to its recommendations. Participation by organizations and agencies chosen by NIMH ensured support by influential health and welfare groups, and the report could later appear to reflect near unanimous professional opinion. Despite the criticisms directed at its emphasis on inpatient services, the report did receive widespread approval. It was used as the basis for the mental health program developed later by the AMA, and the APA declared that it "agrees with and urges the implementation of the basic objectives." The National Association for Mental Health urged support of the program first at a national leadership conference attended by two hundred of the country's most prominent civic leaders, and later at regional leadership conferences in Boston, Miami Beach, Chicago, Dallas, and Tucson. And on the nonprofessional side, official distribution of the published report was made possible by a grant from the American Legion. Thus, it is hardly surprising that the report attracted widespread attention and drew acclaim from vote-conscious politicians.

Equally important, the issuance of the Joint Commission's report coincided with the beginning of a new administration in Washington, headed by a new President who had a family involvement in the problem of mental deficiencies. The cabinet-level committee appointed by President Kennedy cooperated closely with NIMH and there was extensive consultation with the same in-group: NIMH personnel, state mental health officials, and representatives of organizations such as the APA and the National Association for Mental Health. It was no accident that during the course of the committee's deliberations that mental health became linked with mental retardation in the message and draft legislation prepared for the President.

During this same period NIMH and its supporters had succeeded in obtaining more than $8 million in appropriations for planning grants to states to help them develop long- and short-range comprehensive community mental health plans. Such planning efforts not only dramatized areas of need, but also—as they were designed to do—could be expected to expand grassroots support for mental health services.

With this kind of careful development, it is hardly surprising that the progress of the community centers program through Congress should have been so smooth. Given the breadth of the organizational participation in the work of the Joint Commission, small wonder that opposition was all but nonexistent. And it is worth noting that even the partial opposition of the AMA solidified only after its House of Delegates met and overrode its Council on Mental Health rather late in the course of legislative proceedings. In the absence of organized opposition, President Kennedy's commitment to the measure, together with the efforts of congressmen long friendly to all varieties of health legislation, made the success of NIMH and its supportive groups all but inevitable.

Given the additional leverage supplied to NIMH and its surrogates by the construction program authorized by the Act and the growing popular support developing through the comprehensive planning operations, early success in restoring the stricken staffing provisions was preordained. One example of the skillful pressure tactics employed by the mental health enthusiasts to hasten the restoration was supplied by the conference on mental health needs called by the APA and the National Association for Mental Health (one is tempted to list NIMH as a sponsor, too) in early 1965. Carefully selected interested citizens from communities in all fifty states were invited to a two-day meeting at the Sheraton-Park Hotel in Washington, where they could impress important congressmen and the press by their numbers and concern. And at the same time the well-fed and generously wined participants could be inspired to bigger and better efforts on behalf of community mental health by an impressive line-up of governors, highly respected professionals, and Senator Hill, Representative Harris, and Representative Fogarty. It was this kind of sustained effort together with the political climate that produced the crushing defeat for the AMA on medicare that greased the legislative wheels so effectively for the 1965 staffing amendments.

With the provision of federal aid for staffing the new community mental health centers, the bold new program for mental health was complete at the federal level. But the new program focused on the state and local level, so its implementation involved a whole new set of political problems.

IV: URBAN AMERICA

IMPLEMENTATION of the 1963 Act involves a substantial redirection of mental health programs at the local level. The magnitude of this task is illustrated by an important characteristic of America at mid-century— fragmented government in metropolitan areas. As of 1960, two out of three Americans lived in one of the 212 standard metropolitian statistical areas. But this is a far cry from saying that they lived within the jurisdiction of 212 local governments. On the contrary, these areas contained thousands of governments; in no metropolitan community with as many as 300,000 inhabitants was there *one* political unit bearing sole responsibility for all phases of local governmental activity. Though it may be an economic or social unit, the metropolitan area is anything but a governmental unit.

The existence of a host of governments—counties, townships, municipalities, and special authorities of all descriptions—within a single metropolitan community often poses grave problems for the effective performance of governmental functions. The community centers program may be especially handicapped in the achievement of its goal of providing comprehensive mental health services coordinated with other community activities such as education, public health, welfare, and housing. To make matters worse, not only are governments numerous but their boundaries overlap. In many cases, several authorities compete for the same tax dollar. This poses the problem of what unit of government can best assume responsibility for local financial participation.

THE GROWTH OF FRAGMENTATION

The multiplicity of local governments characteristic of the present-day American metropolis is not, of course, a problem which came into existence suddenly, or even recently. The various types of governmental units presently contributing to the metropolitan maze each predate, in some form, the American Revolution.[1]

Early in the seventeenth century, soon after the establishment of the first settlements in America, counties and "towns" or townships were organized as areas of local government. In New England it was the "town" that appeared first. While most of the people actually built their homes within a very small, relatively densely populated area, the surrounding rural territory was nevertheless included within the same political jurisdiction. One government embraced both the thickly populated center and the rural area surrounding it.

In some colonies, notably New York and Pennsylvania, the compact, thickly populated areas tended to separate themselves from the surrounding rural areas, and the distinctly rural area that remained became the township. While these townships did not have much vitality, they remained as clearly defined areas of government. In the South the township never developed at all, and the county became the significant unit for purposes of local government.

Counties were early established in some of the colonies and were organized in most of them before the Revolution, but they varied from one area to another in their significance. In the South the colonial governments established counties and charged them with most of the duties of a general governmental nature. The functions of the county in New England remained meager compared with those elsewhere.

As American civilization pressed westward, finally embracing the whole continent, the institutions of local government developed generally along the lines of the Atlantic Seaboard models. Just as in the East, varying considerations led to the emergence of thriving towns in some places, to strong counties in others, and to many variations of the two. In some cases the state legislatures arbitrarily marked out systems of counties and townships, resorting to various devices to stimulate their growth.

As urban communities developed, the royal governors as representa-

---

[1] See John C. Bollens, *Special District Governments in the United States* (Berkeley and Los Angeles: University of California Press, 1957); Carl Bridenbaugh, *Cities in the Wilderness, the First Century of Urban Life in America, 1625–1742* (2d ed., New York: Knopf, 1955); Ernest S. Griffith, *History of American City Government, the Colonial Period* (New York: Oxford University Press, 1938); Kirk Harold Porter, *County and Township Government in the United States* (New York: Macmillan, 1922). The discussion of the historical growth of various forms of local government which follows is based largely on these four works.

tives of the Crown granted them charters. After the Revolution the state legislatures took over the granting of charters of incorporation. Over the next fifty years an increasing number of self-governing cities, villages, and boroughs organized under special charters with delegated legislative powers were superimposed on the network of township and county administrative units. The democratic movement of the early nineteenth century promoted decentralization of governmental powers and the further multiplication of municipalities.

The most numerous single kind of special service government—the independent school district—also appeared prior to the formation of the United States. Connecticut established them as early as 1766, and other states followed suit later.

This network of parallel and sometimes overlapping jurisdictions was gradually engulfed by the burgeoning urban population. As the population of the cities spilled out over original boundaries, annexation efforts seldom kept up. Often, outmoded governments in the area surrounding the city continued to survive.

The spilling out of the urban population into the surrounding countryside also led to the creation of new jurisdictions. Scores of dormitory suburbs adjacent to the central city were incorporated as new municipalities. Sometimes this was a means of obtaining urban services which the existing county and township governments were ill-equipped to supply; sometimes it was to guard against annexation by the core city. In other cases a community may have wished to control land use through zoning in order to guard against imagined or real threats to its homogeneity, or a high-income area wished to avoid taxation for central city welfare services for which it had no need, or perhaps an enterprise which located in the fringe sought to preserve its immunity from city tax rates by creating a municipality which it could dominate. For whatever reasons, however, the typical metropolitan area today is not a single city but a maze of legally distinct municipal corporations, many of them comparatively new in creation.

While urbanization led to the incorporation of many new municipalities, the plethora of special-district governments now characterizing almost every metropolis was numerically a far more significant result. The creation of independent authorities performing a variety of limited and specific functions, frequently with power to levy taxes, proceeded at such a pace that in 1962 half our metropolitan areas with populations of

300,000 or more contained at least twenty special districts. Thirteen had over a hundred. Responsibility for sewage disposal, mosquito abatement,[2] water supply, and drainage is often assigned to independent special-purpose governments. These and other special districts overlap the boundaries of the counties, townships, municipalities, and school districts. While urban sprawl was certainly not the only factor leading to the multiplication of special-district governments, in most cases their creation was a direct result of the need to supply answers to pressing problems occasioned by the multiplicity of independent governments encompassed by the spreading metropolis.

Other factors also contributed to the creation of special districts. Constitutional or legislatively prescribed tax and debt limits often restricted the efforts of general-purpose local governments to meet the increased needs of the urban masses they served. Or existing local governments may simply have lacked authority to perform a needed function. Special districts were frequently utilized to overcome such obstacles.

As a consequence of the steady growth and increasing urbanization of the population, then, the urbanites of contemporary America are no longer simply "city dwellers." The city dweller of yesterday is a "metropolite" today, but in governmental terms there is no metropolis. Rather, myriad independent, overlapping, and frequently competing local governments crisscross the urban map. Governmental fragmentation has become the rule, not the exception, among the ever-growing metropolitan complexes that are more and more typical of the United States.

TYPES AND NUMBER OF LOCAL GOVERNMENTS

Although the characteristics of metropolitanism are still the subject of much debate, as early as 1900 the federal Bureau of the Census began classifying some areas as metropolitan and reporting population statistics for them. In 1950, as a consequence of a move to standardize the areas utilized by various federal agencies in publishing general-purpose statistics, the "metropolitan district" previously used in the Census of Population yielded to the "standard metropolitan area" established by the Office of Statistical Standards in the Bureau of the Budget. The criteria for delineating these areas were revised in 1958, and in 1959 they were designated "standard metropolitan statistical areas."

[2] This is the term used, whether or not it is accurate.

A standard metropolitan statistical area (SMSA "is a county or a group of contiguous counties which contain at least one city of 50,000 inhabitants or more or 'twin cities' with a combined population of at least 50,000." In addition to this central county, contiguous counties are added to the SMSA if they are socially and economically integrated with the central county. In New England, standards for inclusion are applied to cities and towns, rather than counties.

Although there were 212 SMSA's in the United States in 1960, the term "metropolis" is more commonly reserved for the great cities and their surrounding satellite areas. Such urban giants are becoming more and more typical of the United States, and it is these areas that create the most pressing, and the most challenging, problems for government. In 1960 over half the population of the United States lived in SMSA's encompassing 300,000 or more people, and it is urban concentrations of this order, henceforth referred to as metropolitan areas, that are the focus of this study. Except in the cases of New York–Northeastern New Jersey and Chicago–Northwestern Indiana, each of which is treated here as a single unit,[3] the Budget Bureau's area definitions have been employed. However, because of the special problems of comparability posed by Honolulu's island location and heavy concentration of military personnel and facilities, and by Washington's governmental uniqueness, these two metropolises have been omitted from consideration. There are, then, for present purposes 75 metropolitan areas.

According to the 1962 Census of Governments, there were in the United States that year 91,185 "local governments"—counties, townships, municipalities, independent school districts, and other special-purpose authorities. Of that total, 12,287 fell within the 75 metropolitan areas under scrutiny. As shown in Table 1, the number of governments in these 75 metropolises varied widely. Chicago–Northwestern Indiana had the highest total with 1,170 and Richmond the lowest with 5; the rest ranged all up and down the scale. Figures for the total number of governments, however, fail to give a clear picture of fragmentation in large metropolises. Table 1 shows that five different types of governmen-

---

[3] The New York–Northeastern New Jersey "standard consolidated area" includes four SMSA's—New York, Newark, Paterson-Clifton-Passaic, and Jersey City— but is treated here as one metropolitan area. The Chicago–Northwestern Indiana "standard consolidated area", including the Chicago and Gary–Hammond–East Chicago SMSA's, is considered here a single metropolitan area.

Table 1: Governmental Fragmentation in Large Metropolitan Areas, 1962

Metropolitan Area* (Grouped Regionally)	Number of Governments by Type						Governments per 100,000 Inhabitants	Per Cent of Metropolitan Population Residing in Largest Single City
	Counties	Municipalities	Townships	School Districts	Special Districts	Total Local Governments		
Northeast (20)								
New York–N.E. New Jersey	12	292	102	399	307	1112	7.5	52.7
Philadelphia	7	140	199	331	286	963	22.2	46.6
Pittsburgh	4	189	119	261	233	806	33.4	25.1
Albany–Schenectady–Troy	4	29	48	80	87	248	37.7	19.7
Syracuse	3	39	56	71	59	228	40.4	38.3
Allentown–Bethlehem–Easton	3	35	50	65	58	211	42.9	22.0
Harrisburg	2	29	45	70	57	203	58.8	23.1
Wilkes–Barre–Hazleton	1	37	36	71	23	168	48.4	18.3
Buffalo	2	26	37	46	42	153	11.7	40.8
Utica–Rome	2	32	45	38	36	153	46.2	30.4
Boston	...	17	59	2	47	125	4.8	26.9
Rochester	1	11	19	22	27	80	13.7	54.3
Wilmington	2	14	11	36	10	73	19.9	26.2

Providence–Pawtucket	...	8	24	1	39	72	8.8	25.4
Hartford	...	2	20	...	26	48	9.1	32.9
Worcester	...	1	19	2	20	42	13.1	57.7
Springfield–Chicopee–Holyoke	...	5	12	1	18	36	7.5	36.5
Bridgeport	...	3	4	...	19	26	7.8	46.9
Baltimore	4	11	...	...	8	23	1.3	54.4
New Haven	...	2	8	...1	10	21	6.7	48.8
North Central (20)								
Chicago–N.W. Indiana	8	271	137	375	379	1170	17.2	52.3
St. Louis	5	163	46	105	120	439	16.5	36.4
Minneapolis–St. Paul	5	105	51	86	14	261	17.6	32.6
Detroit	3	80	52	96	10	241	6.4	44.4
Kansas City	4	56	15	116	30	221	21.3	45.7
Omaha	3	27	...	59	102	191	41.7	65.9
Milwaukee	2	42	14	86	5	149	12.5	62.1
Cleveland	2	75	11	41	6	135	7.5	48.8
Louisville	3	57	17	18	34	129	17.8	53.9
Cincinnati	3	68	12	35	10	128	12.0	46.9
Dayton	3	39	37	35	10	124	17.8	37.8
Wichita	1	17	28	38	26	110	32.1	75.7
Youngstown–Warren	2	20	39	38	6	105	20.6	32.8
Grand Rapids	1	11	23	53	2	90	24.8	48.8
Columbus	1	26	17	17	4	65	9.5	69.0

Table 1: (continued)

Number of Governments by Type

Metropolitan Area* (Grouped Regionally)	Counties	Municipalities	Townships	School Districts	Special Districts	Total Local Governments	Governments per 100,000 Inhabitants	Per cent of Metropolitan Population Residing in Largest Single City
Flint	1	13	18	27	2	61	16.3	52.6
Indianapolis	1	23	9	12	14	59	8.5	68.3
Canton	1	19	17	17	3	57	16.8	33.4
Akron	1	18	14	18	3	54	10.5	56.5
Toledo	1	10	12	10	9	42	9.2	69.6
West (13)								
San Francisco—Oakland	5	58	...	143	192	398	14.3	26.6
Portland	4	30	...	109	231	374	45.5	45.3
Los Angeles—Long Beach	2	95	...	141	110	348	5.2	41.9
Seattle	2	46	...	43	190	281	25.3	50.3
San Bernadino—Riverside—Ontario	2	24	...	101	123	250	30.9	11.3
Fresno	1	15	...	85	107	208	56.8	36.6
Denver	4	31	...	21	149	205	22.1	53.2
San Diego	1	11	...	51	77	140	13.6	55.5

	A	B	C	D	E	F	G	H
Sacramento	1	5	...	21	82	109	21.7	38.1
Phoenix	1	17	...	55	28	101	15.2	66.2
San Jose	1	16	...	46	25	88	13.7	31.8
Tacoma	1	18	...	23	40	82	25.5	46.0
Salt Lake City	1	9	...	4	16	30	7.8	54.3
South (22)								
Dallas	4	74	...	60	28	166	15.4	62.7
Tulsa	3	33	...	75	13	124	29.6	62.5
Fort Worth	2	42	...	36	9	89	15.6	62.2
Oklahoma City	3	32	...	46	5	86	16.8	63.4
Atlanta	5	45	...	9	25	84	8.3	47.9
Houston	1	25	...	21	35	82	6.6	75.5
Beaumont–Port Arthur	2	13	...	16	19	50	16.3	39.0
Birmingham	1	30	...	6	7	44	6.9	53.7
San Antonio	1	15	...	16	11	43	6.3	85.5
Orlando	2	18	...	2	19	41	12.9	27.7
Tampa–St. Petersburg	2	26	...	2	10	40	5.2	35.6
Fort Lauderdale–Hollywood	1	24	...	1	12	38	11.4	25.0
Miami	1	27	...	1	3	32	3.4	31.2
Knoxville	3	9	...	...	16	28	7.6	30.4
New Orleans	4	14	...	4	10	31	3.4	69.2
El Paso	1	4	...	7	5	17	5.4	88.1
Memphis	1	6	...	...	8	15	2.4	79.3

Table 1: (continued)

Number of Governments by Type

Metropolitan Area* (Grouped Regionally)	Counties	Munici- palities	Town- ships	School Districts	Special Districts	Total Local Governments	Governments per 100,000 Inhabitants	Per cent of Metropolitan Population Residing in Largest Single City
Nashville	1	7	...	...	7	15	3.8	42.7
Mobile	1	8	...	1	2	12	3.8	64.5
Jacksonville	1	5	...	1	4	11	2.4	44.1
Norfolk–Portsmouth	2	4	...	...	3	9	1.6	52.7
Richmond	2	1	...	...	2	5	1.2	53.8

* "Metropolitan Area" means the Budget Bureau "Standard Metropolitan Statistical Areas" having 1960 populations of 300,000 or more with two qualifications: New York–Northeastern New Jersey and Chicago–Northwestern Indiana are each considered single metropolitan areas, and Honolulu, Ha., and Washington, D.C., are omitted.

Source: Governmental units figures were obtained from Census of Governments: 1962, Vol. I (Governmental Organization), Table 15. Population data were obtained from Census of Population: 1960, Vol. I, Part A, Table 1–33.

tal units—counties, townships, municipalities, school districts, and special districts—are included in the totals in varying combinations.

Examining the 75 metropolises as to the various types of local jurisdictions in 1962 reveals that 166 county governments were included, ranging from 0 in 7 metropolises to 12 in New York–Northeastern New Jersey. Clearly it is impossible to talk about an average, or typical, metropolitan area with respect to the number of counties. Municipalities comprised a little less than a fourth (2,891) of the local governments included in the 75 metropolises,[4] varying from 1 in the case of Worcester and Richmond to 292 in New York–Northeastern New Jersey. While there were no township governments[5] in any of the Southern or Western metropolitan areas, all save Baltimore and Omaha in the Northeast and North Central regions had units of this type. The number included ranged from Bridgeport's 4 up to Philadelphia's 199.

The single most numerous type of governmental unit in the large metropolitan areas, as in the nation as a whole, was the independent school district. Almost a third (3,925) fell into this category. While there were independent school districts in 9 metropolitan areas, they were common to all regions of the country, ranging in number up to New York–Northeastern New Jersey's 399. Other special districts such as health, parks, fire protection, urban water supply, and sewage were almost as numerous as school districts. There were 3,823 special-service governments in the 75 metropolises, 31.1 per cent of total governments. The number in each metro ranged from 2 to 379. The great majority of these special-district governments were single-purpose units.

REGIONAL VARIATIONS IN FRAGMENTATION

Just as the figure for the total number of governments hid differences in the types found in the metropolises, considering the metropolises as a national group obscures notable variations from one part of the country to another. The distinctiveness of the South when contrasted with other

[4] According to the Census of Governments this term includes "all governmental units officially designated 'cities,' 'boroughs,' 'villages,' and—except for New England, New York, and Wisconsin—'towns' " (U.S., Bureau of the Census, *Census of Governments: 1962*, I [*Governmental Organization*], 2.)

[5] The category "township" includes "governments officially known as 'towns' in the six New England states and in New York and Wisconsin, and some 'plantations' in Maine and 'locations' in New Hampshire, as well as units officially termed 'townships' in other areas having this type of government" (*ibid.*, p. 3).

parts of the country and with the United States as a whole is perhaps the most outstanding regional variation.[6] As Table 1 shows, Southern metropolises were, as a group, markedly less subject to a proliferation of jurisdictions than were the urban complexes located elsewhere. Moreover, with the exception of counties, each type of governmental unit was less abundant in the South than elsewhere.

Special districts present a particularly striking regional variation; their abundance in the West is as noticeable as their relative scarcity in the South. The average number of special districts in Western metropolises was more than double the national average; special districts usually accounted for more than half the total number of governments in the West and less than a fourth in other parts of the country. Another regional variation meriting special attention is the total absence of township governments in the South and West.

RECENT CHANGES IN THE EXTENT OF FRAGMENTATION

The significance of the fragmentation just described depends in part on the trend. While the total number of local governments in the United States showed a marked decrease between 1957 and 1962, the number in the 75 metropolises increased. It is true that on an adjusted basis school districts in the 75 metropolises decreased (although not as rapidly as in other parts of the country), but the marked increase in other types of governments more than offset the reduction in independent school districts. In fact, as can be seen in Table 2, the number of governments other than school districts increased by 1,359, an average of 18.1 per metropolis.

Just as the number of governments of various types included in metropolitan areas varied regionally, the extent and nature of the changes between 1957 and 1962 differed considerably from one part of the coun-

---

[6] Three modifications of the Census Bureau definitions of "region" have been employed throughout this discussion. Honolulu, Hawaii, and Washington, D.C., have been omitted from consideration and consequently are not included in the West and South as defined for present purposes. Baltimore, Md., and Wilmington, Del., have been included in the Northeast rather than in the South; Louisville, Ky., is counted as North Central and not Southern. Since in our view Wilmington and Baltimore are more akin to the cities of the Northeast and Louisville to those of the North Central, they have been included in those regions even though the states within which they exist—if considered in their entirety—might properly be described as Southern.

try to another. As shown in Table 2, while the number of school districts decreased in each region, the degree of reduction varied markedly. The only change in the number of county governments occurred in the Northeast as the result of the abolition of authorities of that type in New England. Municipalities grew in number in each region, but only slightly in the Northeast. In the North Central region, on the other hand, the increase was marked. Special districts increased in all four regions, accounting for most of the overall growth in governmental units.

While the picture varies from one part of the country to another, the changes between 1957 and 1962 in the number of local governments lead

Table 2: Increase or Decrease in Number of Governmental Units in Metropolitan Areas Between 1957* and 1962, by Type of Government and by Region

	Change in the Number of Government Units in Large Metropolitan Areas				
Type of Government	North-east (20)	North Central (20)	South (22)	West (13)	Total United States (75)
Total local governments	528	−45	22	148	653
Counties	−7	. . .	. . .	. . .	−7
Municipalities	12	114	60	47	233
Townships	−11	−16	. . .	. . .	−27
School districts	−169	−329	−49	−159	−706
Special districts	703	186	11	260	1160
Local governments excluding school districts	697	284	71	307	1359
Local governments excluding school and special districts	−6	98	60	47	199

* 1957 "governmental units" figures used in the preparation of this table were adjusted to take into account redefinitions of SMSA's occurring between 1957 and 1962; consequently, the increases and decreases reported here represent actual additions or deletions of governments within the geographic limits of metropolises as defined in 1962.

Source: "Governmental units" figures used in the preparation of this table were obtained from U.S., Bureau of the Census, Census of Governments: 1957, Vol. I (Governmental Organizations), No. 1: Table 14, No. 2: Table 3; and Census of Governments: 1962, Vol. I (Governmental Organizations), Table 15.

to one inescapable conclusion. A multiplicity of governments is not only typical of our metropolitan areas, but the jurisdictional tangle has been worsening. Whatever one may conclude from the fact that the number of local governments in the nation as a whole has been shrinking rapidly, the fact remains that they have been increasing in the metropolitan areas. It is instructive to compare the formation of new local governments within the 75 metropolises with what has been happening elsewhere. The number of municipal governments within the 75 metropolises increased 8.8 per cent between 1957 and 1962, while the number elsewhere rose only 3.8 per cent. The number of special districts outside the metropolitan areas rose 23.3 per cent, but the number within increased by 43.6 per cent. Furthermore, the elimination of school districts within the metropolises was achieved at less than half the rate that it was elsewhere. In short, not only are metropolises constantly pushing outward to envelop already existing governmental units, it is also these areas where old governments have been disappearing most slowly and new ones appearing most rapidly. As the great urban complexes, already accounting for half the population, steadily grow even more dominant, their governmental organization, already fragmented, is becoming more and more a crazy-quilt of overlapping jurisdictions.

This, then, is the general pattern of governmental fragmentation in the leading metropolitan areas of the United States. Further, as Table 1 shows, even when cast in terms of governments per 100,000 population, the large metropolitan areas are still beset by multiple jurisdictions. However, the mere existence of a large number of separate governments in a metropolitan area does not preclude the possibility that the great majority of the people in the area might live in a single municipality. But, again as shown in Table 1, in more than half of the larger metropolitan areas less than one half of the people resided in any one city and in only nine did the central city of the area contain as much as two-thirds of the population.

SELECTED AREAS FOR STUDY

Ideally, an examination of the consequences of governmental fragmentation for mental health would involve all 75 metropolises and a wide range of issues, but the scarcity of resources forces one to settle for less. This study was limited to an inquiry into the impact of fragmentation on mental health programing in six metropolitan areas. Although their selection was inevitably conditioned by the availability of researchers for the field work, the choices made were designed to provide significant variation in regard to certain factors thought to have relevance for the handling of mental health problems. These variables included region, size and density of population, rate of population growth, ethnic and racial composition, age distribution, educational levels, and income distribution. Other variables entering into the selection process were the degree of governmental fragmentation and the political climate for social welfare services. No claim is made that the six areas finally selected (Boston, Syracuse, Houston, New Orleans, Minneapolis–St. Paul, and Seattle) constitute the best sample of all metropolitan centers. One can assert, however, that the selections are suitably dispersed across the range associated with each variable.

This dispersion can be quickly sketched. There is one selection from each of the four principal regions of the nation, with two from the regions (Northeast and South) where subregional differences seem greatest. With respect to size of population, an early decision was made to eliminate the extremes. Accordingly, the areas of New York–Northeastern New Jersey, Chicago–Northwestern Indiana, and Los Angeles–Long Beach were excluded because of their great size and complexity, while the smaller areas were excluded because they were not metropolitan enough. The result was a set of moderate- to large-sized metros, ranging from a population of 619,367 in Syracuse to 2,589,301 in Boston.

Population growth of the metropolitan area and of its central city was another factor taken into account in the selection. All but one of the 75 metropolises grew in population from 1950 to 1960, but their rate of expansion varied from slight to more than 100 per cent. The central cities generally grew less rapidly than the metropolises, and more than one-third of them lost population in the fifties. But here too there was great variation, some central cities declining by 10 per cent or more, while others had more than a 100 per cent increase. The six areas selected for study reflect these patterns reasonably well. For example, Houston as a city and as a metropolitan area is growing by leaps and bounds; Boston, on the other hand, has experienced little growth in recent years. In Minneapolis–St. Paul the largest city was declining, though less rapidly than Boston, while the metropolitan area continues to expand. And in Seattle and New Orleans both central cities and suburbs are growing, but less rapidly than in Houston.

American metropolises vary in population density almost as strikingly as they do in rate of expansion. For reasons of history and geography, the large metropolitan areas range in population density from less than 100 persons per square mile to more than 3,000; their central cities range from less than 3,000 persons per square mile to more than 10,000. The selections are reflective of this spread. Thus Boston is the second most densely populated metropolitan area; Syracuse is one of the least densely populated.

American metropolises also differ considerably in many other demographic respects. Among those which could be important in the planning of community mental health services, both administratively and politically, are the ethnic and racial composition of the population, age distribution, educational levels, and income distribution. These factors were taken into account in the selection process, and as shown in Table 3, the six metropolises chosen provide considerable variation in regard to each.

In respect to the development of community mental health programs, perhaps one of the most important variations from one part of the country to another is the political climate for social welfare services generally at the state and local level. Although it defies precise measurement, that climate will greatly influence the probabilities of developing the kinds of support, both political and financial, necessary for any significant expansion of publicly supported mental health programs. In some parts of the country there exists a strong tradition of local pride and initiative in social services, while in other parts the state government commonly bears most of the responsibility. Moreover, some states have long been noted for their progressivism and general hospitality toward extensive social welfare activity, while others have been reluctant to provide anything other than the minimum in the way of governmental services. In the selection of areas for study, an attempt was made to provide some variation in this regard.

Finally, and central to this study, the extent of local governmental fragmentation was a very important criterion in the selection process. By total number of governments, by number of general-purpose governments, by number of governments in relation to population, by the percentage of the population living in the largest single municipality—in each instance American metropolises range all up and down the fragmentation scale. A perusal of Table 4 will reveal the extent to which these six metropolitan areas selected for intensive study vary according to sev-

Table 3: Characteristics of the Population in Selected Metropolitan Areas

| Population Characteristic | Metropolitan Area | | | | | | Median of Large Metropolitan Areas |
	Seattle	Boston	Minneapolis–St. Paul	Syracuse	Houston	New Orleans	
Per cent nonwhite	4.8	3.4	1.8	2.6	20.1	31.0	
Per cent foreign born or of foreign parentage	26.8	41.8	25.0	24.7	8.9	8.1	
Median age	30.2	32.0	28.1	29.5	27.1	28.5	30.5
Median annual income (dollars)	6,896	6,687	6,840	6,405	6,040	5,195	6,439
Median number of school years completed (population 25 years old or older)	12.2	12.1	12.1	11.4	11.3	9.5	11.1

Table 4: Governmental Fragmentation in Selected Metropolitan Areas

Fragmentation Pattern	Metropolitan Area						Median of Large Metropolitan Areas
	Syracuse	Minneapolis–St. Paul	Seattle	Boston	Houston	New Orleans	
Total local governments	228	261	281	125	82	31	89
Local governments per 100,000 inhabitants	40.4	17.6	25.3	4.8	6.6	3.4	13.6
Local governments excluding school and special districts	98	161	48	76	26	17	33
Local governments excluding school and special districts per 100,000 inhabitants	17.5	10.9	4.3	2.9	2.1	1.9	4.9
Per cent of population residing within largest single city	38.3	32.6	50.3	26.9	75.5	69.2	46.9

eral possible measures of governmental fragmentation. It is obvious that by each standard the six areas present a considerable range from most to least fragmented. Syracuse, it appears, is the most consistently fragmented of the large metropolitan areas selected while New Orleans is uniformly among the least.

To what extent will governmental fragmentation hinder the rerouting of mental health efforts contemplated by the community centers program? Governmental fragmentation may be characteristic of the present-day American metropolis, but does it necessarily pose problems for effective government? Does the very existence of a large number of independent jurisdictions within what economists and sociologists call a metropolitan area necessarily create governmental difficulties? Will the politics of implementing the 1963 Act be significantly affected by the pattern of local government in metropolitan America? The field studies that follow will attempt to determine the actual impact of fragmented government on mental health programing in six very different metropolises.

TWO : THE METROPOLITAN MILIEU

V: HOUSTON

CLIFTON McCLESKEY

THE HOUSTON METROPOLITAN AREA, at the time of this study coterminous with Harris county, is in southeastern Texas, adjacent to the shal-
low waters of Galveston Bay near the Gulf of Mexico. Settlement of
the locale began before the successful termination of the Texas War
for Independence in 1836, but by 1890 the population totaled only
about 37,000. From that point on, however, the growth rate was little
short of phenomenal, ranging up to 50 per cent in each census period
and reaching a high of over 90 per cent in the decade 1920 to 1930. Undoubtedly many factors contributed to this growth, but two of the most
important were the development of substantial oil production and the
opening in 1914 of the Houston Ship Channel, a 50-mile dredged
shipping lane from the Gulf of Mexico, capable of bringing all but the
largest ocean-going vessels to the port of Houston. The new port soon
became the principal one in Texas for handling the state's cotton, grain,
and beef exports, as well as a shipping center for petroleum and its
products.

ECOLOGY

The coming of the Second World War added fresh momentum to the
growth and development of the Houston area, as military establishments
and defense plants brought people by the thousands. Unlike some areas
thus affected, metropolitan Houston was able to weather the end of war-
time activity without any loss of economic impetus. As a result, the 1940
population of 529,000 had increased to 1,243,000 by 1960, and the indications are that the growth rate slowed little if any in the 1960s. To a
greater extent than in the other metropolitan areas in this study, the pop-

I wish to acknowledge my great indebtedness to Professor Sol Tannenbaum for
his assistance in planning and conducting the interviews which constitute the
foundation of this study.

ulation of the SMSA is concentrated in the central city, Houston, which had 75 per cent (938,000) of the total in 1960.

Other municipalities in the area include Pasadena (59,000), Baytown (28,000), Bellaire (20,000), West University Place (15,000), and Galena Park (10,000). There are numerous smaller cities as well.

As might be expected from the rate of population growth, employment in the Houston area has generally been at a high level, even when the economy of the entire nation has turned downward. The largest categories of employment in 1960 were wholesale and retail trade (21.7 per cent); manufacturing (21.6 per cent); and transportation, communications, and public utilities (less than 10 per cent). The preeminence of wholesaling in metropolitan Houston is not characteristic of the nation as a whole, and least of all the Northeastern states. Too, the level of manufacturing employment in the Houston area is well below that of many older metropolitan areas.[1]

The implications of this are reinforced by the high (46 per cent) rate of white-collar employment in metropolitan Houston. Low manufacturing and high white-collar employment mean, among other things, fewer union members and a greater preponderence of managerial and professional workers. These economic patterns help to explain why Houston is dominated by the middle class and its values.

Middle-class ascendancy is also evident in the very high percentage of single-unit dwellings (84 per cent) and of owner-occupied dwellings (65 per cent). The tremendous physical and social mobility of the area is suggested by the fact that the persons in 38 per cent of all occupied dwellings had moved there within the two years preceding the 1960 census, and that almost half of all available housing in that year had been constructed in the preceding decade. The relative availability of cheap land and an affinity for automobiles have combined to spawn residential subdivisions located at progressively greater distances from the central city. The area is thus characterized by "urban sprawl," a high proportion (94.5 per cent) of "urban" population, and yet a relatively low

---

[1] It should not be supposed from this that historical influences on the Houston economy are no longer important. The port of Houston is still a major contributor to the economy and the long-standing identification with the oil industry has continued. Oil and gas production, refining, and transportation have continued. But, while oil and oil men are still quite important, they are losing some of their salience due to the depressed condition of crude oil production, the decrease in refinery and petro-chemical employment due to automation, and the rise of other elements of an industrial and commercial economy.

population density (727 persons per square mile). The kinds of social services likely to have high priority are therefore new streets and freeways, drainage, water, and sewage systems, new school buildings, etc.

Several other facets of the Houston metropolitan area deserve to be mentioned. As Table 3 in Chapter IV reveals, the Houston population is somewhat younger and the educational level somewhat lower than is found in the other metropolitan areas studied. Examination of population origins makes clear that the phrase "a nation of immigrants" and all that it implies has little relevance for the Houston area. The same table shows that the percentage of foreign stock is only 8.9 per cent; of the remainder, about 28.4 per cent were born in a state other than Texas.

But, though metropolitan Houston does not have the immigrant groups that Northeastern states have, it does have two sizable minority groups in the Negroes and Latin Americans. In 1960, the nonwhite population (virtually all Negro) was 20.1 per cent of the total population, up from 18.5 per cent in 1950. The census data on persons with Spanish surnames suggest that the Latin American population is around 6 per cent of the total. Thus, more than one-fourth of the area's population is composed of these two distinctive minority groups. The dispersal pattern of Negroes within the SMSA conforms to the pattern of other large metropolitan areas, for close to 90 per cent of the total Negro population is concentrated in the central city (Houston) and several sizable suburbs did not report any significant Negro population at all in 1960. As is generally true elsewhere, the Negroes and Latin Americans in Houston rank near the bottom of the socioeconomic ladder, measured in terms of education and family income. Almost a fifth of Negroes and two-fifths of Latin Americans twenty-five years of age and older in 1960 had not completed the fifth grade, compared with less than 10 per cent for all classes. Approximately 43 per cent of all Negro families and 28 per cent of Latin American families were earning less than $3,000 in 1960, compared with 18 per cent for all families.

POLITICS OF HOUSTON

Partially as a result of these socioeconomic conditions, politics in the Houston metropolitan area can best be described as unstable. There is a deep and fundamental cleavage along liberal and conservative lines, but the division is even enough so that other factors sometimes appear to be decisive—personality, name, incumbency, and so on. The situation is further complicated by the fact that there are in effect three parties, each attempting to maintain its own organizational apparatus; liberal Democrats, conservative Democrats, and Republicans. The Republican candidates for national and state offices have shown considerable and durable strength. Harris county voted overwhelmingly for Eisenhower in 1952 and 1956 and gave Nixon a majority in 1960; the Republican candidate for governor in 1962 eked out a majority as well. At the local level, however, Republicans are in the position of being able to offer competition but not enough strength to win partisan elections. As a result, their local victories have been mostly in connection with municipal offices, all of them filled by nonpartisan elections.

The conservative Democrats, whose chief difference with the Republicans is the tactical one of how best to realize the conservative goals they share, have generally been most successful in local elections for county, school, and municipal offices, although even there they do not have a monopoly. Thus, from 1960 to 1964 conservatives enjoyed a 6–1 majority on the Houston school board, but two liberal victories in 1964 brought their edge down to 4–3. Liberal Democrats hold some local offices, and in legislative and statewide elections they have often been able to match the showing of conservative candidates. For example, six of the twelve representatives in the state House of Representatives from Harris county in 1965 were liberals and six were conservatives, although there may be one or two on each side less deserving of the affixed label.

The situation thus is one of great competitiveness among the interested groups, with the main lines of division ideological in nature. Each has its own peculiar advantages and handicaps. The Republican Party, with its strongly conservative orientation, is unquestionably helped by the configuration of forces that make up the "conservative climate" associated with Houston. But the setting is in a one-party tradition, a one-party state, and the GOP has found this a difficult hurdle to overcome. Conservative Democrats are of course strengthened by the "conservative climate" of the community, and by the fact that they have traditionally controlled state and local affairs; recruiting candidates and workers, financing campaigns, and so on, are all made easier by the attribution of power. The growth of the Republican Party, however, with its more frankly conservative ideology, has drained off some conservative activists as well as voter support. The liberal Democrats have made repeated efforts to weld together a coalition of white liberals, labor union members, Negroes, and Latin Americans; but the potential has not been fully realized.

Mention of Houston's "conservative climate" perhaps demands some further comment upon that phenomenon. Its manifestations are not too difficult to depict. There is a sharp distrust of programs and policies of the national government. It is true that this distrust is of a carefully calculated type, for there has been no serious objection to federal aid for the freeway system, for the Port of Houston, for flood control and drainage programs, for airports, and many other activities, but such programs as aid to education, urban renewal, and milk and lunches for school children have met heavy resistance. Desegregation has been a slow and meager process, although there has been no defiance of the courts once the orders have been given, and a certain amount of desegregation in the private sector was accomplished without the necessity of judicial action. Social services are generally starved for funds; libraries, police protection, social work, charity hospital care, and so on are apt to compare poorly with the services available in other metropolitan areas. There are the "political education" courses provided by large firms for their employees, presented ostensibly as a nonpartisan civic educational function but carrying varying degrees of conservative content. And, of course, there is the activity of various ultra-conservative groups in the Houston area—the John Birch Society, Christian Anti-Communism Crusade, Young Americans for Freedom, etc. At times encouraged and abetted by civic groups and public officials, the ultra-conservatives have made Houston one of their strongest centers. While their greatest contribution has been to nourish and keep alive the spirit of conservatism, they have on occasion affected public policy and elected one of their own to public office.

THE GOVERNMENTAL SYSTEM

Turning from the political to the governmental system, one can begin by noting the three varieties of local government in Texas: county, municipal, and special district. The 254 counties in Texas still operate under the legal fiction that they are administrative subdivisions of the state, having only those powers and responsibilities assigned to them by the state constitution, statutes, or administrative action. Although there is no general power in county government to legislate for the health, safety, and morals of the community, it usually is not difficult to persuade the legislature to pass local bills authorizing specific counties to undertake new programs. In reality, then, there may be considerable discretion in the hands of county officials, and they are popularly regarded as local officials rather than as state administrators—a viewpoint facilitated by the fact that they are chosen at the local level, usually by direct election.

In addition to the traditional services of collecting taxes, building roads, keeping public records, and so on, Harris county also supports such programs as libraries, charity hospitals, veterans' services, and a psychiatric diagnostic center, to mention only a few. These and other programs are financed principally by the ad valorem property tax. Although the tax *rate* is at the maximum allowed, county revenues can be increased at will by officials through an increase in the assessment ratio (representing 20 per cent of true value).

Harris county, like all counties in Texas, is governed by a congeries of elected officials who preside over more or less independent departments. Included among these are the sheriff, tax assessor-collector, county clerk, treasurer, county attorney, as well as justices of the peace and constables, but by far the most important officials are the four county commissioners (elected from each of the four precincts into which the county is divided) and the county judge. As the county commissioners court, these five persons approve the budget, schedule bond elections, appoint the nonelective department heads, and generally control the finances of the county. The court has no formal authority over the various department heads, even those it appoints, but informal authority—buttressed by budgetary powers—is exercised by varying degrees. Each member of the court has individual responsibilities as well. For example, each commissioner administers the county road and bridge program in his precinct and serves as liaison to the court for certain agencies. Thus, one commissioner is unofficially the man to whom the county building superintendent looks for guidance, another is responsible for overseeing the County Welfare Department and its director, and so on. The county judge, who is the presiding officer of the commissioner's court, and who in addition functions as liaison for his designated agencies, is also a judicial officer, and in that capacity he is responsible for handling lunacy and commitment proceedings. Politically, the Harris county commissioner's court has been dominated by conservative Democrats for some time, but the person serving as county judge since 1958 has been classified as a liberal.

Unlike counties, municipalities in Texas have the legal status of public corporations. Cities and towns over 5,000 population may if they wish adopt a home-rule charter enabling them to structure and empower their government as they desire. Municipalities unable or unwilling to adopt home-rule charters are governed by the provisions of the "general laws" regarding the structure and powers of such municipal corporations. In practice, both the home-rule and the general laws cities use one of the three most common types of municipal government (council-manager, mayor-council, and commission).

There are twenty-six municipal corporations lying wholly within the Houston metropolitan area; several small ones lie partially in the area and partially outside it, and hence are not considered further here. Many of these municipalities are of fairly recent origins, no less than thirteen having been incorporated in the past fifteen years. Many of these municipalities are little more than legal ghosts, having a corporate existence but possessing no corpus of functions and services. Part of the explanation is to be found in the fact that for some of them the chief reason for creation seems to have been a desire to prevent annexation by another municipality, or to provide protection for property through zoning ordinances. Almost half of the municipalities have no zoning ordinance, including the three largest cities—Houston, Pasadena, and Baytown. All three have a record of active and aggressive annexations.

Not all of these twenty-six municipalities levy taxes, but of those that do, most found the ad valorem property tax their mainstay, providing somewhere between two-thirds and three-fourths of their total revenues. According to a 1961 study, only three of the general laws and none of the home-rule cities used the maximum permissible tax rate.[2]

The assessment ratios vary widely from one municipality to another, but none was over 69 per cent. Thus, although comparisons are difficult, it seems reasonably clear that these cities, towns, and villages have not exhausted their tax sources, although they may very well have gone as far as their voters are willing to go.

The situation with respect to special districts in Texas is one of flexibility to the point of chaos. The basis for their creation is a variety of authorizing statutes, or sometimes state constitutional amendments; approval of voters in the proposed district is usually but not always required, and occasionally the legislature itself will create a special district.

[2] Glynn Tiller, "A Profile of Municipal Government in Harris County, Texas," Unpublished M.A. thesis, University of Houston, 1963, Chapters 1, 2, and 6.

The functions and powers of a given district are of course dependent upon which of the several authorizations is utilized, as well as upon the wishes of those who are designing the district. Lacking the tie to the state that the county has, and lacking the cities' spectrum of functions that make citizens more aware of their presence, the special districts in Texas tend to be rather obscure and unsupervised governmental agencies.

So far as the Houston metropolitan area is concerned, the 1962 Census of Governments shows a grand total of fifty-six special districts, of which all except three had property tax powers. The single most numerous variety is school districts, of which there were twenty-one in 1962. Of the twenty-three single-function districts, thirteen were for water supply and six for natural resources. There were twelve multi-function districts. As a group, the school districts are of the greatest importance, both in terms of the number of persons affected and in terms of the amounts expended each year. Two of the nonschool special districts are important enough to warrant mention: the Navigation District, which has jurisdiction over the Port of Houston, and the Harris County Flood Control District, which is countywide in area.[3]

From this brief profile it can be seen that Houston is in many ways the archetype of the new American city. There is a rapidly growing, highly mobile population, with a high proportion of the labor force employed in white-collar occupations. There are present and potential tensions arising from a sizable number of impoverished and poorly educated Negroes and Latin Americans. Politics in Houston has become a three-way struggle with considerable ideological content between conservative Democrats, liberal Democrats, and Republicans, in about that order of strength. Some eighty-two governments, mostly municipalities and special districts, exist in the area.

STATE STRUCTURE OF MENTAL HEALTH SERVICES

Some idea of the level of mental health services available in Texas can be gleaned from Table 1, prepared by the state Mental Health Planning Committee; it shows the psychiatric services available in Texas and the six metropolitan areas having a population of 300,000 or more. Even when

[3] Harris county voters in November 1964 approved the creation of a countywide mosquito control district, and in November 1965 they finally approved—after three previous rejections—the formation of a countywide hospital district.

Table 1: Psychiatric Resources in Metropolitan Areas of Texas with 300,000 Population or More, 1963

Standard Metropolitan Statistical Area

Psychiatric Resource	Houston	Dallas	San Antonio	Ft. Worth	El Paso	Beaumont	Total	State Total
Psychiatrists	82	80	59	37	14	5	277	436
General hospitals accepting psychiatric patients	7	4	4	5	3	3	26	58
Private mental hospitals	2	2	0	0	0	0	4	5
State mental hospitals	1	0	1	0	1*	0	3	12
U.S. government hospitals	1	1	0	1	0	0	3	6
Resident treatment, children	0	0	0	0	0	0	0	3
State schools for mentally retarded	0	1	0	0	0	0	1	6
Full-time outpatient clinics	5	9	3	2	1	0	20	32
Part-time outpatient clinics	1	1	1	0	0	0	3	8

* Not a state hospital in ordinary sense; see below, p. 98 for clarification.

Source: Research Memorandum Number 2, Office on Mental Health Planning, Jan. 24, 1964 (Austin: Mental Health Planning Committee), Table 1863–B1.

due allowances are made for the limitations of the data on which it is based, it is unmistakably clear that Texas has lagged considerably behind the other states. Such a list by no means exhausts all mental health resources, but it does include the most obvious ones. Although these six metropolitan areas have 44 per cent of the state's population, the only state mental hospital within their boundaries is at San Antonio. Yet four of the five *private* mental hospitals and almost 60 per cent of the psychiatrists are found in these six metropolitan areas. Similarly, twenty of the thirty-two full-time outpatient clinics and three of the eight part-time clinics are located in these six metropolitan areas. The figures for residential centers for children and state schools for mentally retarded show the same curious imbalance—virtually none in the largest cities. Seemingly, the private sector of mental health has made a better adjustment to population patterns than has the public sector.

Although the state may not care to locate its facilities in the largest metropolitan areas, it does provide most of the residential care available to the mentally ill and the mentally retarded. The provision of care for the mentally ill is one of the oldest social services undertaken by the state of Texas, going back to the earliest years of its existence. Despite this historic commitment, the actual handling of mental illness by the state left much to be desired, and its mental hospitals suffered from all the handicaps and disabilities characteristic of state mental hospitals across the nation in the first half of the twentieth century. Reform in Texas began in 1949 with sweeping administrative changes, followed by a greatly expanded capital improvement program in the early 1950s and by the adoption of a new Mental Health Code in 1957.

Until 1949 the status of the state hospitals was perhaps symbolized by the fact that they, and other eleemosynary institutions, were under the administrative authority of the Board of Control, the state's purchasing agency. In 1949 the mental hospitals and eleemosynary institutions were put under the jurisdiction of the newly created Board of State Hospitals and Special Schools. Another reorganization was undertaken in 1965 as a result of the state mental health planning efforts, when a Department of Mental Health and Mental Retardation was established.

Only one of the six state mental hospitals is located in a large metropolitan area (San Antonio). Closely associated with these six institutions are three geriatric centers, which take only patients transferred from the mental hospitals upon determination of their treatment needs. Each of the hospitals and centers serves the population in a specified geographic district. Thus, Houston patients must be sent to Austin State Hospital, 160 miles away. The six mental hospitals and the three geriatric centers have a bed capacity of slightly over 14,000. Occupancy rates tend to be high, as indicated by the annual report for 1962–1963, which showed 15,921 patients in the various institutions on August 31, 1963. Four outpatient clinics are operated in conjunction with the mental hospitals at Austin, Terrell, Big Spring, and Wichita Falls. Their first obligations are to serve furloughed or discharged patients from the hospitals, and the vast majority of their patients are of this type; others residing in the geographical confines of the district may also be treated, however, depending upon the availability of staff. Patients are charged from nothing to $10 per visit, depending upon their ability to pay. As Table 2 indicates, the treatment capacity varies greatly from one clinic to another.

Table 2: Outpatient Clinics Operated by the Board of State Hospitals

Outpatient Clinic Operated by Board	Patients on Books, 8/63	Patient Treatment (Fiscal Year 1962–1963)
State hospital-related clinics		
Austin	1,033	3,951
Big Spring	62	1,943
Terrell	354	2,658
Wichita Falls	23	169
Not state hospital-related		
San Antonio	898	7,424
Dallas	714	7,639
Fort Worth	426	2,742
Harlingen	222	1,901

Source: Annual Report for the Board for State Hospitals and Special Schools, Fiscal Year 1962–1963, pp. B–54, 55, Austin, Texas.

In addition to the hospital-connected clinics, the board also operates adult mental health clinics. The centers in Dallas and San Antonio began operating in 1958; those in Fort Worth and Harlingen in 1962. As with the state hospital-related clinics, these have a responsibility to help care for patients furloughed or discharged from state hospitals. It appears, however, that they put greater emphasis on help for other types of patients, for only about a third of their referrals are from state hospitals. Services are limited to those who cannot afford private care, with fees set according to ability to pay. The number of patients and the number of treatments given is shown in Table 2.

Mention should also be made of the Houston State Psychiatric Institute, although it will be discussed more fully in connection with Houston mental health resources. First opened in 1957, and operated under the auspices of the Board of State Hospitals and Special Schools strictly as a research institution, HSPI furnishes a wide range of services to a very limited number of carefully selected patients. The board also has nominal responsibility for a child clinic and day hospital at Galveston, but it is actually operated under an interagency contract by the University of Texas Medical School there.

One should also note a recent innovation by the board, viz., contracting with local hospitals or clinics to provide care for persons who would otherwise be sent to one of the state hospitals. These contractual arrangements have been put into effect in El Paso, Beaumont, and Lubbock, all cities located quite some distance from the nearest state mental hospital. Judging from the reduced admittance rate at the state hospitals, the contractual plan has been a successful one, and expansion to other cities is planned.

State care of mentally retarded persons began much later than care for the mentally ill, going back only to the World War I period. For much of the ensuing time, the special schools for mentally retarded persons were treated pretty much as stepchildren, but the late 1950s and early 1960s saw a considerable improvement in their situation. Three new schools were established, old ones were expanded, and operating budgets almost tripled. The mental retardation division of the Board of State Hospitals and Special Schools operated six schools with a total of 11,500 patients. Despite the expanded effort, there is still a waiting list of over 500 persons. Since less than 5 per cent of the patients admitted are discharged, the long-range projections are for continuing pressure upon facilities.

Until 1965 the mental health authority was the commissioner of health, who directed the separate state Department of Health. Despite his designation as mental health authority, the commissioner was not able to develop a major role for his agency in mental health. The mental health division (subsequently transferred to the new Department of Mental Health and Mental Retardation), was one of five divisions in the Preventive Medical Services branch, which was in turn one of seven departmental branches. The state never appropriated any funds for the Division of Mental Health, and it subsisted solely on grants from the National Institute of Mental Health. In 1964–1965 there was a budgeted staff of eight professional and eight clerical workers but not all of these positions were filled.

Functions of the Mental Health Division included educational and information programs, research and epidemiology, and community services (essentially technical and administrative consultation plus some limited financial assistance to local mental health agencies). The limited nature of the assistance thus available is indicated by the division's report in 1964 that forty-eight of the state's fifty-eight local health departments had services related to mental health, and of that forty-eight, the Division of Mental Health had provided funds and technical assistance to six. Another set of figures revealed that the aggregate budgets for nine community clinics during the two-year period ending June 30, 1964, was $641,000, of which state funds for six of them represented about 8 per cent.

In terms of intrinsic importance, probably the mental health responsibilities of the Texas Education Agency are second only to those of the Board of Hospitals and Special Schools. The Division of Special Education administers the program of state assistance to local school districts to enable the hiring of special education teachers. Types of special classes include those for the mentally retarded and emotionally disturbed. Funds were allocated in 1963–1964 to provide over 2,684 teachers for 73,319 pupils. Of these, over 1,700 teachers were for the purpose of handling almost 22,000 mentally retarded children—both those classified as educable and those classified as trainable.

Although still in the pilot stage, the state assistance for classes for emotionally disturbed children is perhaps the most portentous of the lot. First set up by the legislature in 1963, the classes in Houston and elsewhere were designed to explore the possibilities and the problems inherent in such classes. The maximum number of students involved is only sixty-five, but it should be noted that this discussion refers only to the classes for the emotionally disturbed that are financed under this program; the school districts themselves may also finance additional classes. The results of the first year were so encouraging that modest expansion of state support was provided by the legislature in 1965.

A second very significant activity in mental health under the auspices of the TEA is through the federally financed vocational rehabilitation program. Unlike the special education programs, which are essentially state grants to the local school districts, the field work in vocational rehabilitation is carried on by the state agency itself by means of the area offices and counselors distributed across the state. The field staff for the vocational rehabilitation program consists primarily of counselors. No psychiatrists or clinical psychologists are employed by the division in a treatment capacity; such services are instead purchased from other agencies or institutions—state, local, or private.

There are several other state agencies involved in the mental health effort to some greater or lesser degree. For example, the Texas Youth Council is responsible for approximately 3,000 juveniles cared for in four correctional schools and for the administration of juvenile parole programs (only the most populous areas have parole officers). While one could plausibly argue that a great part of the work done by the agency is of its nature mental health, there are as well direct services available to its wards. No inpatient beds are maintained since psychotic juveniles are transferred to the facilities of the Board of State Hospitals and Special Schools, but diagnostic and a limited amount of treatment work is done.

The Texas Commission on Alcoholism counsels, carries on educational and informational duties, and stations counselors in the mental hospitals, the tuberculosis, hospitals, and in the state prison system. Since all of this is to be done with an annual appropriation of less than $250,000, it is not hard to see that something less than comprehensive coverage results.

Still another portion of the responsibility for mental health services belongs to the Child Welfare Services Division of the Department of Public Welfare. The division is responsible for child care and welfare for children who live away from home and those who may live at home but who are delinquent or are emotionally disturbed. The division spends some $2 million annually on this program with a caseload of some 6,000 children. While only 178 of these are classified as mentally ill, many of the remaining ones (neglected children, unwed mothers, etc.) would be likely to be in need of help. Although the division has a psychiatric consultant, children who are mentally retarded or emotionally disturbed are not treated but are referred to public and private treatment agencies.

The foregoing describes the more salient agencies involved directly in the mental health endeavor at the state level. There are others, of course: the services to the handicapped (including mentally retarded and mentally restored) of the Texas Employment Commission; the diagnosis and treatment facilities of the prison system; the counseling work of the Commission for the Blind; the psychiatric and psychological help given students in the state colleges and universities; and so on. However, these agencies and their activities are either so peripherally involved, or so limited in their contribution, or serve such a specialized population, that further pursuit along these lines seems unnecessary.

STATE AGENCY RELATIONSHIPS

With this somewhat extended review of agency structure at the state level now completed, it is possible to focus on the critical question of their relationships. Basically, there are three sources of information bearing on that question: agency heads and their top assistants, persons at the middle management level, and knowledgeable persons outside the state agencies under consideration. It soon became clear that responses from the first group, and to some extent from the second, were affected in two ways by the existence and work of the state Mental Health Planning Committee. First of all, the committee's composition was such that it brought together people from most of the state agencies interested in mental health, many of them the agency heads. It was not always possible to know when these respondents were describing relations *before* the formation of the committee and when they were describing relations growing out of its work. In the second place, many of the interviews took place at a very critical stage in the Planning Committee's operations just after the first psychiatric consultant and chief architect of the committee had been replaced. There was considerable reluctance on the part of agency heads to say anything that might conceivably affect the course of events.

Despite these difficulties it was possible to come to some conclusions about agency relations. First of all, it was generally agreed that agency relationships have not been overtly hostile or unfriendly. In a state where funds for social services are always insufficient, there inevitably is a certain amount of scrambling for the available money, but there were no indications that this went beyond acceptable limits, or that the fragmentation of agencies had greatly exacerbated it. In particular, there is nothing to indicate that the failure of the state to provide funds for the Mental Health Division was in any way related to agency rivalry.

Second, the amount of agency interaction appears normally to be quite limited. Knowledgeable respondents spoke repeatedly of the lack of communication and coordination, with a distinct tendency for each agency to go about its program planning with little or no consultation with others. One particular case referred to involved parallel planning by the Board of Hospitals and Special Schools and the Mental Health Division for clinic services in the same geographic area, neither being apprised of the other's plans. While most agencies were not so deliberate in their aloofness as the Texas Youth Council, they did not seem greatly troubled by the relative isolation that exists.

Third, such formalized cooperative efforts as have been undertaken, although few in number, seem to have produced satisfactory results. The chief instrument is the interagency contract. By such a contract between the Board of State Hospitals and Special Schools and the Regents of the University of Texas, the operation of the Moody State School for the Mentally Retarded was turned over to the Galveston Medical School in September 1963. Similarly, the Commission on Alcoholism has a contract with the Hospital Board for the placing of counselors in certain of the mental and tuberculosis hospitals. The vocational rehabilitation division of the Texas Education Agency similarly contracts with the Hospital Board for placing counselors in the hospitals. Thus, although the interagency contract is sometimes a cumbersome and frustrating device, it appears from these examples to have some possibilities for wider application.

But by far the most important linkage between mental health agencies —and this is the fourth and crucial finding—is provided by the personal relationships and contacts, particularly at the middle management level. These ties are very often professional in origin, but in some cases they stem from the fact that a person may have been employed by two or three different agencies during the course of his career. But whatever the origin, there is no mistaking the great importance of these informal ties. It is likewise clear that they contribute to the impression of good relations between agencies, because they facilitate a certain amount of "bootleg" work in the disposal of individual cases requiring assistance from other agencies. For example, one agency head indicated his belief that interagency relations were good and gave as an example his success in getting prosthetic aid from another agency for a legless youth in his care by merely picking up the telephone.

One should not minimize the importance of services thus exchanged, nor of the communication thus brought about. Nevertheless, there are several worrisome aspects. For one thing, the pattern described may get in the way of a better structuring of relations, because of the tendency to deal with special and specific problems rather than confront broader issues, and the tendency to overlook the limited and ad hoc character of these relations. The interactions are most likely to occur at levels below that of agency heads, where there is a considerable amount of personnel turnover; thus the quality of relations is apt to vary with an agency's personnel situation. Finally, despite a contrary assumption on the part of some agency heads, it is very much to be doubted that all or even most problems with interagency facets can be successfully handled on this informal basis. Rather, it appears that a certain amount of conscious or unconscious screening or referrals takes place, so that other agencies are called upon only when there is some likelihood of their being able to provide help.

MENTAL HEALTH ACTIVITIES IN HOUSTON

The mental health services available in Houston, like those at the state level, tend to be quite limited. A basis for overall comparisons is hard to establish, but a 1960 study reports the efforts of local community councils in twenty-three selected American cities to portray the health, welfare, recreation, and central planning services *available to or for local residents* from any nonprofit, relatively permanent source. Although each of the local councils defined the geographic area covered, standardized categories and definitions of services were established, including federal, state, and local governmental as well as voluntary endeavors. Services available to local residents (e.g., state hospitals) were included, even if they were not physically located in the area.

Even when due allowance is made for the shortcomings of these comparative data, it is clear that Houston offered very few services. It ranked twenty-second out of the twenty-three cities in per capita expenditures for health, welfare, and recreation services in 1960; it ranked nineteenth in health services alone. It hardly comes as a surprise, then, that the per capita expenditures for mental health services placed

Houston at the bottom of the group ($2.24 for Houston, compared with $7.78 for all twenty-three cities). Although that study is now several years old, there is not much to indicate any significant improvement in Houston's ranking.[4]

In describing these limited services in Houston, it is perhaps wise to begin with those that are related to state agencies previously mentioned. Although there are no state mental hospitals in the area, the Board of State Hospitals and Special Schools (and its successor, the Department of Mental Health and Mental Retardation) does operate the Houston State Psychiatric Institute (now known as the Texas Institute for Mental Science).

While its research and training orientation force HSPI to be selective in admissions, it nevertheless constitutes one of the most important resources in the area. It offers inpatient care (forty-three beds in 1964) and there is a follow-up clinic for persons discharged from state hospitals. There are also two outpatient clinics, one for adults and one for children. But clearly HSPI-Baylor is the major source of professional talent available for other agencies in the community. It has further importance in a leadership capacity.

The Texas Education Agency similarly is an important provider of service to the Houston area. In 1963, some 306 special education units were provided for mentally retarded children in Harris county schools, as well as two of the state's six pilot classes for emotionally disturbed children. The vocational rehabilitation program operated by TEA is also important in metropolitan Houston. Basically, its objective is to provide through contractual arrangements for those persons who are mentally retarded or emotionally disturbed and who are not eligible for help from other agencies.

Mental health services provided by other state agencies in the Houston metropolitan area are virtually nonexistent. The Welfare Department's local staff has important responsibilities, disbursing some $15 million annually to approximately 20,000 families, but little of this is directly related to mental health. Indirect involvement of the Welfare Department in mental health problems occurs, of course, in cases such as the aged who need guardians before they can be con-

---

[4] Research Bureau, Houston Community Council, "Income and Expenditures: A Comparative Report for Health, Welfare, and Recreation Services in 23 Cities" (Oct., 1963), Tables 1, 2, and 3.

tinued on old age assistance and the dependent children who are receiving aid because the father is mentally incompetent. But the Welfare
Department serves principally as a referral agency in cases of this
nature, seeing its role as that of determining eligibility rather than providing treatment or financial assistance to those who are themselves
emotionally disturbed or mentally retarded. As for the Mental Health
Division in the state Health Department, its resources are so meager
that when spread over the entire state any Harris county services would
be exceedingly minute. The state Commission on Alcoholism has no
office in the area.

Scanty as these state services to the Harris county population may
seem, they compare favorably with the mental health activities carried
on by the various local governments. As befits its status as the only
general government with areawide jurisdiction, Harris county is perhaps
doing the most in the mental health field. Its principal activities relate
to: the county Psychiatric Diagnostic Center; the county school board
and its psychiatric-psychological services to local school boards; and,
until November 1965, inpatient and outpatient facilities at the city-
county charity hospital.

The Psychiatric Diagnostic Center originated in the Second World
War when a Psychiatric Department operating in conjunction with the
Juvenile Department was set up. In 1954 space in a vacated county jail
was made available and a Psychiatric Ward divorced from the juvenile
program was organized. Improved facilities were obtained in the old
city-county charity hospital (Jefferson Davis Hospital) when a new
hospital was put into service in 1963, and the Psychiatric Ward was
renamed the Psychiatric Diagnostic Center.

It cannot be emphasized too strongly that the center serves only a
diagnostic function. Its clientele is limited to those persons ordered to
undergo psychiatric examination by a justice of the peace or the county
judge (who plays a key role in the operation of the center) as a result
of complaints lodged with those officials. Admissions to the center
in 1963 totaled 1,600, of which some 915 were ordered committed to
one hospital or another. Fewer were placed in nursing homes or with
a guardianship agency. There is a staff of forty-three (1964 figures) and
an annual budget of about $317,000, drawn entirely from the county's
general fund.

A second area of county activity is the county school superintendent's program for providing psychological and psychiatric services to the school districts of Harris county. The county school board and the superintendent appointed by it are supposed to supervise common school districts (as distinct from independent districts) but only one such district has survived in Harris county. As these administrative responsibilities disappeared, the county school board and the superintendent found it desirable to undertake new roles or face abolition. Fortunately for them, they were armed with a small earmarked tax levy that yields around $175,000 annually. Accordingly, several services are now offered to the various independent school districts, including small but significant mental health services.

The psychiatrists concentrate on helping teachers to recognize and understand the emotionally disturbed child and to apply certain techniques of help. Children are seen primarily in connection with that objective and for illustrative diagnosis. No treatment as such is provided; those needing it are sent on to other agencies, if available. An estimated 100 to 125 children a year are handled in this fashion. In addition, some 250 children a year are given various psychological tests. All of the county's nineteen independent school districts utilize these services at one time or another except the largest, the Houston Independent School District. In a county with 350,000 scholastics the small number of children handled makes the program seem a trifle pathetic, but its real value is presumably in the better preparation of teachers to handle their problem children. Certainly the teachers and special education supervisors who were interviewed felt that the county superintendent was providing real help for them.

The county was formerly involved in mental health activity as well through its contribution of 35 per cent or so of the funds for the operation of Ben Taub Charity Hospital (the city of Houston provided the other 65 per cent). The establishment of a hospital district in late 1965 changed the governing and financial structures, but little else. The entire medical program of the hospital is closely tied to Baylor University College of Medicine, which staffs the hospital and supervises its training program. Despite these ties, it is abundantly clear that the psychiatric services at Ben Taub are essentially of a stopgap nature. The inpatient facilities consist of a total only of twenty-seven beds, mostly for emergency and acute treatment. There is a rapid turnover in patients, for the ward is simply not geared to long-term treatment. The outpatient clinic, which is serviced by eleven or twelve residents, is similarly limited in its services.

Other than the county, the public schools are the only local government offering significant mental health services. Most, though not all, of the county's nineteen school districts provide some psychological evaluation and psychiatric consultation of their own, in addition to that made available through the county school superintendent's office, although the amount and quality of such services is apt to vary considerably. The Houston Independent School District relies entirely on its own resources. In addition to a consulting psychiatrist attached to the Health Services Division, the HISD has twelve psychologists and two administrators working in a Psychological Services Division. A substantial portion of their work is group (educational) testing, but a certain amount of individual testing is done as well. Since the district has some 218,000 pupils enrolled, there should be no illusions about the comprehensiveness of the services.

Perhaps the most significant mental health effort made in the public school system involves classroom and instructional services. In 1963–1964, there were 306 classes for mentally retarded children in the county. Since the local districts' outlay is confined to classes in excess of the state allocation, and to administrative and capital outlays, there is some question as to how much credit the local schools are entitled to for such effort. In addition, there are several classes for emotionally disturbed children. Five of these (one a state-supported pilot class) are in the Houston Independent School District, although the 1963–1964 school year began with only four of them staffed. Approximately forty pupils are involved, having been chosen because of their record as under-achievers and as disruptive of regular classes. Thus they are not psychotic or even violently disturbed, but are rather those for whom an eventual return to regular classes is deemed possible.

The local government programs for mental health in the Houston metropolitan area are pretty well exhausted when the efforts of the county and of the school districts have been recounted. To be sure, there are some very trifling activities; one or two doctors in the city health department's well-child clinic may be concerned with the emotional as well as physical health of the children and parents, and local judges may employ a psychiatrist in connection with judicial proceedings before them, but these are happenstances, not programs.

Given the nature and the meagerness of the mental health endeavors of local government in Harris county, the question of the relationships of the agencies involved is largely an academic one. Since the schools are providing essentially evaluative and diagnostic services, the great need is for treatment facilities for those who need help. But local governments do not provide such services. (It is apparently unthinkable to refer school schildren to the charity hospital for psychiatric care.) The school districts and the county school superintendent's office have apparently developed good relations but for very limited purposes. While there was ample evidence that here, as at the state level, professional ties contribute greatly to good communication among the persons in the various school districts dealing with mental health problems, the help that can be given to each other is infinitesimal. Conceivably the county Psychiatric Diagnostic Center and the charity hospital psychiatric ward and outpatient clinic could interact fruitfully, but apparently they do not. In a word then, there really are no significant interrelations among local government agencies.

When one turns from publicly supported local programs to those that are privately supported, a much greater range of services is found. Their consideration can perhaps best proceed under the headings of (1) inpatient services, (2) outpatient services, and (3) other services.

Houston's private inpatient services are to be found in two mental hospitals and in four general hospitals. Each of the two mental hospitals has around forty beds each; both have numerous affiliated psychiatrists but none as paid staff members. Hedgecroft, a nonprofit institution, was chartered as a mental hospital in 1960. Bellhaven Hospital is a private, proprietary institution created in late 1963. The importance of patient fees for Hedgecroft and Bellhaven means that both, but particularly the latter, serve principally middle- and upper-class Anglo-Americans.

Not all the local general hospitals offer inpatient psychiatric care, but the four that do so provided approximately 125 beds in 1964. The largest psychiatric ward (51 beds) is provided by Methodist Hospital. The ward is financed entirely by fees. Although about the same overall size as Methodist, Hermann Hospital has no separate psychiatric unit as such. Some 20 beds in the charity wing are set aside for patients who were admitted for other reasons but who need psychiatric care; all of these cases apparently involve the medically indigent.

The psychiatric ward at Memorial Baptist Hospital (900 beds total, in four locations) consisted of 48 beds in 1964, with expansion to 70 contemplated the following year. Admission policy is such that most cases entering the ward are comparatively mild, and virtually all of the ward is open. The small number of inpatient psychiatric cases at St. Joseph's Hospital, operated by the Sisters of Charity of Incarnate Word, were housed in general surgical and medical wards until completion of remodeling in 1965 when a 34-bed psychiatric ward was provided.

The venerable Child Guidance Center is unquestionably the most important provider of private outpatient service. First established in 1929, the center is financed primarily by the United Fund, with about 8 to 10 per cent of its annual expenditures derived from patient fees scaled to ability to pay. There is a six-month waiting list for the agency's services, and the number waiting for help would be far greater if many referral agencies had not given up attempting to get prompt treatment for patients. Although open to patients from all income levels and of all races and ethnic origins, in practice most patients are from middle- and upper-class Anglo-American families. The center provides individual counseling and treatment, but also emphasizes group therapy for children and for their parents. A number of full- and part-time psychiatrists, psychologists, and social workers are employed by the center, but it has experienced considerable difficulty in keeping all staff positions filled.

Another source of service is the Junior League Out-Patient Department in cooperation with Texas Children's Hospital. The relationship is a contractual one for the operation of eighteen or nineteen specialty clinics for the training of pediatricians. Two of these clinics, plus a day-care program discussed below, are related to mental health: one is a mental evaluation clinic for the mentally retarded, and the other is a child-family clinic for children with behavioral problems.

Mention might also be made of the outpatient clinic for alcoholics operated under the auspices of Methodist Hospital but staffed and served by the Houston State Psychiatric Institute. Designed as a research project, the clinic has a balanced staff of professional personnel. The treatment program consists of group therapy, with most patients from middle-income groups. It is necessary as well to call attention to the outpatient clinic at Hermann Hospital. Since the clinic is open only one-half day a week and sees only six to eight patients each time, all of them medically indigent, it can hardly be said to constitute a major resource for the community.

The category of "other" mental health services includes most obviously the more than eighty psychiatrists located in the Houston area. The proportion of time devoted by each to private practice varies tremendously; some have no private practice, others have nothing else. Extrapolations of responses to a questionnaire sent in early 1963 to sixty psychiatrists in the area by a Community Council Committee indicated that around 8,700 different patients were seen each year, almost two-thirds for treatment and most of the remainder for diagnosis only. Roughly 70 per cent of all cases were handled on an outpatient basis. While the extent of overlap, if any, of these with other figures reported in this chapter is not clear, it can easily be concluded that most psychiatric care in the Houston area is provided by private practitioners. Interestingly enough, over half of the respondents reported that they could take additional cases for treatment if some satisfactory financing system were available.

Still another approach is that represented by the Family Service Bureau. It is an old agency, having originated as the United Charities in 1904. The changes in its program over the years provide mute testimony to the changes in American society, for many of the services performed by the agency in its early years are now entirely the responsibility of public agencies. It now offers a number of activities related to mental health, particularly family counseling, the provision of homemaker services, and family life education. The largest percentage of cases are drawn from middle- and lower-income groups; a little over three-quarters of all cases are of the Protestant faith. Negroes are served; indeed, several of the social workers and homemakers employed by the agency are Negro.

And then, of course, there are several agencies and programs touching in some way on mental health whose impact is so slight, and which are so devoid of distinctive character, that even a brief summary is not warranted. Still, a mention of some of them might be useful for illustrative purposes. Such agencies as the Vocational Guidance Service, Jewish Family Service, Catholic Family Services, Day Care Association, Florence Crittenden Home, Faith DePelchin Home, and a number of others grapple daily with mental health problems along with the other social ills drawing their primary effort. Some of them provide a limited amount of counseling, some employ psychiatric consultants a few hours a month to guide the social workers and staff.

Their programs are apt to be such that separation of mental health aspects is difficult, and hence the quantity of their services is as hard to judge as the quality. Surely it can be said, however, that their collective efforts represent a significant part of the total mental health services available to the community, and this total is so woefully small that the surface has hardly been scratched.

The nature of the relationships among private agencies is not an easy one to portray. There is certainly much to indicate a generally supportive relationship, but this varies somewhat according to several coloring factors. One of these, most noticeable among family service agencies with relatively minor mental health involvement, stems from religious differences in the sources of agency support and in the clientele. Another seems to originate in assessments as to the effectiveness of an agency. For example, there was considerable open criticism of the Child Guidance Center that apparently grew out of the feeling that the center had not developed the services expected of it. And, as would be expected, the investigation uncovered some instances of nonsupportive behavior or attitudes that relate most directly to personality conflicts.

Still, the prevailing air is one of support, and it is worth considering why this should be. No doubt the feeling of being beleaguered and the solidarity it engenders would be important. It may also be related to the paucity of services; when resources are so desperately scarce, poor relations with potential sources of help may be a luxury no agency feels able to afford. Working relations, it appears, are pretty much in the hands of social workers rather than the mental health professionals, which means that locally, as at the state level, the role of vocational and professional ties is quite important. Thus, while the Community Council and its various committees represent the formal communications machinery, it is not the most important link.

The matter of communications is worth additional comment. The general feeling, with certain exceptions, seemed to be that communications among private agencies are generally good. In any case, it appears that specialization was perhaps as much a villain as fragmentation in impeding the circulation of information. For example, there was some indication that communications *between* the various professions (social worker, medical, etc.) was much poorer than communications *among* the members of a given profession in different agencies. It also appeared that good communications were not to be taken for granted; the best-informed persons were those who worked at it. Those who did not soon drifted out of the communication stream. Finally, the question might very well be raised: Even if the communication system generally is good, from the standpoint of the distribution of information, is it necessarily an efficient one, i.e., does it function with minimum inputs?

The statement that private agencies are generally supportive does not mean that they work closely together in policy planning and in program development. Although the Community Council is the formal coordinating body, its effectiveness appears to be somewhat limited. There appear to be at least three reasons for this. First of all, the Council is not equipped with sufficient formal sanctions to compel such cooperation. Apparently, there is a tendency for each agency to plan its program, and then to confront the council with a *fait accompli*. Second, the composition of the council militates against strong controls, because almost every agency is equally represented, without regard to size and importance. Third, there is the matter of the social worker's approach to policy making and to group relations. Perhaps because they are accustomed to working with poorly defined authority, the social workers tend to meet difficult situations by negotiation and moral suasion rather than by authority and clear-cut decisions, attempting to avoid whenever possible conflict situations. The result is hyper-caution and timidity.

The third level of government involved in the Houston–Harris county mental health effort is the national one. Of all the federal agencies so involved in the area, surely the most important one is the Veterans Administration, which operates a 1,250-bed general hospital in Houston. It, of course, draws patients from a much larger geographical area, but in early 1963 about 50 per cent of those receiving inpatient psychiatric care were residents of Harris county. All of these psychiatric patients are adults; about 18 to 20 per cent are Negroes. The Veterans Hospital, of course, serves a special population.

The various psychiatric wards provide around 420 beds. Normal stay for the psychiatric patients averages about 60 days, which means that there are some 1,260 cases a year. Applying to this the estimate that 50 per cent of these are Harris county residents, some 630 persons in the metropolitan area will each year receive such service. For comparative purposes, it will be noted that this is equivalent to about *70 per cent* of the total number of persons committed each year to the state mental hospitals from Harris county.

One other federal agency providing mental health services deserves mention. The U.S. Public Health Service has an outpatient clinic in Houston to provide medical services to merchant seamen and to members of the armed forces and their dependents. Some 1,100 patients each month receive care of one sort or another, but the number receiving psychiatric and psychological help is reported to be quite small. Acute alcoholism is the major category of cases in the mental health field for the clinic, with perhaps six to eight patients a month being hospitalized. These, and the small number of narcotics cases, are sent to the U.S. Public Health Service Hospital at Fort Worth, which specializes in mentally ill and narcotics cases. Apparently the general practitioners at the Houston clinic attempt to treat whatever mild cases of mental disorder present themselves. One gets the impression that the really severe cases requiring inpatient care are disposed of by transfer; less severe cases are handled on a catch-as-catch-can basis.

AGENCY RELATIONSHIPS

It is particularly difficult to get evidence bearing on the relationship of federal and state mental health agencies, and the generalizations offered here are pieced together out of numerous and varied fragments, a disproportionate share of which were gathered at the state level. Their relations seemed to be deeply colored by two general conditions: First, the political climate in Texas has been characterized by a considerable amount of states' rights thinking, complete with a tendency to regard Washington agencies with suspicion if not outright dislike. Second, there is nevertheless a desire to utilize federal funds to ease the pressure on the state treasury (year in and year out, about 25 per cent of all funds spent by the state of Texas are obtained from the federal government). To satisfy the latter urge requires primarily certain legal and financial relations, and the former condition does not encourage going beyond that. The relationship can thus best be described as a "correct" one, satisfying all formal niceties but not going much beyond.

Further, it can be said that, despite their financial contributions, federal agencies have not exerted continuing influence on state mental health programs. It is by no means certain that state agencies would welcome or permit more leadership in program implementation from federal agencies, but in any case there was little evidence of this being attempted. There are, of course, legal as well as political limits to what could be done by federal officials, but these limits do not appear to have been crowded.

When one turns to the local level, it is necessary to deal more in their potential relations with federal agencies, since there are not the same extensive financial-legal ties found with state agencies. Nevertheless, federal and local relations are colored by the same two factors. Local aversion to federal programs in general is, if anything, stronger and the financial urge weaker than at the state level. Both private and public local agencies sometimes fail to avail themselves of the federal assistance in mental health that could be obtained, although the degree of abstinence varies greatly from one agency to another. One of the most fascinating, and slightly incredible, aspects of this is the periodic search in the community for an agency willing to undertake participation in a given federal program. There does appear to be a somewhat greater effort on the part of federal administrators at this level to provide leadership and implementation support, although this may be because the widely used demonstration research programs facilitate such efforts.

But the generalizations above do not hold for the relationship of local agencies to the Houston Veterans Hospital, which has in several ways been integrated into the community. It is a teaching hospital for Baylor College of Medicine, and staff members often hold double or triple appointments in medical institutions. Mental health professionals—psychiatrists, psychologists, and psychiatric social workers—serve on numerous local agency boards, including the health section of Community Council, and they have repeatedly been entrusted with leadership responsibilities. There are perhaps several explanations for this. The VA Hospital is an important resource, despite its somewhat specialized clientele; it is the single largest reservoir of professional manpower; there is no longer any serious question about the legitimacy of its services. It may be, however, that the single most important factor is that it is engaged in providing direct services and hence is in a much better position to develop a network of interactions, to engage in exchanges, as it were, than are federal agencies not involved in providing direct services.

The relationships between state and local governments are essentially confined to those growing out of provision of direct mental health services; there is no financial nexus in the form of cash payments flowing in either direction. Houston field offices of the state agencies operating in Houston appear to have been as well integrated into the community as local ones, although that may not be saying a great deal. They seem to have been accepted in their local roles, handling referrals, serving on study groups and on local boards (including Community Council), and, in the case of Houston State Psychiatric Institute, playing a very important leadership role. Local personnel seemed generally understanding of the handicaps and program limitations under which their state counterparts operate. The only clear case of local dissatisfaction with a state agency had as a target the director of a state mental hospital, for reasons related mostly to his personality.

It must be repeated, however, that these generalizations apply to the agencies that interact in the provision of direct services. When a state agency is not so involved, relations with local agencies are apt to be minimal and casual. One can speak safely of good working relations between state and local agencies, but otherwise there is little interaction. It is particularly lacking when it comes to mutual aid in program development and implementation, for the policy-making processes in Austin and in Houston seem to be entirely unrelated. One suspects that a prime factor in this pattern is the patience born of long frustration in attempting to stretch too-scanty resources, a situation as common for state agencies as for local ones. Certainly the local people most impatient with the level of services were the least tolerant of state agencies.

The relationship of local private agencies to local public agencies is, of course, one of the most important. Certain points stand out clearly. While there are no widely publicized rifts, the private agencies have a rather low regard for the public ones in the field of mental health. The public sector provides very little in the way of services needed by the private social work agencies. The latter are not dependent on public programs; quite the reverse is true. The social work agencies thus find themselves handling tasks that elsewhere have long since been deputed to public agencies. This resentment is exacerbated by the view widely held among private agencies that certain of the public agencies, e.g., the county Welfare Department, or the Juvenile Division, are not even doing what it is in their power at present to do. There is as well the consideration that public local agencies respond to political forces beyond the reach of the private sector; the Juvenile Division, for example, is controlled by the state district judges. Finally, there is the matter of professional standards. The private agencies complain that the local public agencies lack qualified staff and the complaint appears to be well founded.

In concluding this review of mental health structure and agency relationships, there are three overarching findings that need to be stated. First of all, it appears that many difficulties originate in the fact that, while patients typically have more than a single problem, each of the various agencies often is equipped to deal with only one type of problem. This necessarily requires a great deal of shuttling of patients from one agency to another if any attempt is made at comprehensive care. For any population, the number of patients lost in the process would be sizable, but a mentally ill person is especially prone to disappear in the interstices.

Second, the available evidence suggests strongly that an important factor in agency relations is that of professional ties. Relations seemed better when physical proximity and/or responsibility for direct services facilitated the development of professional associations among personnel. It seems that the poorest relations were in evidence at the levels where there was little opportunity for professional linkages to develop.

Third, between all levels, and between agencies at a given level, there are significant communications problems. People find it very hard to stay informed on what other agencies, at the same or at different governmental levels, are doing. The fragmentation of agencies clearly contributes to this, but of equal if not greater impact is specialization—the child specialist in child psychiatry does not know what is being done in adult psychiatry, for example. The paradox is more than apparent. The professionalization that helps to tie like-minded people together in different agencies operates at the same time to separate people within their own agency, or to produce more specialized agencies.

COMMUNITY INFLUENCE AND MENTAL HEALTH

Any attempt to describe the place of mental health programs and agencies in the system of community influence necessarily requires some consideration of the overall structure of power in Houston. Unfortunately Houston has not been subjected to intensive community power structure analysis. And since findings from Dallas, or Atlanta, or New Haven cannot be safely applied to it, the implication is that nothing can be said at present about the situation in Houston. But the needs are sufficiently great to justify "making do" with the scanty materials at hand. Published materials are extremely limited, whether one turns to journalism or to scholarly writing. In the interviews conducted for this study, questions were often asked about the respondents' perception of general community power, where they seemed to have some credentials as observers or participants. These results are complemented by the writer's own impressions, built upon observation over a period of five years and sharpened by occasional discussions with politicians, scholars, and interested citizens in the area.

Perhaps the most important conclusion bears upon leadership structure. If the pattern of community decision making is viewed as a point along a continuum ranging from elitism to pluralism, it seems very unlikely that Houston would be located near the elitist pole. Such evidence as there is indicates a structure of power and influence tending toward pluralism.

The relevant evidence includes, first of all, the existence of a sizable number of competing centers and bases of power in the community. There is the business and industrial elite, with its power base in money and jobs. There is the Negro elite, with its base in bloc voting and the possibility of "direct action" tactics. Organized labor constitutes still another center of power, with its economic and political leverage. There is a communications elite, grounded in the need of a complex community for the lubricant these persons possess. There is the elite founded upon the professions, notably medical and legal, and their place in society. And one should not ignore the political elite—the public officials, party leaders, and activists—whose power is based on the following they have developed within various interest groups and within segments of the electorate. Needless to say, the power and influence of each of these varies greatly, but there are sufficient examples that might be submitted to justify the conclusion that each elite is capable of exercising some power and influence.

Another feature supporting a pluralistic assessment of power in Houston is the ease of access into the Houston political system. Possibly because of economic and social opportunities that abound, and possibly because of the problem of incentives and rewards for political action, many persons with capacities for effectiveness as leaders or workers, are not drawn into the political system. The result is that the needs of the political system are so great, and the talent available so limited, that individuals and groups may readily penetrate the system.

One might also note the heavy reliance on elections to decide public issues. Popular elections for the choice of county, municipal, and special district officials, the necessity of voter approval for the recurring bond issues, and the frequency of referenda for decisions on particularly troublesome issues leave no doubt of the availability of elections as an instrument of mass participation. It is true that the proportion of adults taking advantage of the numerous electoral opportunities is small (voter turnout as a percentage of the potential electorate is at a peak of 40 to 45 per cent in presidential elections; it is far below that level in local elections). While low turnout rates admittedly reduce the amount of popular influence on public affairs, the participation of forty to fifty thousand citizens and the opportunity for participation of several times that number make it difficult to disregard the pluralistic ramifications of these elections.

Finally, one might argue in support of the pluralistic assessment that neither the interviews nor the writer's five years of reasonably close attention to the Houston scene support an elitist interpretation of power and influence in Houston. The available information on a wide range of decisions—firing of school superintendents, United Fund budgets, school desegregation, municipal elections, proposals for zoning, bond issues and tax increases, municipal water supply, the county Domed Stadium, financing of the charity hospitals—all seems to support the proposition that in the Houston metropolitan area a pluralistic system prevails.

Although its pluralism is the most important aspect of the Houston structure of leadership, there are other dimensions that bear mention.

One of these is the communications process, made doubly significant by the existence of that pluralism. From the little evidence at hand it appears that the various centers and subcenters of power and influence do not always communicate well with each other. This may be due in part to the large number of such centers and the consequent difficulty of linking them all, and to the number and complexity of the issues involved. It may be due in part also to the high ideological charge imported to some issues, which tends to impede candid and informal exchange. The doubtful quality of leadership may be another contributing factor. In any case, the communications system seems to be inadequate, with certain portions—the mass media—forced to carry an impossible burden.

Another dimension that bears notice is the lack of established leadership within the various competing power centers. In some cases, this means that there are rival contenders for the leadership positions, with none able to establish hegemony (the Negro community would be an example of this tendency). Such a situation complicates decision making, since one can never be sure of the credentials of the participants. In other cases, there may be persons who are accepted as leaders but who are not in fact very competent in their leadership roles if competence is judged in terms of the capacity to influence their own followers as well as other leaders in the decision-making process. It appears that leadership recruitment suffers from the competition for the time and energies of those with the necessary potential. For this tendency there may be several explanations. In a community where physical growth and economic development have been incredibly rapid, there inevitably are opportunities for persons of mediocre talents to rise to positions unattainable to them in a more competitive situation. The possibilities of this happening are increased when, as is the case in Houston, the social system by its values, traditions, and educational subsystem does little to equip persons to provide the kind of leadership needed in the new society. Closely related to both these factors is the need, in a rapidly changing society, for extraordinary amounts of leadership as new organizations form and as old ones adapt. Where the process of change is so great that the process of institutionalization never catches up, better than average leadership will be required.

One question remains to be raised in connection with the issue of general power and influence in Houston: How has it been affected by political fragmentation? One encounters here the same need for empirical verification and the same necessity for a stopgap assessment. It would seem very probable that fragmentation has contributed to the pluralism discussed above in at least three very important ways. One, it has helped to produce a variety of centers of political power—the county government, the school districts, the municipalities, and so on. Second, there is a tendency for social and economic groups to form along the geographic lines of a number of these political entities. Thus, when the various Chambers of Commerce within the county do often interact in supportive ways, they are organized along the geographical lines of the larger cities and may often be involved in competition with each other for reasons relating to the needs of their particular community.

It seems likely also that political fragmentation adds to the difficulties of decision making in a pluralistic system because it inevitably introduces a host of jurisdictional questions. Of course such questions may also arise in the absence of fragmentation, as in a hierarchical system such as found in the bureaus of an administrative agency, but in fragmented communities, unlike bureaucracies, there is no established authority for resolving the issues. Similarly, fragmentation contributes to the problem of insufficient leadership resources, by adding to the number of power centers that must be "staffed" with leaders. In a less fragmented system, some activities now requiring considerable leadership could be handled hierarchically.

Finally there appears to be this consequence of fragmentation: a tremendous amount of mobilization is necessary to influence any decision. A system as fragmented as that of Houston has such a potential for friction that leaders may be unduly preoccupied simply with maintaining the status quo. Even if they are not, the investment in time and energy necessary for change is apt to discourage all but the most strongly motivated. This should not be taken to mean that nothing ever gets done—the growth of the Houston metropolitan areas is proof enough to the contrary—but it does mean that more difficult and controversial matters are hard to handle properly.

In trying to relate mental health to the general structure of power and influence, it is perhaps best to begin by recalling that social welfare programs have on the whole fared poorly in the Houston metropolitan area. As previously reported, Houston ranked twenty-second out of twenty-three selected cities in its per capita expenditures for health, welfare, and recreation services in 1960. Its per capita expenditures for mental health of $2.24 were the lowest in the group, comparing very unfavorably with the $7.78 reported for all cities in the 1960 study.

Since the starved condition of social services in Harris county is generally recognized and deplored by professionals and by lay persons interested in the various facets of such services, it seems fair to conclude that the social welfare agencies in general have not found the key to influencing the community's power structure(s). And since mental health is one of the most inadequately supported of these social services, it seems equally fair to conclude that those responsible for it are even less able to influence community leadership. Undoubtedly there are several reasons for this, which are more or less common to all communities. The fact that mental health's clientele group by its nature cannot be effectively organized and the apathy of the general public toward mental health services are two reasons. It seems likely, however, that the lower levels of service in Houston are also affected by the local patterns of influence on behalf of mental health.

There are basically two groups in Houston with interests ranging over the spectrum of mental health needs and policies. One of these is made up of the psychiatrists, who are organized into a Houston Psychiatric Society. It was rather generally agreed that the society had not in fact been very influential. Several factors apparently contribute to this. First, the society and its members are bound by the code of ethics of the medical profession, which in Houston is construed in such a restrictive fashion that any public leadership by a physician is discouraged. Second, the psychiatric fraternity still has a relatively low status with others in the medical profession and it cannot always get a serious hearing easily. Third, most of the psychiatrists in Houston are engaged in private practice and hence are not oriented toward seeking community action, since they can progress in their careers and feel that they are rendering important services without any organized programs. Finally, it might be that at some points in time the relatively more liberal and progressive outlook of psychiatrists has hampered the functioning of the society vis-à-vis the medical society and other conservatively oriented power structures. Whatever the reason, the Psychiatric Society has not been able to play any large role in shaping community action in mental health, although some of its members have struggled valiantly.

The second all-encompassing group working on behalf of mental health is the Mental Health Association. There was rather complete agreement that it was the responsibility of the local Mental Health Association to educate the public and its various leadership structures, a consensus formalized by action of the Community Council, it might be added. There was almost equally widespread agreement that the Mental Health Association had failed to meet this responsibility. The handful of respondents who were not critical of the MHA in this regard were mostly those who turned out in several respects to be poorly informed, or those who were themselves under fire for failure to meet mental health responsibilities. The criticism ranged from disgusted references to people who "do nothing except sit around and talk" to allusions to the agency's staff and its deficiencies, but there could be no mistaking the widespread dissatisfaction with the MHA's failures in mobilizing community support. Insofar as general status and influence were concerned, the board of the MHA was considered to be a very good one, including as it did several very distinguished names. However, authoritative sources indicated that some difficulty was experienced in retaining good members and in getting actual work out of more than a handful. An attempt was made to examine in some detail the Mental Health Association board, but the returns of the self-administered questionnaire devised for that purpose were so poor as to preclude any use at all of the results.

In addition to these two groups with their broad range of interests, there are several agencies with a substantial enough interest in mental health to be considered as actual or as potential influences. It is impossible to examine the place of each of these in the system of community influence, however. One of the most important, the Houston State Psychiatric Institute, will be taken up below in connection with the discussion of leadership in the mental health community, but here the question concerns the relationship of mental health groups to the general community and its elites. Consequently, the Child Guidance Center, an agency important to one sector of mental health, will be used as a case study.

The board of the center was selected for closer examination regarding community influence partly because of its apparently high status and partly because it was one of the few voluntary agencies devoted exclusively to handling mental health problems. As the study progressed it became clear that the Child Guidance Center, while conceded to be engaged in a quality program, was subject to considerable criticism from professionals and from referral sources because of its limited intake. Such considerations remind one that there is no basis for supposing that these findings are typical for all voluntary agency boards. However, responses from persons outside the Child Guidance Center regarding agency boards and their influence tend to confirm the results of the Child Guidance Center investigation.

What follows is drawn partially from a questionnaire designed for use with the Child Guidance Center board, and partially from interviews with persons outside of the CGC, as well as with the president and the executive director of the agency. Since only eleven of the thirty-six CGC board members returned usable questionnaires, not much weight can be given to them. However, the responses do suggest that the board members saw themselves as having only a modest amount of influence with political, business, and opinion leaders. While the majority of the respondents felt that the board had been somewhat effective in furthering the cause of mental health in the community, there was an even division on the question of the board's effectiveness in furthering the agency's objectives. Interviews with persons outside the CGC revealed a widespread belief that it has a "blue-ribbon" board, judged in terms of the status and of the personal commitment of some of its members. However, it was also generally believed that the potential of the board for advancing mental health in general and developing the CGC program in particular was not being realized.

From bits and pieces of evidence that came to hand, it appears that the failure of the Child Guidance Center to influence community leaders is not an atypical case. None of those interviewed in the course of this study was inclined to believe that mental health agencies and boards could exert significant influence on the various power centers.

Many agencies, some of them only partially involved in mental health programs, were said to have difficulty in getting influential people actually to work on behalf of the agency. The tendency apparently is for a small number of persons on each board to do most of the work, and this group does not change much in composition over the years. There was also a feeling among some of the respondents that persons of stature and prestige are often too busy to do more than lend their names to an agency, and hence the people who do most of the work are often in the second echelon. In some instances, of course, agency boards themselves, for political or ideological reasons, would refuse to undertake to get community support for a program. However, the most common failing was lack of aggressive leadership rather than the hostility of board members toward mental health objectives.

If there is no institutional or group capacity to influence the community's elites, there is still a possibility that particular individuals with an interest in mental health might have such a capacity. This possibility was investigated and discounted. There are a number of persons who have a particular interest in mental health and who have played important roles within the mental health community. However, it does not appear that these persons have tapped community power on behalf of mental health. The reasons are no doubt varied and obscure, but, whatever the explanation, the evidence available makes clear that these individuals have had little success in moving the community and its leaders to any kind of frontal assault on mental health problems.

It thus appears that the mental health community has not been able to reach in an effective manner the leaders of the general community. It is important to consider why this is so, and particularly to ask whether or not fragmentation is a causal factor. There could be no greater mistake than to imagine that fragmentation is the sole, or even the primary, cause of this state of affairs. There are too many other forces at work, some of which have already been touched, to permit such a conclusion. It does appear, however, that fragmentation contributes to the difficulty of exerting community influence on behalf of mental health in several important ways.

First of all, vertical fragmentation in terms of local, state, and federal divisions complicates matters, for in Texas the state is considered to have the responsibility for handling mental illness. It is no doubt hard enough to persuade community leaders to act when their responsibility is clear; it is doubly difficult to do so when it is not. Even those who might concede that the state is doing a poor job are apt to hesitate to accept the proposition that the local community should therefore carve out a greater role for itself.

There are also the consequences arising from fragmentation along a horizontal plane at the local level. For one thing, it leads to agency proliferation. It impedes the development of a mental health "community," if by that term one means a group whose members share certain values and objectives and whose interactions are of such a type and degree as to make them interdependent. As is pointed out elsewhere, there is relatively little interaction and interdependence among local mental health agencies.

This same type of fragmentation complicates the development of unified leadership. The number of agencies is so great that matters of common interest cannot be handled on an informal basis, yet no formal organization linking them all has emerged. There is, of course, the health section of the Community Council, but it includes more than just mental health, and in any case it is not composed of the type of persons needed to approach community leaders. There is also a coordinating committee with representatives from psychiatry, psychology, and social work, but it is concerned with professional standards and relations rather than with taking the initiative in program development. It has already been noted that the Mental Health Association has not been able to perform effectively its function of community information and education, but even if it had been discharging that responsibility successfully, it still would not have been able to bring all agencies together, to plan and develop programs, and to persuade community leaders to implement these. Even its strongest critics would not be likely to charge the association with such responsibilities. Thus, when one asks who in Houston speaks for mental health, the answer must be "everybody and nobody." Leadership responsibility has been lost among the welter of agencies.

Local fragmentation, then, has impeded effective communications among agencies, has contributed to the failure to develop authoritative methods for allocating responsibilities in mental health, and has prevented emergence of the unified leadership in mental health that is made even more necessary by the pluralism of the Houston community.

Decision Making in Mental Health

Everything said thus far is prefatory to the question of how things get done in Houston insofar as mental health programs are concerned. First, the formal machinery for the coordination and planning of mental health programs will be considered. It will not take long, however, for planning is an extremely limited function in the Houston area. There are city and county agencies concerned with the physical development of the area (subdivision platting, street and highway programing, etc.), but there is *no* public agency with responsibility for planning social services. Such planning as there is, is entrusted to the Community Council of Houston and Harris county.

The organization, financing, and functions of the local Community Council are probably quite similar to what exists elsewhere. Financed primarily through the United Fund, the Houston council is composed of representatives from more than 120 agencies. Included among them are representatives from 4 federal, 9 state, 6 county, and 6 municipal agencies, plus the Houston Independent School District. The private agencies represented cover pretty much the entire field of social and civic agencies, ranging from the American Association of University Women to the Medical Society to the YMCA's and the YWCA's.

The council attempts to provide four types of services: coordination and planning, health and welfare information, personnel administration and consultation, and research. The coordination and planning function, the only one of interest here, is carried on through three formally constituted sections, each composed of delegates from member agencies plus appointed individuals: (1) family and child welfare, (2) recreation-informal education, and (3) health. Planning associates, generally with a background in social work, are assigned to work with each section and the agencies that fall within its jurisdiction. Mental health functions are handled by the health section.

Although community planning is universally conceded to the Houston Community Council, there are several reasons why it has not been able to discharge that responsibility. One is its lack of sanctions. Agencies not dependent on the United Fund for financial support—most notably public agencies, but some private ones as well—could not be expected to heed the council very closely, since it has no authority over them. But even agencies supported wholly or partially by the United Fund are not subject to positive control because of the subordinate and dependent relationship of Community Council to the United Fund. No attempt was made to explore in depth the relationship between the United Fund Budget Committee, which passes on agency requests, and the Community Council, which prepares an evaluation for the Budget Committee, but few persons and agencies are worried about Community Council invoking financial sanctions if they do not conform to its planning outputs.

The Community Council is also handicapped in its planning and coordinating function by its inability to tap the power structures of the community. It is preponderantly composed of second- or third-echelon people, and those who do have access to power are not always active. Given the emphasis on representation from the various component agencies, a heavy proportion of professionals, particularly social workers, is inevitable.

This, in turn, may contribute to another difficulty, the operating philosophy of the council. Even its top officials do not visualize the council as a leadership organ; the emphasis is rather on functioning as a forum for all views. The reliance is on development of a consensus among the agencies involved, rather than on pointing them toward improved services in a forthright fashion. The chief weapons in this kind of coordination/planning are personal contact, indirect suggestions, planted ideas. Bold and aggressive leadership, the preparation of plans and programs beforehand, and techniques of coercion are all eschewed. When staff members have on occasion pushed hard, their fellows as well as the member agencies have seen this as a lack of understanding of how things are properly done.

It is only too easy to criticize the council and its staff for a lack of positive leadership, but in all fairness one must grant the possibility that this operating philosophy is founded on past experience, and that the bland consensus approach is all that is practicable in the Houston context. Whatever the origins may be, the consequences are a failure to come to grips with the community's problems.

This is easily seen in the history of the most recent mental health study. A study completed in 1957 was by 1960 considered out-of-date, and the local Mental Health Association asked Community Council to conduct a new study. Council approved and a forty-three-member Mental Health Services Steering Committee was set up under the auspices of the health section of the council. By 1964 the committee was ready with a report. It consisted of eleven mimeographed pages, four of which dealt with the committee's origins and composition, and summarized the twenty-one recommendations covered in the remaining seven pages.

The first thing one notices about the report is that no hard data are offered to support the very general recommendations. For example, the second recommendation deals with psychiatric beds, but neither existing beds nor planned additions are reported, although the committee had such data at its disposal. Neither are estimates of future need provided. To say only that it is necessary "to maintain a constant awareness of the need for additional psychiatric beds" appears to be a flight from rather than an exercise of planning.

Furthermore, the assignments of responsibility to agencies are hopelessly vague and meaningless. To say that the development of a part-pay after-hours clinic is the responsibility of "Houston Psychiatric Society, clinics in general hospitals, Child Guidance Center, Houston State Psychiatric Institute, Houston Psychological Association, National Association of Social Workers, Harris County Medical Society, Mental Health Association" is to accomplish nothing except possibly to point toward the need for another committee. In fact, a committee to study the problem of getting a part-pay clinic was subsequently appointed.

There are other indications of the approach of the Community Council—or at least its health section—to the planning and coordinating process. The hard data which the study committee had to work with were supplied by the various subcommittees rather than by the council's research bureau or by other staff members. The amount of empirical data actually compiled was small. Any reasonably competent researcher could have defined the problem as authoritatively and with as much detail on the basis of no more than at most a few weeks of full-time analysis. Recommendations and assignments of responsibility are operations requiring considerable consensus-building, and hence if done properly they might necessitate several months of work. However, it is hard to escape the conclusion that these recommendations and allocations could have been prepared with far less time and effort.

In short, a process supposedly involving forty-three people that covered four years from inception to completion produced results that would be ridiculous if they were not so implicitly tragic. Given the time and opportunity, almost any member of that committee working individually could have prepared a more effective report. It is as awesome as it is worrisome to see how a group process could so impede the exercise of individual initiative and judgment.

The Houston Community Council, as has been indicated, is unable to perform satisfactorily the two essential functions: (1) matching known and projected resources against estimated needs; and (2) authoritatively allocating responsibility for action to meet anticipated demands. If the effectiveness of the council is so limited in the planning process, how then is it decided what is to be done and by whom?

As far as the private sector is concerned, the answer seems to be that each agency plots its own course on the basis of its own determination of needs and of resources. At some point, not necessarily in the earlier stages, Community Council will be consulted, particularly if United Fund financing is being sought, but its approval is not a prerequisite to the inauguration of a new program or the organization of a new agency. No doubt the council could effectively abort any proposed action that clearly and greatly overlapped the program of some other agency, but such a proposal is unlikely simply because there is plenty of room for new programs without trespassing on areas already staked out. Furthermore, the council, perhaps in recognition of its own weakness as well as of the vast blank areas of program, tends to go along with the proposals that come its way.

The public agencies are even more independent of any central coordinating authority. Each has, of course, its policy-making authorities to whom it is responsible, but they are not as a group working in conjunction, and each policy-making body is inclined to act with little or no reference to other agencies or authorities.

The lack of any central agency for the allocation of responsibility in the mental health field in Houston is not without some advantages, particularly from the standpoint of encouraging innovation in programs. However, it does tend to dissipate interest and resources, and makes it impossible to establish any kind of planned priorities for combating mental illness. That these are unfortunate consequences of fragmentation and dispersal is made clear by the one concrete recommendation of the Mental Health Services Study Committee:

Establish a permanent structure of inter-organizational communication and mutual planning between the mental health service organizations, appropriate professional groups, public officials and concerned citizens. Because of the constantly changing nature of the Mental Health problem, it is recommended that a coordinator be designated to serve as a community planning advisor for mental health.

The council's executive board handled the recommendation in what is probably a firmly established tradition: it approved the principle of the recommendation, but with the proviso that financing from outside the United Fund–Community Council structure would have to be obtained. More than a year later no funds had been found for that purpose, nor had there been any developments with respect to the recommendation for permanent structure for communication and planning.

Turning now to the question of leadership within the mental health community, one finds one principal and several secondary sources. The major source is clearly the Houston State Psychiatric Institute (and Baylor Medical School's Department of Psychiatry; the two are virtually synonomous). The respondents almost invariably pointed to HSPI and its staff as being in the forefront of any action in mental health, and one's own observations confirm this. The case studies reported below do not reveal this HSPI role, but there is an explanation for this seemingly contradictory finding. First of all, this role for HSPI is a rather recent one, beginning before the installation in 1962 of the present director, who, unlike his predecessor, has encouraged community involvement for the institute's staff. Second, the ways in which HSPI exerts influence do not lend themselves to being reported as "case studies."

One has only to recount some of the activities of the institute and its staff which are outside its regular research and training programs to gain an appreciation for its contribution. It provides the psychiatric staff for the county Psychiatric Diagnostic Center and (as does Baylor Medical School) for the psychiatric services available at the city-county charity hospital. HSPI furnishes consultants for the county school superintendent's program of psychological services for school districts, and for the various school districts that provide services beyond what the county superintendent offers. Where relevant to their function, most private social agencies buy a few hours of psychiatric consultation each month, and HSPI is the chief provider. It has developed a training program in cooperation with the Child Guidance Center and is similarly engaged with the Junior League Out-Patient Clinic and Texas Children's Hospital. The outpatient clinic for alcoholics at Methodist Hospital is staffed and served by HSPI. Institute personnel are involved in the management of two small local foundations in the mental health field. The list could be extended even further, but the point is surely clear: the Houston State Psychiatric Institute comes close to omnipresence.

Involvement is not necessarily policy leadership, and the institute staff would probably be the first to admit that they have not been able to move many mountains. The institute is undoubtedly handicapped in trying to play any kind of leadership role by its status as an administrative unit of a state agency, particularly when the state office has at times been less than enthusiastic about community involvement. It is no doubt limited as well by the fact that it is a relatively new institution, still occupied with a host of internal administrative and organizational problems. And, of course, there is the intractability of the community and its institutions. One cannot honestly state that the Psychiatric Institute has been a highly successful leader in mental health, although it does overshadow all others.

The secondary leadership sources seem to fall into three main categories. One of these is the civic-minded lay leaders. Although they have often been pioneers in the mental health field, they have not as a general rule attempted any leadership of the entire mental health community. Rather, they have channeled their energies where mental health is concerned into the affairs of one or two agencies, where their contributions are often considerable. While they include some of the finest members of the Houston aristocracy, they have not demonstrated much capacity to mobilize that class, just as they have not been able to lead on a broad mental health front.

Another type of secondary leadership comes from a small number of professional persons. This type obviously overlaps with HSPI, but it includes others as well. Some are affiliated with the VA Hospital or other institutions, but many are engaged primarily or wholly in private practice. Even among those in this category who are connected with institutions, leadership has been an individual matter rather than an institutional one. In their efforts these persons have often been limited by their relative youth and inexperience and by the demands made upon them professionally, so that their overall contribution has been less than might have been expected.

The final type of secondary leadership for the Houston mental health community might be termed "external." It would include such diverse sources as the Hogg Foundation, the U.S. Public Health Service, the Ford Foundation, and the Department of Labor. By encouraging the community to look at certain needs and problems, and often by providing financial assistance, external leadership has made itself felt with increasing effectiveness in recent years. Indeed, these external authorities are, next to HSPI, currently providing the most important leadership for Houston, particularly if one judges by the stimulation of interest and beginning action on unmet needs.

In concluding this discussion of leadership sources, three points perhaps need to be stated. First, it will be noted that the list does not include a category composed of public officials, either state or local. This is perhaps unfair to the one public official who has displayed a real interest in mental health (County Judge Bill Elliott). Unfortunately, his politics have not endeared him to other county leaders or to the business community and consequently he has not always been very effective. In any case, one exception does not justify a category and no public official was found, with this exception, who has attempted to lead in the mental health field.

Second, there is a conspicuous lack of leadership from professional organizations. None of them, including the local psychiatric society, or the psychological association, or the nursing association, has played much of a role.

Third, inherent in what has been said to this point is the suggestion that a major transformation has been occurring in leadership patterns. It appears that individual leadership, whether from civic-minded lay persons or from professionals, is declining in relative importance. What is emerging is a period of institutionalized leadership. Conceivably this is connected with broader patterns in American society, although it could just as easily be a local manifestation, confined to the mental health field.

It might be worthwhile to try to illustrate these generalizations with case studies of local decision making, although it must be emphasized that they do not rest on such evidence alone. The cases selected involve relatively minor decisions, for the obvious reason that no major ones have been made in Houston in recent years. It hardly needs to be said therefore that a different pattern might emerge if and when larger decisions are made. Furthermore, these cases shed no direct light on the forces that operate to keep major decisions from coming before the community. And, of course, one can never be sure of the extent to which cases chosen in this fashion are typical, though there certainly was no conscious bias in their selection. Despite these limitations, the brief studies presented below should contribute to an understanding of the decision-making process in the Houston metropolitan area insofar as mental health is concerned.

The Contract with the Board of State Hospitals and Special Schools for the Treatment for Indigent Patients at Ben Taub Hospital. It will be recalled that the city-county charity hospital (Ben Taub Hospital) operated a twenty-seven-bed psychiatric ward and an outpatient clinic. Before 1966, the financial condition of the hospital steadily worsened, and the unwillingness of either the city or the county to increase support, plus the failure to secure the voters' approval of a hospital district, led to a desperate search for additional funds.

At one point there was some consideration of abandoning altogether the psychiatric services at Ben Taub. Before any such action got underway, however, the mayor of Houston decided to seek financial help from the state for psychiatric and tuberculosis services, hoping to persuade it to meet its existing constitutional and legal responsibilities for these services. Under the mayor's leadership, a delegation consisting of the mayor, the county commissioner, who serves as "liaison man" for the hospital, the administrator of Ben Taub Hospital, and the chairman of the Ben Taub Hospital board visited Governor John Connally in Austin in mid-April 1965 to seek help. The governor pointed to the contractual arrangements by which the Board of Hospitals and Special Schools has been paying for locally provided mental health services in El Paso, Lubbock, and Beaumont for indigent patients otherwise destined for the state hospitals. (One can ask why the Houston authorities needed the governor to tell them of a state program that was generally familiar to those in the mental health field in Houston.) It appears that the governor did not intervene with the Board of Hospitals and Special Schools on behalf of the Houston group, but when they took their request to that board they obtained approval of a contract providing $85,-000 for the three months of June, July, and August. (The Board for State Hospitals and Special Schools, it will be recalled, was to go out of existence at the end of that period.) It has been impossible to ascertain with certainty the role of two persons associated with the state board. One is the chairman, who happens to be a fairly prominent Houstonian, and the other is a Houston psychiatrist who had been serving for several months as assistant director of mental health and hospitals. One of the principal figures in the board approval was apparently the director of mental health and hospitals, Dr. Ruilman.

All indications are that the entire matter was developed by the public officials involved, with the mayor playing the leading role. The psychiatrist who heads the hospital's psychiatric ward was not party to the negotiations and was acquainted with it only after it was an accomplished fact. Similarly, the Houston Psychiatric Society and the Mental Health Committee of the Harris County Medical Society were not kept informed of developments, possibly because the entire matter developed very rapidly and time apparently did not permit consultation with all interested parties and groups. One of the four persons involved in the contract negotiations stressed that under normal conditions all of the relevant groups would have been consulted.

While one should not underestimate the importance of finding a means of getting a potential quarter of a million dollars annually from the state for psychiatric services at Ben Taub, it is entirely possible that this will do little to change the level of services available. The local money that previously supported the inpatient and outpatient services may simply be diverted to nonmental health needs of the hospital. In that case the chief consequence will have been to change the method of financing essentially the same services previously offered.

The Establishment of Southmore House. Southmore House was established in 1964 as a half-way house for narcotics addicts on leave from the USPHS Hospital at Fort Worth and on parole from state and federal correctional institutions. The idea of such a house for Houston originated with the director of vocational counseling and training at the Fort Worth Hospital, who was greatly concerned with the high rate of recidivism at the hospital. That official sought out someone in the Houston area who would be willing to undertake the establishment and operation of a half-way house, and who was qualified to design a proposal to get the federal funds available for research-demonstration projects of this sort. The executive director of the Houston Vocational Guidance Service (a United Fund agency) was approached and subsequently agreed to play such a role.

Not much information is available on the first step, which was to persuade the Vocational Guidance Service Board to agree to organize a half-way house under its auspices. After considerable soul-searching as to whether or not this was a proper function, and after a local survey which showed that community agencies by and large refused to try to work with narcotics cases, the VGS Board agreed to sponsor the project.

The next step was to enlist the support of the numerous officials and agencies in the area whose cooperation would be essential to the success of the project. Contact was made with every relevant agency, including the narcotics division of the local police department, the local office of vocational rehabilitation of the Texas Education Agency, the Houston State Psychiatric Institute, one of whose staff members was deeply involved in designing the project, the local office of the Texas Employment Commission, the county judge, the county adult probation department, the YMCA, the state Board of Pardons and Paroles, and so on. The Harris County Medical Society and its Mental Health Committee were also consulted. A great deal of effort went into enlisting the support of these agencies, not only by expounding the merits of the project but also by putting a representative of each one on the agency's board. All of them pledged support. While there were one or two instances in which the agency's pledge was interpreted rather narrowly when the time came to honor it, no one withdrew support once the project got underway, and generally the agencies' responses were quite favorable.

It took more than a year to get the project organized and approved, the principal delay being caused by the problem of raising the local share, which was 15 per cent of the total; the remainder came from an HEW grant. The United Fund was not even approached in search of financial assistance. Eventually the necessary funds were raised from certain wealthy individuals and from foundations.

It seems clear that the two principal figures in the establishment of Southmore House were the Public Health Service official at the Fort Worth Hospital who inspired action and who worked in Washington to ensure the HEW grant, and the executive director of the Vocational Guidance Service, who personally developed the local organization and support. While the Board of the Vocational Guidance Service could have refused to allow the project under its auspices, it is doubtful that its disapproval would have blocked action. Some other springboard could no doubt have been found. The cooperation of the related agencies was essential, of course, but since the number of persons involved in the project would never be large, no major commitment of resources was required of any one of them. It is worth noting that the Community Council was not drawn into planning and organizing the project, although it undoubtedly was informed of it. The director of the Vocational Guidance Service was the principal organizing force and assumed full responsibility for obtaining agencies' cooperation, although members of his board also helped in this respect.

Once the project was established, it was found necessary for staff members of Southmore House to conduct meetings with personnel in all the cooperating agencies, the police departments, the employment service, and so on, to inform them of the project and what would be needed from them. An initial effort was made to rely on agency heads and executive personnel to communicate this information to their subordinates, but it was soon found that intra-agency communications were so poor that it was necessary for Southmore House to deal directly with personnel in the agencies who would be involved in working with the House residents in order to ensure their familiarity with what was expected of them.

The Suicide Prevention Center. In January 1964 a psychologist who was not a member of the Houston Psychological Association and did not possess the Ph.D. persuaded the Full Gospel Men's Association and the Junior Chamber of Commerce to support a Suicide Prevention Center. In the initial stages, two psychiatrists were also associated with the project. When the center came to the attention of the Harris County Medical Society, it asked its recently established Mental Health Committee to examine the proposal. The committee did so and, primarily on the basis of the involvement of the two psychiatrists, recommended to the Medical Society that it endorse and participate in the project. The Medical Society endorsed the center but declined to participate. The two psychiatrists took this as a rebuke and withdrew from the project.

In the meantime, the Harris County Psychological Association had become concerned with the center, and particularly with the qualifications of the psychologist who was involved and who became the dominant figure after the withdrawal of the two psychiatrists. The question apparently came before the Liaison Committee, which had been organized in 1958 or 1959, with representatives from psychiatry, psychology, and social work. The committee, which is particularly interested in questions of professional ethics and conduct having interdisciplinary aspects, was instrumental in having the matter brought once again to the Medical Society and referred to its Mental Health Committee. When it was discovered that the project was essentially a lay operation, with no medical or professional direction, the Mental Health Committee recommended that the Medical Society withdraw its endorsement. This was done, and soon the two lay groups helping to support the center terminated their support. The center closed shortly thereafter.

DECISION MAKING AT THE STATE LEVEL

It should be amply clear by this time that the most important decision making in mental health has involved the state rather than the local community. Even so, as seen earlier, the state has been a poor provider of mental health services, although its record with respect to a number of other social services may be no better. Mental health problems and issues simply have not been of great importance in Texas politics.

It seems advisable to conceive of decisions at the state level as the product of four sets of interacting forces, the first and most important of which is the state legislature. Power in both houses tends to center around the presiding officers. They are, of course, neither omnipotent nor omnipresent, and hence a certain amount of influence devolves upon their respective lieutenants, upon committee chairmen, and upon certain individuals set apart by their legislative prowess or bloc leadership. Second only to the presiding officers are the persons who dominate the appropriations process, the chairmen of the appropriations committees and their ranking members. Indeed, so many major decisions have been made in recent years by the conference committees for appropriations that even the presiding officers have looked askance at them.

There are two formal devices for tying some of the top legislative leaders together. One is the Legislative Council; the other is the Legislative Budget Board. Both are composed of the lieutenant governor and the speaker plus several appointees from each house. The Budget Board is especially influential, since the legislators have generally shown more affinity for the legislative budget than for the one prepared by the governor's office, and since the chairmen of the committees handling appropriations and revenue and taxation must be included among the members.

Although mental health policy has not been a major issue in the Texas legislature, several decisions important to that field have been made in the past twenty years or so. These include two far-reaching reorganization acts, one in 1949 and one in 1965, a complete revision of the mental health code in 1957, and the establishment of the Houston State Psychiatric Institute the same year. To a considerable extent the role of the legislature in such decisions has been its traditional one of mediating between conflicting interests and views originating outside the legislature. The alternatives are thus developed externally, and the legislature chooses and compromises among them.

There are several reasons why it is hard for the Texas legislature to rise above that method of operation, some of them inherent in representative assemblies, some of them shaped by the Texas system. Among the latter would have to be included rapid turnover of members, particularly in the House, and the lack of adequate staff services for committees and for individual members. In spite of such handicaps, some of the most important leadership in mental health programing at the state level has come from within the legislative branch. Legislatively inspired search for new approaches, encouragement and pressure for innovation, and guidance in the legislative process have been particularly noteworthy in certain instances.

The element of uniqueness in each situation makes it difficult to generalize about the contributions made by various elements to mental health policy making. It appears that the chairmen of the standing committees involved are seldom active in identifying problems or devising solutions. But, though they are inclined to wait for proposals and counterproposals to be brought to them and their committees, they typically are in the vanguard of efforts to work out a viable measure. They are valuable as well from the standpoint of rounding up votes, perfecting strategy, and generally shepherding the measure through the legislative maze. Still, though it would be difficult to pass a measure without their cooperation, the committee chairmen do not stand out as leaders in mental health policy making.

The same point can be made even more emphatically where the

presiding officers are concerned. It is essential not to incur their disapproval, since each has a very considerable veto power, but there is little to suggest any direct and important role for them in mental health decision making. There are too many other policy areas of greater concern.

Both the Legislative Council and the Legislative Budget Board have been variously involved in mental health efforts. The council did considerable spadework in connection with the 1957 Mental Health Code, although the Budget Board and its staff, particularly the director, were more influential. There was no attempt to plumb the interaction of the board, the executive director whom it appoints, and the staff which he directs, nor to ascertain the sources of their motivation for the improvement of mental health policy making. It may be significant that such leadership has been provided by those within the legislative branch who are most intimately acquainted with state agencies and their programs. If so, the nude and screaming women observed by a budget examiner in the mid-1950s in one state mental hospital and the patient sleeping on the floor in another may have contributed more than is realized to the development of leadership in the mental health field.

The second of the four principal forces involved in policy making at the state level is the governor. The Texas governorship is considered to be a weak office, weaker than the chief executive in any of the other most populous states and in some of the less populous as well. His powers are at their lowest in executive and administrative functions, for there are more than 130 separate and independent agencies and the governor has no formal control over any of them. His chief source of administrative influence arises from his power to appoint most of the agency boards, but the extensive use of six-year staggered terms, and the lack of any removal power, limit the value of appointments. Persuasion, then, is likely to be his chief administrative technique.

But considerable influence can still be wielded, particularly when coupled with the governor's legislative and political power. The governor benefits from his role as party leader and as the dominant political figure in the state, but his greatest opportunities—and greatest pitfalls— lie in his relations with the legislature. A governor who is skilled in the use of his constitutional weapons, notably the veto power and the appointive power, and who further knows how to turn his political position to good advantage, may be able to exert great influence on policy questions. As might be expected, the record of governors in dealing with the legislature varies considerably.

What force have governors customarily exerted, administratively, politically, legislatively, with respect to mental health? The record suggests that they have provided very little positive leadership. Significant developments within the administrative agencies concerned seem to owe little if anything to the governor or his staff, although it must be remembered that this administrative position would not in any case facilitate such efforts. No Texas governor has carried the fight for better mental health services to the public in the same way that issues of education or water resources or tourist development have been carried. No governor has cared for a major confrontation with the legislature on the question of mental health services, although Governor Allan Shivers came close in 1951 when a special session of the legislature was pushed to provide funds for capital improvements in the state mental hospitals.

Nevertheless, the governor is a key figure in the decision-making process. Although his office has seldom been the initiator or promoter of proposals for better mental health services, it has not blocked the efforts of others, and indeed at times it has provided important assistance in getting legislative action. If one imagines the spectrum of interest to run from bitter opposition to avid support of improved services, then Texas governors would have to be located in the middle.

The third set of forces to be considered in decision making at the state level involves the administrative agencies. There are several reasons why agencies are generally considered not to be of great importance. Perhaps the principal reason is the paralyzing concern with the legislature, for it is to that branch rather than the weak chief executive that administrators look for approval and guidance. The volatile and unpredictable nature of legislative politics often leads administrators to play safe by doing nothing to disturb the status quo. Too, the agencies suffer from the extensive use of part-time boards and commissions. While actual administrative power often gravitates to the executive directors appointed by these plural executives, the necessity of board approval of policy and program changes divides responsibility and provides sometimes a real bar to leadership, and sometimes an excuse for inaction. Finally, both upper and lower reaches of the state bureaucracy suffer from a lack of administrative vitality and quality traceable to the state's antiquated personnel policies, poor pay, lack of a merit system, and so on.

These generalizations about state administrative agencies apply mostly to those involved in providing mental health services. The Board for State Hospitals and Special Schools, which administered the state mental hospital program as well as the special schools for the mentally retarded, overshadowed all others at the state level in the field of mental health. No major changes in program have come about although there were some modest steps, most notably the development of outpatient clinics connected with the hospital system, and the contractual arrangement with local governments in a few areas to provide treatment in those communities for patients who otherwise would have been sent to the state hospitals. The available evidence suggests strongly that this leadership in innovation stemmed from the administrators rather than from the board members although certain individuals on that board undoubtedly encouraged such steps. It might be noted also that the agency enjoyed the support and encouragement of the legislative leaders in this period, partly because of the high esteem in which the executive director was held by key figures in the legislature.

Even this modest kind of leadership has been absent from other administrative agencies. For example, the Texas Education Agency was an innocent bystander to the efforts to produce the program of pilot classes for emotionally disturbed children which it was assigned to administer. The Welfare Department has avoided any involvement in mental health issues. The Division of Mental Health in the Health Department had no innovative record of which to boast and was so devoid of influence that no state funds were available for its operation. The Commission on Alcoholism has drifted along for years. The Texas Youth Council has been aggressive and effective in seeking support for its general functions, but not so much in connection with its mental health services.

The fourth set of forces to be considered as part of the decisional process in Austin is made up of interest groups; there is some reason to suppose that they may be more influential in Texas than in some states. The incoherence of the party system, the high cost of political campaigns in such a large state, the weakness of the chief executive, all seem to open unusual opportunities for group influence. Additional influence comes from the fact that the more conservative groups have come to play an unusually important role in the politics of the conservative faction of the Democratic Party, which has effectively controlled state government for many years.

In assessing the impact of groups on decision making in mental health, mention must be made of the negative influence of the powerful conservative groups such as the Texas Manufacturers' Association, the Chamber of Commerce, oil and gas companies, utilities, contractors, banks, and so on. There is no discernible opposition to mental health services as such, simply a concern to limit state undertakings, whether in education, or welfare, or mental health. This concern is rooted partly in ideological opposition to the expansion of what might loosely be called "the Welfare state," and partly in practical concern to hold down state expenditures and the taxes necessary to pay for them. Interestingly enough, mental retardation programs have benefited considerably from the support of certain lobbyists and other persons with important group connections, apparently due to their own personal concerns.

What of the ultra-conservative groups which the state has a reputation for harboring? The distaste of such groups as the John Birch Society for mental health programs is clearly evident to anyone who has even cursorily examined their literature. It is known that they have had considerable impact in local communities in opposing such activities as fund raising for the Mental Health Association, the use of counselors in public schools, and psychological testing programs. However, no evidence was uncovered of the ultra-conservative groups' having been involved or influential in any state-level decisions. There was some concern about their potential for unpleasantness, a concern strong enough to produce greater caution and to influence strategy in minor ways.

There is no doubt that the Texas Medical Association with its Mental Health Committee is the most important of all groups directly concerned with mental health. Since its role unfolds fully in the case studies reported below, not a great deal needs to be said at this point except to note that the influence of the Texas Medical Association is greatest when it is attempting to block or to modify action. To get positive action is far more difficult for the association. Although there was a clear consensus among those interviewed on the importance of the medics, it was surprising how much resentment of them was uncovered among others in the policy process—conservatives as well as liberals.

The impression should not be given that the Medical Association is the only voice of the profession. There is a state psychiatric society, but it is weak and impotent, except when its own leadership is a part of the Medical Association leadership. There is at least one subgroup of psychiatrists, however, who do carry weight—the faculty in the medical schools, and particularly the heads of the psychiatry departments. Some of the nonmedical administrators and the legislators evidently appreciate the medical educators a great deal, partially because they are often at odds with the official position of the Medical Association.

What of the other professional groups, the psychologists and social workers? Although both have state organizations, neither has a paid staff at the state level. Their influence is apt to be minimal and exercised through indirect means. The impotence of the psychologists is in part related to the absence of a professional licensing law. Since the Texas Medical Association has been responsible for blocking attempts to get such legislation, there is an understandable coolness between certain elements in the two groups.

The Hogg Foundation must be mentioned in any consideration of mental health groups. It is in some ways a hybrid creature, a privately supported foundation that is legally and administratively a part of the University of Texas. In the past the Hogg Foundation has oriented itself largely toward broadly defined research in mental health areas. A recent change in policy has turned the foundation more in the direction of action programs, in the form of pilot-demonstration projects with built-in evaluation features. As a chief source of research support within the state, the Hogg Foundation naturally developed good ties with the psychiatrists, psychologists, and social workers, particularly those in the field of education but also those involved in state and community programs. As a part of the University of Texas, the foundation is prohibited from any lobbying activity, but it is doubtful that this constitutes any real handicap, since its activities behind the scene involve it very much in the policy-making process. The Hogg Foundation and its long-time director, Robert Sutherland, are generally regarded as very influential, although not as much so as the Medical Association.

By contrast, the Texas Association for Mental Health is viewed as a group with little influence. This may be an unduly pessimistic view, but the association did not commit itself officially to lobbying activities until 1963. Prior to that time its chief role had been as a service organization, raising funds for special projects, doing referrals, publishing and distributing materials, and the like. As such, the association worked closely with most, but not all, agencies related to mental health. Indeed, at times the association functioned as an outlet for views which could not be expressed officially by the state agencies themselves. It seems likely that a limited amount of influence was acquired thereby. For example, the association apparently played a crucial role in obtaining the necessary legislation for the six pilot classes for emotionally disturbed children set up in 1963, and in funding that program. In view of the fact that it has had guidance from the Hogg Foundation and some of its leaders are prominent lay persons, the association would seem to possess at least an intermediate policy role. And yet, respondents in the administrative agencies and in the legislature generally regarded the TAMH as a weak organization, as much a front for the state hospitals as anything else.

While it is very desirable to illustrate and supplement these generalizations about decision making at the state level with case studies, there is no denying the shortage of recent decisions of a magnitude to make them useful. It appears best to report briefly what is known of certain events in 1956–1957, and then to concentrate on the origins, formation, and functioning of the state Mental Health Planning Committee and on the passage of the 1965 act reorganizing mental health services.

The 1957 Decision against Bricks. When the budget requests for the 1957 session of the legislature came in from the Board of Hospitals and Special Schools, a major item was funds for building a large state hospital in the Houston area. The Legislative Budget Board's reaction was that too much emphasis had been put on bricks and not enough on treatment and restoration. On the advice of the lieutenant governor, chairman of the Budget Board, presiding officer of the state Senate, and a man with close ties to powerful groups in Austin, the Budget Board approached the Texas Medical Association "hat in hand," asking it to sponsor an objective study of state mental health services. The association was cooperative. Some difficulty was encountered in funding the study, but the necessary money was finally obtained from a prominent south Texas businessman, H. E. Butt, and Dr. Francis Joseph Gerty was brought in from Illinois to conduct the study. Although Gerty's report did recommend a small hospital in the Houston area, it was largely oriented to community-based care and to research needs. At about the same time, the American Neurological Society conducted a study of the Austin State Hospital, which pointed out some glaring deficiencies.

When the legislature convened in January 1957 the Budget Board arranged for a plane to fly key figures to Michigan for a week to study some valuable but expensive work being done at a clinic there. The attempt was to convince the legislators that high daily cost of patient care could be good economy in the long run. It evidently succeeded, for the decision was soon made to reject the building program of the Hospital Board and to turn funds instead into hospital staff and research.

What was described as a "knock-down, drag-out" battle was fought with the Hospital Board on this issue, but, armed as it was with Gerty's report, the Neurological Society's study, and the evidence accumulated on the Michigan trip, the Budget Board won its case. The major result was that the legislature authorized the establishment of the Houston State Psychiatric Institute rather than another mental hospital. There were also top-level administrative changes soon after in the hospitals and special schools, which weakened the previous emphasis on custodial care. The pattern of limited administrative innovation in mental health service in the Department of State Hospitals and Special Schools began subsequent to this. Looking back, those who were involved feel that the state turned an important corner in 1957 in the handling of mental health programs.

The Origins of the Mental Health Planning Committee in Texas. As clearly as can be determined, two unrelated processes represent the ultimate roots of the mental health planning effort in Texas. Even before Congress had completed action on the 1963 Mental Health Centers Act, the AMA Mental Health Congress in October 1962 had asked the Texas Medical Association, the Texas Neurological Association, and the Texas Association for Mental Health each to get five of their best people together on the subject of mental health planning. The group of about fifteen persons was asked to begin making preparations for a plan with respect to mental health services in Texas.

Apparently on their own initiative, and independent of this group, the staff of the Division of Mental Health in the state Health Department had begun preparing a planning grant application even before final action was taken by the United States Congress. The two lines of action converged when Commissioner Peavey turned to his Mental Health Division for assistance with his role in the AMA-related group. A planning grant application was submitted to NIMH. There is no indication that any state agencies with mental health responsibilities except the Health Department and the Department of State Hospitals and Special Schools were involved in the preparation and submission. More importantly, the proposal was taken to the Texas Medical Association, where it was approved only after vigorous discussion.

The Formation of the Mental Health Planning Committee. The plan submitted to and approved by NIMH called for a four-member executive committee, a seventeen-member steering committee, and a hundred or so members of the general planning committee. The membership of both the steering committee and the executive committee was determined by what had already taken place. Commissioner Peavey was designated as chairman of the executive committee, Dr. Ruilman as cochairman, with Sutherland and west Texas County Judge C. L. Abernethy as the other two members. The steering committee was composed of seventeen persons, including the members of the executive committee. An effort was made to persuade both the speaker of the house and the lieutenant governor to serve on the steering committee, but both refused.

An early analysis set forth the principal questions to be dealt with by the general Planning Committee, and it was decided to organize the general committee into task forces, each of which would be grappling with one of these broad questions. The selection of personnel for the Planning Committee became then primarily a matter of finding persons who could contribute to the work of a given task force.

The reservoir from which these persons were chosen was a file of some three to four hundred names obtained from members of the executive committee, the steering committee, and interested groups and organizations. The staff of the Division of Mental Health worked up a basic fact sheet on each—geographical area, standing in community, offices held, reasons for inclusion, and so on. The executive committee and Dr. Spencer Bayles, who became the first coordinator for the Planning Committee, then attempted to match task force needs with the available personnel. The formal invitation to serve on the general committee went out over the signatures of Drs. Peavey and Ruilman, and there was as well a cover letter from Governor Connally, obtained only with difficulty at the last moment. The rate of acceptance was good, with only about 10 per cent of those invited refusing to serve, but among the refusals were several conservative political and community leaders who could have helped the committee a great deal. The general committee eventually numbered 110 persons, in addition to the 17 on the steering committee.

Although the executive committee had been advised by the director of the Legislative Budget Board to pick experts on mental health, "idea men," and politicians, the process by which names were obtained and the conception of the task forces as problem-solving groups led to a heavy emphasis on mental health experts. Almost 60 per cent of the 127 Planning Committee members were professionals.

Broken down in another fashion, the list reveals that there were at least 45 state officials and employees and 38 persons connected with educational and research institutions. No more than 6 of the 38 physicians lacked institutional affiliations, and no more than 20 of the total of 127 members were totally without professional or institutional connections. A look at the 16 Houstonians on the committee lends emphasis to the point. There were 7 physicians (including the chairman of the state Board of Health, and the director of HSPI), 2 psychologists, 2 social workers, 1 hospital administrator, 1 architect, the county judge who handles legal commitments to the state hospitals, the publisher of one of the city's two principal newspapers, and 1 businessman. Only the last three or four could be said to be representatives of the general community rather than the field of mental health. Due to the large number of state officials and employees, there was disproportionate representation from Austin, but otherwise there was probably as broad a geographical distribution as could be effected, given the emphasis on mental health professionals.

Two aspects of this process are worth singling out for comment. First, the Health Department played the leading role, despite its very minor responsibilities in the state mental health programs. The reason, of course, is that the commissioner of health, as the mental health authority for federal purposes, received the planning grant. Too, the staff of the Division of Mental Health in the Health Department staked a claim to a role by its early involvement, and in any case it constituted the only available source of staff services in the early stages of the planning endeavor. Second, the political leadership of the state was not drawn into the formation of the Planning Committee, except indirectly through the director of the Legislative Budget Board staff and the governor's budget director. As seen above, the speaker of the House and the lieutenant governor declined to serve. An effort was made to draw in several influential businessmen, including a west Texas publisher and an east Texas industrialist, but they too refused. The governor's budget director was pressed to obtain names from Governor Connally, but he presented only one or two. A deliberate decision was made at an early point not to ask the governor to appoint the entire Planning Committee. The principal reason given was the apparent lack of interest on the part of the governor. It would serve no useful purpose here to attempt to fix responsibility for the failure to interest the state's most important officials in this new approach to mental health services, but there is no doubt that their disinterest added to the committee's problems.

The Functioning of the Mental Health Planning Committee. Although a general evaluation of the state Mental Health Planning Committee is not in order here, it is possible to discuss several aspects of its functioning that help to illuminate the process of mental health programing at the state level.

There were, first of all, problems of leadership and of staff work. Particularly in the early and intermediate phases of the committee's work, Drs. Peavey and Ruilman, the two state officials most directly affected, were not able or willing to provide much leadership. The first psychiatrist-coordinator, Dr. Spencer Bayles, was commuting on a part-time basis from his Houston practice. The members of the general Planning Committee were interested in their work and turned out in surprising number, but a perusal of the minutes of their task force meetings reveals an aimlessness and a lack of focused discussion. The structure of the committee added to the leadership problem. In the design stage there was an attempt to get the steering committee members designated as task force committee chairmen, but they refused to agree to this. Each task force was instead left free to choose its own chairman at its first meeting. This also posed problems of another sort, for the task force chairmen were concerned that they and the committee members were simply window dressing, and that the steering committee was going to write the final plan on its own. This suspicion was only partly allayed by inviting all task force committee chairmen to the meetings of the steering committees.

The drift of the work sessions may also be related to weaknesses in the utilization of staff. The Planning Committee staff on the whole did an excellent job of marshaling data, but this was not digested or synthesized before being distributed to committee members. The result was a mass of data that few knew what to do with and even fewer read in entirety. Too great an analytic and interpretive load was put on the general committee members.

The problems of leadership were compounded at a critical point by the departure of Dr. Bayles from the post of psychiatrist-coordinator as a result of his having become involved in a political conflict with an influential legislator who had good connections with the Texas Medical Association, the speaker of the house, and the governor. The executive committee was given to understand that Bayles had to go or the project was dead. Drs. Peavey and Ruilman at once took the lead in having him replaced by Dr. Moody Bettis, who had only recently been appointed professor of community psychiatry at the Houston State Psychiatric Institute. Coming as it did only a few months before the plan was to be completed, the change undoubtedly created problems. It also altered the leadership stituation, because both Peavey and Ruilman came to play a greater role in the work of the Planning Committee. The latter's involvement brought the mental hospital people into the forefront of what had been mostly a Health Department undertaking until that time.

Another illuminating aspect of the Planning Committee effort came shortly after the turnover in the office of psychiatrist-coordinator. Drs. Peavey and Ruilman apparently then effected an agreement on legislation relative to administrative organization of mental health services, stipulating that the Health Department would give up its Division of Mental Health and any claims to mental health jurisdiction to the Board of Hospitals and Special Schools, or its successor. The board in turn would cede to the Health Department the tuberculosis hospitals for which it had responsibility. Very little is known about the way in which the trade was arranged. Obviously the two administrators had to be sure that their respective boards would agree, and no doubt there was consultation with an eye to the likelihood of getting the necessary legislation. The whole question of tuberculosis control and treatment was under consideration by a separate group concerned about the then existing fragmentation in tuberculosis programs. Case finding was vested in the Health Department, hospital care was handled by the state hospitals, and aftercare was back in the hands of the Health Department.

Thus, the transfer made a great deal of sense from the standpoint of administrative rationalization of both tuberculosis and mental health services. It did mean that the Planning Committee was in effect committed to a course of action that otherwise might not have been recommended. It also meant that any program of community mental health services would be administered by the same people responsible for the state mental hospitals. The suspicion in some quarters that state mental hospitals would not look favorably on a program to decentralize mental health services inevitably raised doubts and questions.

A third and perhaps the most revealing development involved the Planning Committee's proposals for administrative structure. At a meeting of the steering committee and the task force chairmen in September 1964, a preliminary decision was made to recommend that the mental health services of the Health Department and the State Hospitals and Special Schools Department be transferred to a new department to be called the Department of Mental Health. A nine-member board would be created, with no designation of membership categories—the feeling was very strong against a medically dominated board. The reasoning reflected not only the opposition of some members of the Planning Committee to medical domination but also a belief that the legislature would not agree to it. There would also be a commissioner of mental health, who would be chosen by the board and who would have to be a psychiatrist. There would as well be a strong professional advisory board, but membership on it would not be limited to the medical profession alone.

A meeting with the mental health committee of the Texas Medical Association had been scheduled for a week later, and at the steering committee meeting there were some (most notably Drs. Peavey and Ruilman) who felt that it would be a mistake to go to the TMA committee with firm recommendations. They should instead go to consult and to listen. However, with the backing of the psychiatrist-coordinator, Dr. Bettis, the steering committee and task force chairmen decided to lay their recommendations before the TMA committee.

At the subsequent meeting, Dr. Talkington evinced some doubt as to the recommendations from the Planning Committee and said that the TMA committee had decided the night before, apparently on his urging, not to offer any opinion on those recommendations. A member of the TMA committee who was also on the steering committee (and also a member of the Board for State Hospitals and Special Schools) urged a resolution of approval of the Planning Committee's recommendations; he left the meeting thinking a consensus had developed in support of that proposal. However, parliamentary procedure was invoked and the motion was forced to a vote by the members of the TMA committee. With a key man missing, the vote was 3–3; the chairman, Dr. Talkington, cast a negative vote to kill the motion and break the tie. At that point Drs. Ruilman and Peavey indicated to the group their willingness to accept a medically dominated board, which was contrary to the Planning Committee recommendation.

In the days that followed, there was considerable maneuvering and negotiation to get the TMA committee to reverse its stand. The top leadership of the TMA was prevailed upon to lend some indirect support for the Planning Committee position, and influential persons in the field of psychiatry stepped in to effect a compromise. It was finally agreed that the recommendation of the Planning Committee would specify that three of the nine members of the new Mental Health Board would be physicians, at least one of them a psychiatrist. The provision for a psychiatrist as commissioner of mental health was retained. It was recommended as well that a medical committee be established by statute, composed of six psychiatrists, two general practitioners, and one pediatrician. The medical committee would have some significant duties, including selecting three psychiatrists, from among whom the board would appoint the commissioner of mental health. There was also to be created a Mental Health Advisory Council, which would apparently be an interdisciplinary group. Thus there was some gain for the TMA group, but the results stopped short of the medically dominated board they sought.

The Creation of the Texas Department of Mental Health and Mental Retardation. The compromise recommendations of the state Mental Health Planning Committee were embodied in H.R.3 and S.148, identical bills introduced in the Texas legislature in late January 1965 by Representative W. H. Miller of Houston and by Senator Bruce A. Reagan of Corpus Christi. Both were seasoned legislators in good standing with legislative leaders and with a legislative record in the mental health–mental retardation field.

Judging from the internal evidence, these bills were intended as vehicles for further action rather than as finished products. In any case, a number of changes were made once the bills had been considered by the legislative committees to which they were consigned. Some committee amendments reflected the tensions described in the preceding case study between the lay leaders and the Texas Medical Association. In general, the medics were the losers, for committee amendments to the original bill deleted the requirement that three members of the proposed state Mental Health Board had to be physicians and removed the provision for a medical committee to help choose the commissioner of mental health. They also diluted the original provisions for a medical advisory board.

Finally, some committee amendments reflected an entirely new set of concerns: the place of mental retardation programs. The state mental retardation planning effort had been an entirely separate one, and the state Mental Retardation Planning Committee had not completed its work in early 1965. Yet the legislation being considered was of vital importance for the special schools, since they were included in the proposed administrative reorganization. Accordingly, a number of committee amendments reflected the belated entry into the policy sphere of those concerned with mental retardation. The changes made at the committee stage ranged from the relatively inconsequential (but doubtless highly symbolic) one of broadening the name of the new agency (Department of Mental Health and Mental Retardation) to a bifurcation of administrative structure below the level of the commissioner of mental health. The result of the latter was specification of posts of deputy commissioner of mental health and of deputy commissioner for mental retardation—a continuation of the administrative division that had existed in the old agency, although the commissioner of mental health would be in a stronger position than the previous executive director. However, the mental retardation group failed at this stage to win an amendment changing the qualifications for commissioner of mental health so as to permit the appointment of a nonmedic with "proven administrative experience and ability." Because of a particular person as well as because of a principle, the group continued this fight at later stages.

In the committee stage of consideration there had been close cooperation between the House and the Senate committees, so much so that they reported identical committee substitutes for the original bills. The decision was made to "run" with the bill in the House first, and on March 4 it was brought to the floor for a second reading. An amendment to the committee substitute was offered by a veteran legislator (Gene N. Fondren) with ties to the House leadership. He upheld the mental retardation groups by moving to change the qualifications of the commissioner of mental health in order to allow a nonmedic to be appointed. Over the strong objections of Representative Miller, the bill's manager, the Fondren amendment was adopted after motion to table failed by a 91–45 vote.

On March 10, H.R.3 came up for its third reading and final passage. An amendment, apparently conceived by Miller, was offered by Representative Willis J. Whatley (Houston) that created a third deputy commissioner's post for research and training and deleted the requirement that the deputy commissioner for mental health had to be a board-certified psychiatrist. After its adoption without difficulty, Representative Bob Eckhardt, a long-time liberal leader from Houston with ties to the more community-oriented psychiatrists there, offered an amendment to undo the Fondren amendment adopted on second reading. Eckhardt had done his work well, and by a vote of 96–44 the House reversed itself and restored the committee's specification that the commissioner of mental health had to be a physician. Thus amended, the bill passed the House 139–1 and was sent to the Senate.

There H.R.3 was referred routinely to the Committee on State Affairs on March 15. Since the committee had previously considered an identical Senate bill, it was able to recommend on the following day passage of H.R.3, which was then set for floor action on March 17 by unanimous consent. When it was taken up, the fight over the qualifications of the commissioner broke out again, and an amendment to H.R.3 that would allow a nonmedic to occupy the post was beaten by only one vote. The very considerable interest that existed is indicated by the somewhat unusual circumstance that every senator was present and voting on the proposed amendment, which lost 15–16. Senator Reagan, the Senate leader for the bill, then won quick acceptance of an amendment restoring the original committee specification that the deputy commissioner of mental health had to be a board-certified psychiatrist. The measure was then given its third reading, passed, and returned to the House for action that would reconcile the slightly different versions that had been passed.

Representative Miller, the House manager of H.R.3, was willing to accept the Senate changes, but before he could get floor action the chairman of the House Appropriations Committee, who had not previously been involved, unexpectedly intervened to demand that the House refuse the Senate changes and hence force the bill to a conference committee, his apparent concern being to delete the medical requirement for the commissioners. A round of conferences and negotiations that involved those in the forefront of the mental health planning effort, those in the mental retardation field, and officials who were leaders in the legislative process (including the speaker of the house and the governor—or rather his emissary) finally produced a compromise. The chairman of the House Appropriations Committee would not force the bill to conference if a new bill were introduced to provide for an executive director who would be the second-ranking official in the agency. On that basis it was possible for the House to accept the Senate's changes, and the bill went to the governor, who signed it into law. (The amendatory legislation that figured in the compromise was never passed.)

The story does not quite end with the governor's signature on H.R.3, because appropriations for the new department still had to be made. The chairman of the Appropriations Committee evidently had not lost his interest in the agency, for its backers both in and out of the legislature were dismayed to find that the committee had revised the administrative structure below the level of commissioner and deputy commissioners in what they deemed an undesirable fashion. The supporters were also quite concerned by the small amount appropriated for the establishment of community mental health and mental retardation centers. Efforts to persuade the governor to use his item veto power to remedy the first set of disappointments were unsuccessful, and so the new agency came into being with something less than a grand entrance, financially speaking.

What can one say in summary about the leadership process just described? First, it seems clear that there was never any doubt about legislative support in general for an act reorganizing state hospitals and special schools, and authorizing the establishment of community mental health centers. Difficulties arose only (1) when the interested parties—those concerned with mental health and mental retardation, the medical society, the psychiatrists, etc.—were unable to agree among themselves, and (2) when the proposals began to compete with other policies and programs for the available state funds.

Second, despite the fact that most controversy during passage involved essentially minor issues, in comparison with the overall import of the bill, there was almost enough heat generated to destroy it. At critical junctures some of the interested parties talked seriously of abandoning the whole reorganization effort. Other key figures, including the governor, were so displeased by the squabbling among the interested parties that they were ready to wash their hands of the whole matter.

Third, it is noteworthy that individual legislators played significant roles. Although they typically were responding to group requests, their interest and strategic capacities at critical points probably saved H.R.3 from unacceptable mutilation or outright rejection. Fourth, although the public officials who had general leadership responsibilities, such as the governor, the lieutenant governor, and the speaker, were unwilling to commit themselves to one side or another in the particularistic disputes, their tacit and sometimes direct support in principle for the legislation did help to bring about compromise and to ensure final passage.

FINANCING MENTAL HEALTH SERVICES

The financing of mental health services in Houston is difficult to discuss in concrete terms both because of the ill-defined boundaries and because mental health services are often intermingled with other services in budgetary and accounting systems that do not permit their segregation. At the state level, at least, there is no difficulty in identifying the source of funds for mental health services since the state treasury is virtually the exclusive source. While there is considerable earmarking of taxes for specific services in Texas government, there is none for mental health. Instead, all appropriations for mental health are made from the general revenue fund on a biennial basis.

In the past, state appropriations for mental health have not been such as to bolster the state's relative position. Expenditures for state mental hospitals were only 1.53 per cent of all state general expenditures in 1964, ranking Texas thirty-ninth in the nation, and the per capita general expense of the mental hospitals was only $2.52—a ranking of forty-ninth in the nation.[5] It is true that mental hospitals are by no means the only measure of mental health services, although in Texas they are the chief such service, but other indices do not put the state in a better light. Thus, Texas ranked forty-eighth in per capita expenditures for community mental health programs and thirty-seventh in scheduled professional man-hours for psychiatric outpatient clinics in 1964.

No doubt some comfort can be derived from the fact that the appropriations for agencies and programs most directly related to mental health have consistently increased in recent years. Thus, appropriations for mental hospitals increased by 30 per cent from $41.75 million in 1960–1961 to $54.45 million in 1966–1967. The budget for Houston State Psychiatric Institute more than tripled in the same period, and funds for community mental health services (state outpatient clinics, contracts with local agencies, and grants-in-aid to local governmental agencies) increased tenfold.

But such figures can be very misleading. When one begins with a near-zero base, large percentage increases can be purchased rather cheaply. Also, while health's share of the state's dollar has been increasing slightly, from 4.35 per cent in 1960–1961 to 4.6 per cent in 1966–1967, the mental health share has been declining. The appropriations for mental hospitals, the Houston State Psychiatric Institute, and community mental health services represented 41 per cent of the total health expenditures in 1960–1961; by 1966–1967 the appropriation for the same mental health services amounted to only 36 per cent. Mental hospitals, HSPI, and community mental health services represented 1.78 per cent of total state spending in the 1960–1961 biennium; in the 1966–1967 budget, they had declined to 1.66 per cent of all state expenditures. From 1960 to 1966 state expenditures as a whole increased by 50 per cent; expenditures for the mental health services just mentioned increased only 40 per cent.

One aspect of the financial pattern that requires comment is the method of state support for locally provided services. At present, the state operates several outpatient clinics, for which $992,020 was appropriated for the 1966–1967 biennium. It has also been involved in a program of contracting with local agencies and clinics for the pro-

---

[5] Joint Information Service, American Psychiatric Association and National Association for Mental Health, *Fifteen Indices* (Washington: APA, 1966).

vision of mental health services to indigent persons who would otherwise be sent to state hospitals. Effective with fiscal year 1966, there were also funds for grants-in-aid to local governmental agencies organized as community mental health centers. For the 1966–1967 biennium, contract funds and grants-in-aid are budgeted together ($1,350,-000 for the biennium), with the share going to each to be determined by the Board for Mental Health and Retardation.

Three methods of supporting community mental health services have thus evolved: state clinics, state contract payments to local agencies, and grants-in-aid. Each method has different consequences and implications, and some of those who have been in the forefront of the fight for community mental health centers are visibly concerned that the method of contractual payments rather than grants-in-aid will be chiefly relied upon in the future.

When the discussion of financing mental health services is shifted to the local level, one is denied the comfort of statistical data, for the agencies are so diverse and the functions so intermingled that comparable figures are virtually impossible to obtain. But the most important question, after all, is not how much is currently provided by local sources but whether it is possible to provide substantial increments, since it is all but universally admitted that the present level of services in the community is too low.

Three sources of funds characterize support in the private sector. One is patient fees. At present this tends to be an either-or proposition. Either a patient pays most if not all of the costs of his mental health services, or he pays little if any. It is possible that patient fees could be made to support a larger share of the total burden without serious damage to some patients' financial situation and without jeopardizing their relations with the agency. This, at least, was the opinion of one respondent, who cited his own experience with a major service organization in Houston which did successfully expand the proportion of funds coming from patient fees. It is supported by some other fragments of evidence. For example, the Child Guidance Center, a United Fund agency, derives only about 8 to 10 per cent of its total funds from patient fees although its clientele has a median income of $6,000 to $6,500 annually. The problem is in part the traditional bias of social workers against the payment of fees for services of the sort rendered.

Another source in the private sector is what might be called "unorganized" philanthropy to distinguish it from United Fund endeavors. Individuals and foundations have in this fashion made significant contributions to the development of services in the Houston area. It seems unlikely, however, that unorganized philanthropy could do much in the long run to carry program expansions of the sort necessary.

What of the "organized" sector of philanthropy, the United Fund? It is already the primary support for several of the most important mental health agencies in Houston–Harris county, such as the Child Guidance Center, the Family Service Bureau, the Mental Health Association, and numerous other agencies with more limited roles. As a very important source of funds raised in the community, the United Fund naturally figures in discussion of the future.

But among the respondents there was rather general agreement that the United Fund could not possibly be expected to raise significantly greater amounts of money for mental health. Its overall increase each year is very carefully calculated in terms of what is thought feasible, and it seems fair to say that the increase is not proportionate to the expansion of problems. Whether this lag is due to the policy process within the Fund or to the resistance in the community is immaterial in this respect. The total United Fund is not going to expand. It also seems unlikely that there will be a redistribution of the available UF Funds so as to make significantly more available for mental health; the process of allocation all but guarantees that such will not happen.

Consideration of local public support for mental health must begin with a review of the existing patterns. Of the municipalities in Harris county, only Houston has supported mental health services financially. This was done until 1966 through contributions to the operation of Ben Taub Hospital, the city-county charity hospital, with its psychiatric ward and outpatient clinic. Heavy pressure on the Houston budget led to repeated but unsuccessful efforts to persuade the county to provide all of the charity hospital's financing. The solution eventually was a hospital district with its own taxing powers, and thus both the city and county withdrew. The voters were not persuaded to approve the district until recently, and hence there is no way of knowing what this augurs for the psychiatric ward and clinic, but a safe guess would be that they will continue to have low priority in the hospital's budget.

It seems equally likely that the city of Houston will not develop any great budgetary enthusiasm for mental health services. The political climate is largely responsible for this situation. It is true that Houston currently levies property taxes at a rate that could not be increased without a referendum and a favorable vote, but it assesses taxable property at only about 40 per cent of market value. Legally, then, city revenues could be increased by 250 per cent. If some city services are starved—and police, recreation, library, and other services as well as mental health are—it is because the city's officials are unwilling to order the increase in assessments necessary to provide adequate financing. While one should never underestimate the importance of conservative ideology and opposition to the social service state, as well as the reluctance of homeowners to pay additional taxes, it seems very likely that the Houston business community is an especially powerful force for discouraging expanded city services. After all, two-thirds of the city's revenues are derived from the property tax, and a sizable part of Houston's property taxes are derived from business and industry. Approximately 33 per cent of the gross assessed value of real property in Houston, and a much larger proportion of the total assessed value of personal property, are owned by business and industry.

Leaving aside its former contribution to Ben Taub Hospital, the county's role in mental health servicing includes some $317,000 annually to support the county Psychiatric Diagnostic Center and probably not more than $35,000 annually for psychological services administered by the county school superintendent's office. The first is financed from the county's general revenue fund supported by the ad valorem property tax; the county superintendent has an earmarked property tax to rely on. The county is in a different position from the cities with respect to the property tax because it serves as the collection agency for the state property tax as well. Since the same valuation is used for both county and state property taxes, the county commissioners are under great local pressure to keep assessments as low as possible in order to minimize state taxes. There are statutory ceilings for county tax rates, of course, and these plus the political ceiling for assessments operate to keep county expenditures low. Even so, the Harris county tax valuation ratio (20 per cent) is one of the higher ones in the state. Numerous proposals have been made to overcome the handicap imposed by the coupling of state and county tax valuations, but to no avail. Until it becomes possible to increase the county valuation without increasing the state property taxes as well, it will be exceedingly difficult to expand county services in any field, including mental health.

The financial situation at the local level, public and private, can be summed up as follows. While the community undoubtedly has the total resources sufficient to allow a greater investment in mental health, it would be very difficult to expand substantially the present level of community support. State funds would have to provide the backbone for any sizable mental health program. In any federal-state-local financial arrangement, the local share is apt to be about what it presently invests in mental health. In particular, while community mental health centers may be possible in Houston, the necessary local support will be achieved simply by redeploying the funds presently available.

It might be well at this point to explain the basis of this pessimistic view of the situation at the local and state level. Leaving aside general political and social forces such as the prevailing ideological conservatism in Texas and in Houston, there are four salient determinants of the fiscal patterns under consideration. One of these is the tax structure. Although students of public finance have concluded that a broad-based tax such as income or sales tax is essential to allow state and local governments today to meet their emerging responsibilities, not until 1961 did the state of Texas levy a general sales tax. It still has no income tax. At the local level, the principal reliance was on the property tax until a municipal income tax was authorized in 1967. The property tax has not been pressed to its legal limits, for the assessment ratio is invariably well below 100 per cent although tax rates are typically at or near the legal ceiling, but it suffers from the same administrative and economic limitations that caused state governments to seek other sources of revenue. It also suffers from political limitations.

A second determinant is an alleged constitutional limitation that has probably impeded state mental health programs of assistance to local governments. Article 16, Section 54 of the Texas constitution requires the legislature to make provision for the custody and maintenance of "indigent lunatics" at the expense of the state. Article 3, Sections 50 and 51 prohibit the pledging of the state's credit to any person, association, or corporation, including municipal corporations. Another clause of the latter section authorizes a tax levy for pensions for Confederate veterans and their widows, and adds, "The legislature shall have no power to make any grants, or authorize the making of any grant of public moneys to any individual, association of individuals, municipal or other corporations whatsoever."

Doubts raised by these provisions that the state could legally make grants to local governments were not swept away until 1967. At the time the Mental Health Planning Committee completed its work in the summer and fall of 1964, the task force on legislation produced a majority report which interpreted the state constitution to bar state grants-in-aid to local governments. If the state were to support such services, it would have to organize and administer them. The chief architects of that interpretation were an assistant attorney general and the general counsel of the Texas Medical Association. Although a minority report based on the views of a University of Texas law professor was filed that argued that there was no constitutional issue, the majority of the task force carried the day in the general Planning Committee. Hence the recommendation was made in the final plan that a constitutional amendment be submitted to the voters to permit state grants to local governments. This approach was apparently welcomed by the attorney general, who preferred not to render an official opinion in order to avoid antagonizing one side or the other.

But, as it happened, the attorney general's office was required to construe the same constitutional provisions in another case involving an entirely different kind of service. The result was an official opinion that such payments could be made, thus clearing the way for legislation to that effect in the mental health field. Since the attorney general's opinions are not legally binding, there was still the possibility of a judicial action to forestall state grants-in-aid to local governments, and a constitutional amendment was therefore initiated and adopted in 1967 that established the legality of state grants to local governments for mental health services.

Another determinant, closely related to the first, is the competition for available resources. With the exception of the program of the county school superintendent, which is financed by an earmarked tax, all public support, local and state, is drawn from general revenue funds. Given the limited tax funds provided by the tax system just described, it is to be expected that there would be an intense scramble for them. In competition with highways, public schools, and welfare services, mental health is apt to come in a poor second. The reasons are not hard to find. Mental health services do not reach a broad stratum of society, and effective group support has been difficult to mobilize. Furthermore, there has been little effective leadership. This may be partly due to the lack of enthusiasm of the medical profession for mental health programs, and it may also be due to chance and the vagaries of history. Also, there does not seem ot exist among mental health activists the zeal and commitment that would lead to aggressive action.

Lack of zeal is accompanied sometimes by divisions within the mental health ranks. In Houston the psychiatric services at Ben Taub suffer from orientation of the Baylor College of Medicine staff toward teaching rather than service. Hence, no really strong pressure has been exerted to expand and improve mental health services there beyond the level necessary for instruction. Friction between Baylor and the Harris County Medical Society is another contributing factor.

Finally, there is the factor of fragmentation. One can see it most clearly in two aspects. First of all, there is a widespread belief among local mental health leaders, especially those in official positions, that the care of the mentally ill is constitutionally lodged with the state, and the local governments have no responsibility for such services. Second, at the local level the inadequate financing of Ben Taub could until 1966 be traced directly to fragmentation, and mental health suffers from this. At both state and local levels, it seems quite likely that the proliferation of agencies contributes to the difficulties of adequate financing because support is divided, but this is obviously much more difficult to document.

MANPOWER AND STAFFING

The question of improved mental health services is not one of financing alone—there are formidable staffing problems also. Data from the state Mental Health Planning Committee report indicate that some 360 psychiatrists were located in Texas in June 1964. Of these, 117 were in public practice only, with 236 wholly or partially in private practice (no data were available on 8). The ratio of psychiatrists to the state's total population approximates 1:30,000, compared with a national ratio (1961) of 1:18,000. The same source reported 588 psychologists in Texas, of which 67 per cent hold the Ph.D., 9 per cent the Ed.D., 19 per cent the M.A. in psychology, and the remainder some other type of master's degree. Of the total, a little over half had completed an internship, and about three-fifths were professionally connected with some aspect of mental health endeavor. Forty-nine per cent were connected with some university, 20 per cent worked for the federal government, and 10 per cent for state and local governments.

Details on social workers and nurses are much harder to come by. The Office of Mental Health Planning reported about 865 social workers holding master's degrees or national accreditation, but the number with psychiatric specialization or otherwise involved in mental health is unknown. Of the 30,000 nurses in Texas, it was estimated that only 400 were engaged solely in mental health work, but obviously many others—particularly those in hospitals—are sometimes engaged with psychiatric patients. Nursing care in mental health undoubtedly suffers from the unfavorable ratio of nurses to the population: 170:100,000, compared with a national ratio of 286:100,000 and a recommended ratio of 350:100,000.

While it is difficult to be precise in stating the extent to which present manpower supplies are inadequate, the preceding figures, the difficulty in filling existing positions reported by both state and local agencies, and the respondents' remarks testify to serious inadequacies. The report of the Mental Health Planning Committee carries the same testimony. Since there is not enough staff available for present services, the expansion called for by the concept of mental health centers would obviously make staffing the major problem. For example, the state Planning Committee recommended an initial 21 mental health centers located so that each region served would have a minimum of 100,000 population, with no person more than two hours' driving time from a center. Since the proposal calls for only one such center for the one and a quarter million people in Harris county, the establishment of such centers would be only a first step. Even so, the manpower requirements for the first step can be calculated by multiplying the following staffing recommendations for each center by 21:

    a. a board-certified psychiatrist with administrative experience as director

    b. 2 other psychiatrists (or the equivalent in part-time persons)

    c. 2 psychologists

    d. 6 social workers
    e. 6 nurses
    f. 7 therapists, counselors, and trainers
    g. 36 nursing aides or attendants
    h. "adequate" clerical and administrative and housekeeping staff
    i. 50 volunteers.

Thus, there would be needed 63 psychiatrists, 42 psychologists, 126 social workers, and 126 nurses, and so on for these 21 centers.

It is out of the question for that many additional professionals to be trained with existing facilities. Psychiatry residents are trained at three medical schools and one state hospital, but the present output "is inadequate even to replace the potential wastage of psychiatrists who either leave the state or are no longer able to practice . . . and above all to meet new needs that are developing." Two departments of psychiatry reported that their combined training maximum was forty, but they actually had fifty-four trainees enrolled.

In psychology, there are presently two nationally approved clinical training programs in Texas, with two others being developed. Presently about 15 clinical psychologists are being turned out each year; the estimates are that this should be increased to 50. Expansion of the number of trainees would necessitate considerable increase in funds. There are two schools of social work, with present enrollment totaling 130, the maximum for existing facilities and faculties. Only in the nursing field, where there is a total of 33 schools offering a variety of degree programs, did there seem to be room for expanded training.

But the lack of training facilities is not the only barrier to an increased output of mental health professionals. The investigation conducted by the Mental Health Planning Committee revealed two other key factors: inadequate stipends for trainees and a lack of interest on the part of qualified students. While the latter factor was most in evidence in the fields of nursing and social work, it also entered into psychiatry and psychology. It seems to result from a number of conditions, ranging from a failure to acquaint prospective students with the field and its possibilities, to unattractive salaries and working conditions.

Training persons in Texas is one way of trying to supply manpower for mental health, and it is perhaps the chief method. About half the psychiatrists received their M.D. degree from a Texas school, and about the same number of psychologists of those who responded. Slightly less than one-third of the social workers holding the M.A. or a higher degree in social work had been trained in Texas. But, as these figures make clear, there is as well a heavy reliance on persons trained elsewhere. What could be done to help hold Texas graduates in the mental health professions, and to attract still more from other states? Higher salaries would undoubtedly have the first priority. In mid-1964, psychiatrists in the state hospital system were paid from about $9,000 to $22,000 annually (the latter for positions of administrative responsibilities). Directors of community outpatient clinics who were psychiatrists ranged from $18,000 to $25,000 annually. A chief psychologist in the state system had a salary range of $9,216 to $11,-232; in community clinics, from $8,628 to $10,512. While these scales may not vary greatly from the average across the nation, they are several hundred to several thousand dollars below the salary scales found in the most progressive states.

Proposals to attract and hold more professionals also included providing better opportunities for continued professional growth through such devices as research and educational leaves, training for new specialities, travel to professional conferences, and so on. Expanded fringe benefits were suggested as another worthwhile approach. Though not elaborated, the suggestion for a more favorable administrative climate seems well founded.

Still another approach to the manpower problem is to make better use of the existing supply. It is estimated that one-third of all nurses are no longer practicing their profession; presumably some significant part of this group could be restored to activity. The suggestion was made too that psychiatrists not licensed in Texas and who for one reason or another did not want to bother to try to obtain licenses be allowed to engage in public practice only without the license. Another approach is to make sure that persons are being used to the limits of their capacity, i.e., a Ph.D. in psychology should not be doing what an M.A. can do; a psychiatrist should not be doing work that can be handled by a social worker. It has also been suggested, though not explored in depth, that far better use should be made of such related persons as ministers, teachers, counselors, and so on.

Needless to say, a number of the proposals mentioned in the preceding paragraph would help to achieve some of these objectives, although others would require modifications of professional standards or of relations between certain professions.

Because the manpower universe is necessarily larger than the Houston metropolitan area, it is extremely difficult to treat the local situation separately. The Houston SMSA represented roughly 13 per cent of the state's population in 1960, but in 1964 it had almost 25 per cent of all private psychiatrists, 15 per cent of all psychologists, and a little over 25 per cent of all social workers in the state. Its situation was undoubtedly helped by the fact that one of the state's two existing approved programs in clinical psychology and one of the three functioning departments of psychiatry were located within its confines. There is no school of social work in Houston, but there are three nursing schools. Even so, the survey of the local situation reveals significant unmet personnel needs under the existing programs. There is no evidence to suggest that the training institutions have initiated action sufficient to meet those demands, much less to satisfy the manpower needs for expanded mental health programs.

Nevertheless, certain encouraging developments should be noted. One is the training efforts of the Institute of Religion, a nonprofit corporation organized under religious auspices and located in the Texas Medical Center. Its primary objective is to prepare clergymen to minister to the sick, including the mentally ill. Another development is the extensive use of volunteers that has been built up by the child psychiatry division of the Houston State Psychiatric Institute. Over one hundred have been trained for duties as social work technicians, including conducting interviews. From fifteen to thirty can be found working in the child psychiatry division, with another fifteen to twenty in the Texas Children's Hospital, where several cooperative programs are in effect.

What can be said about the impact of fragmentation on mental health manpower? There seems to be some impact on the recruiting of qualified students, which is said by training institutions to be one of the chief difficulties. Part of the recruiting problem relates to the type of patient, the prevailing salaries, and so on, but there was strong feeling as well that part of the trouble lay in communicating to potential trainees the nature of the opportunities in mental health. The kind of communication required (visiting high schools on career days, meeting with counselors, providing work opportunities, etc.) requires a certain amount of special skill and a considerable amount of organizational and administrative endeavor. One significant impact of fragmentation may thus be the breaking down of agencies into units too small to afford this kind of staff assistance. Of course, one should not try to explain all recruiting failures in these terms, because there are some agencies (e.g., the state hospital system) large enough to afford such personnel which nevertheless have done little in this vein.

It is likely that fragmentation also contributes to the problem by making it difficult to get a comprehensive picture of manpower resources and needs, thus discouraging any coordinated or overall assault on the problem. Such evidence as was uncovered seemed to negate another hypothesis, namely, that fragmentation truncates career opportunities and thus adds to the manpower problem. Apparently the shortage of personnel is great enough that qualified persons can climb without too much difficulty by lateral movement (i.e., get promoted by moving to higher positions in another agency). Of course, in this fashion fragmentation may contribute to other problems with personnel, such as high turnover and lack of identification with the agency or institution.

The manpower situation in Texas and in Houston can be summed up in the following terms: Manpower resources are inadequate for present levels of program and will be even more so if there is significant expansion of services. Considerable inquiry has been made into the several dimensions of the problem, and a number of recommendations have emerged. There is no reason to suppose that there will be any prompt action taken on them. Some attention has been given to the possibility of utilizing more nonmedical professionals, including clergymen and educators, and to the development of more extensive volunteer programs. Still lacking are motivation and aggressive action.

VI: SEATTLE

MORTON KROLL

THE SEATTLE METROPOLITAN AREA is the largest in the Pacific Northwest. In 1960 its population was 1,107,000, as compared to the Portland area's population of 822,000. Seattle ranks well ahead of the other two metropolitan areas in the state of Washington, Tacoma, its adjoining neighbor, and Spokane. It was the third largest metropolitan area in the entire Far West, according to the 1960 census, outstripped only by Los Angeles –Long Beach, and San Francisco–Oakland. Geographically, the Seattle area contains King county and part of Snohomish county to the north.

Seattle and environs enjoy plentiful water and abundant greenery. The metropolitan area is bordered on two sides by large bodies of water, Puget Sound to the west and Lake Washington to the east. The sound provides excellent port facilities, and the lake and the sound are a mecca for water sports. The Olympic Mountains to the west and the Cascades to the east provide a base for tourists, recreation, and forest products industries. The Cascades further contribute to the supply of inexpensive electric power, most of which is supplied to the metropolitan region by a city-owned utility.

ECOLOGY

The development of the Seattle metropolitan area parallels that of other metropolitan areas except that it came later. While Seattle was a mature urban center in 1900, it was not until the late 1940s and early 1950s that settlement began to spread out rapidly beyond the city. Like New Orleans, Seattle's growth patterns were influenced by topographic facts. Puget Sound prevented settlement to the west, and Lake Washington, a long, relatively narrow lake, inhibited the growth to the east. The

I wish to express my appreciation to Professor Donald B. Seney of Denver University for the service he rendered as research assistant during the data-gathering stage of this study. Professors Charles M. Strother and Kenneth McCaffree read the manuscript and made many useful comments.

construction of a floating bridge in 1940 allowed the utilization of the east side area, and from about 1950 it has been the fastest growing section of the region. In a similar way, the completion of a north-south freeway in 1965 has facilitated suburban developments to the north of the city.

The general economic condition of the area lacks vitality and diversity. The primary employers are the aircraft, truck frame, and railroad car industries as well as forest products, port facilities, and allied and supporting establishments. The largest single employer in the area is the Boeing Company, known for its commercial and military aircraft as well as for missiles and space equipment. These are cyclical industries, and on occasion the Boeing labor force has risen or dropped drastically in a single year. Nevertheless, Boeing remains the region's dominant employer and a bellwether of the economic health of the area.

Foreign competition, rising labor and transportation costs, and the use of metal, plastic, and concrete materials in the place of wood have adversely affected the forest products industry. The Port of Seattle has declined in recent years. A lack of leadership may be a factor in the port's malaise, but the major problem is the absence of indigenous industries that depend on large-scale water transportation. The port's decline and what to do about it have been an issue in local elections for a decade.

Seattle serves as regional headquarters for a variety of activities, including such agencies of the federal government as the Civil Service Commission, the Post Office, and the Thirteenth Naval District. The University of Washington School of Medicine and Hospital, along with other hospitals in the area, make Seattle a primary medical service area for the state and for a good part of the Northwest as well. Moreover, the Seattle metropolitan area serves as a psychiatric center to the state.

The University of Washington ranks as the second largest employer in the region. With an institution so massive in facilities, enrollment, faculty, and staff, higher education qualifies as big business in the region. In fields that the community generally regards as noncontroversial, university officials often play important roles. With the exception of the aerospace field its faculty virtually monopolizes the technical and professional expertise in the area.

It is not surprising then that Seattle has one of the most highly skilled labor forces in the country. The 1960 census ranks Seattle first of cities over 500,000 population in the percentage of the work force employed in white-collar occupations—47.8 per cent—although Houston is close behind with 46 per cent. It ranks second in the number of families earning $10,000 per year or more—22.9 per cent of the city's population is in this bracket.

King county, in which Seattle is located, is governed by three commissioners who are selected for four-year terms on a partisan basis. As a rule more active and more willing to exercise their powers than the city fathers, the county commissioners as the administrative arm of the state government are more limited in the scope of their powers.

The metropolitan area has an inordinately high number of governmental units. By 1962, the standard metropolitan statistical area, encompassing King county and southern Snohomish county to the north, had 281 units of government including 190 special districts. The greatest growth in governmental units came between 1950 and 1960, when 59 special districts and 11 municipalities were organized. The metropolitan area is highly fragmented both formally and informally. The only metropolitan governmental unit is Metropolitan Seattle, which is currently empowered to collect, treat, and dispose of sewage. The organization of METRO for this one function came after a long and difficult battle, and it is highly unlikely that METRO will be anything more than an areawide single-function sewage authority, although it was hoped originally that it would be given other functions.

Seattle has a weak mayor form of government. The formal system has been buttressed by a series of de facto weak mayors and strong councils. The outlook and emphasis of the city council and the mayor in recent years has been on the need for balanced budgets and the avoidance of new taxes or assessments. So few differences among council members have reached the public eye that a recent editorial in the *Seattle Post-Intelligencer* stated, "We think a little difference of opinion on the council now and then is a good thing." [1]

The City Council, for the most part, acts as a body to ratify decisions requiring governmental action that have been made in the community. Certain groups or individuals initiate, approve, support, and provide consensus for questions and present a *fait accompli* to the council. One study of the local "power structure" showed that 67 per cent of the key influentials came from the business community. The general philosophy of local government in the area is that it should do as little as possible. Bud-

[1] *Seattle Post-Intelligencer,* March 8, 1965, p. 12.

getary restrictions are, of course, consonant with this attitude. The lack of initiative on the part of the formal policy organs of local government encourages action by a variety of ad hoc and long-standing groups; their extent depends upon the issues and the degree to which they involve the community. For example, the Municipal League of Seattle often initiates studies of local government problems as a prelude to their consideration by the City Council.

Local social service agencies headed by the United Good Neighbors provide a broad spectrum of services that are inadequately handled by public agencies or are not provided publicly at all. Cooperation between local private groups and local government is, on the whole, smooth and intimate. In fact, local government officials appear at times pleased to be relieved of the burdens and responsibilities of providing certain social services.

None of the governments of Seattle, King county, or the other municipalities and jurisdictions within the area could be characterized as aggressive. Each does what is formally expected of it. Several interrelated factors appear to explain the timidity of local government in the metropolitan area. First of all, every unit and level of government in the area suffers from an inadequate revenue base. The state government relies for revenue on the property, sales, and business and occupation taxes as well as various license fees. The property tax cannot exceed forty mills per dollar valuation. The cities in the state are restricted to a maximum of fifteen (occasionally sixteen) mills for their property tax. Statewide, the property tax accounts for about 40 per cent of municipal revenues, the remainder coming from business and occupation, service, and other taxes. The counties are restricted to eighteen mills. Special districts are further limited.

The general social-cultural climate places a low priority on governmental activity. The quality of persons obtaining local office, with a few exceptions, has not been notably high. More important, both city and county leadership have limited themselves to the maintenance of a cautious status quo. Policy leadership, direction, and pressures for change generally come from outside the formal instruments of government.

Thus, metropolitan Seattle presents the picture of a rapidly growing area spread over one county and a fraction of another, containing some 280 units of government. The region depends for its livelihood largely upon aircraft construction, forest products, tourism, and shipping, all of which are cyclical. It has a first-rate state university and is a center for medical services for the Northwest. The social and political realities of the Seattle area, coupled with the budgetary restraints on government at all levels, create a climate within which private groups and private individuals exert an important voice and decisions. Despite the proportion of well-trained and highly paid employees, the area, by most accounts, lacks a cosmopolitan outlook. For example, those arts requiring community support experience continuing difficulties. A good symphony orchestra has had yearly financial problems. A newly formed repertory theater may become solvent, but its future is by no means secure. The Seattle Center, which includes an opera house, playhouse, exhibition hall, sports arena, and other facilities, lacks sponsors. Conservative in social orientation, the formal structures of government show little initiative in tackling social causes, preferring to leave welfare and social services to the private sector as much as possible.

FORMAL STRUCTURES AND
MENTAL HEALTH OPERATIONS

In the Seattle metropolitan area, mental health programs are found in variety, but there is little, on or beneath the surface, that binds them together. Alcoholism is only reluctantly admitted to be associated with mental health. Professional and lay groups involved in mental retardation dissociate themselves from the groups concerned with mental illness. It is symptomatic of the ways in which mental health programs have developed in Seattle that autonomous identification should be strong. Since coordinated planning is required by federal legislation, attempts have been mounted in the state and at county and regional levels to coordinate planning activities. But King county has not been especially successful in the planning process.

Government-supported mental health programs are dispersed through the three levels of federal-state-local government with unpatterned, program-oriented relationships among all three. The primary mechanism of official association is through grants-in-aid flowing from the federal to the state and local agencies, and from the state government to local units. The working relationships which result from this process tend to be limited to specific programs that, often as not, are conducted independently of one another.

The federal government's relations with numerous state and local agencies typify this atomized pattern. Grants-in-aid are provided by the National Institute of Mental Health to the state Departments of Institutions, Health, Public Assistance, Public Instruction, and other state agencies. NIMH funds have, of course, been allocated for specific purposes to programs and institutions operating in the region.

In fiscal 1964, NIMH training grants alone amounted to $939,090. This sum was divided among nine institutions and covered twenty-five separate grants. Thirteen of the twenty-five grants were made directly to the University of Washington, and these amounted to 67 per cent of the amount for training grants allocated to the state. Grants for research for the 1964 fiscal year totaled $349,567. Thirteen of the nineteen grants under this allocation were made to projects at the University of Washington. While it is difficult to assess the precise impact the university has on mental health activities, from these figures one can appreciate its considerable influence on training and research in the state. In only three instances were these grants limited to programs underway in the metropolitan area. Taken as a whole, federal grants-in-aid reveal no great design, or no design at all, for the metropolitan area. Individual research and institutional training grants are rendered on an ad hoc basis, but no overall regional pattern has emerged over the years. Under these circumstances little initiative has been demonstrated by the state, federal government, or the major institutional recipients of grants to build up anything more than the current apparently unrelated collection of grants.

The major direct service federal programs in the mental health field are conducted at the Veterans Administration Hospital and the Public Health Service Hospital. In both installations the services offered are regarded as inadequate by their staff. The Public Health Service Hospital operates with one full-time psychiatrist and a fourth of a secretary's time. Its catchment area is broader than the metropolitan region, although 70 per cent of its patients are from Seattle. As a public health hospital the patient clientele is restricted to American seamen, coast guard, military personnel, Indians, and their dependents.

The continuation outpatient clinic of the VA Hospital is located in the heart of the Seattle city center and has been in operation since 1946. Its purpose is to serve veterans who have service-connected neuropsychiatric disabilities. Its service area is not limited to the metropolitan region, though it does draw heavily from Seattle. Its staff consists of a supervisory clinical psychologist, three psychologists, three part-time psychiatrists, and four psychiatric social workers. At any given time in the past several years, it has been treating about 300 patients.

The federal government's direct services, then, are meager; they are adequate perhaps within the letter of the legal prescriptions of the programs but not adequate to meet the real needs of their clientele as perceived by their staff. Federal services reflect the general problem of publicly supported mental health activities in the region.

To date, principal public mental health activities in the Seattle metropolitan area have been carried out by state agencies. The first state hospital was the Western State Hospital, opened on the grounds of the abandoned Fort Steilacoom in 1871. Eastern State Hospital at Medical Lake opened in 1891 and Northern State Hospital near Sedro Woolley followed in 1911. These hospitals were located in what are considered out-of-the-way rural areas. Until the mid-1950s they offered only custodial care. Today these three hospitals are the major state-supported treatment centers for the acutely mentally ill in Washington.

The state Department of Health came upon the mental health scene with the establishment of its Mental Hygiene Section within the Division of Preventive Medical Services in 1944 to provide early diagnosis of preventable mental illness in returning servicemen. The services of the section were also available to parents of children who had behavior difficulties. As mental health authority for the state of Washington, the Department of Health assumes no direct supervisory or administrative responsibility with respect to local mental health projects, other than in maintaining professional consultation relationships and working with the local groups in terms of making available to them federal Mental Health Act funds. The department's stated goal is to develop preventive or positive community mental health programs in contrast to spending all of its professional time in treating mental and emotional illness. These programs have elements of an epidemiological approach to problems of mental illness.

In the 1950s a revolution took place in the Department of Institutions, which had charge of state mental hospitals as well as penal institutions. Beginning with the 1952–1954 biennium, the Department of Institutions moved from the backwaters to the forefront of professional standards and practices. A Division of Mental Health was established to provide treatment in the state hospitals, do research on mental illness, and engage in preventive programs through community action. The state hospitals shifted their emphasis to treatment. Professionally qualified personnel were brought into the division and within a short period of time it became *the* state agency with a virtual monopoly of professional knowledge and skills in the mental health field. The Department of Institutions became a lively advocate of new programs; in so doing it began to compete with the Department of Health.

Under the National Mental Health Act of 1946 the state Department of Health had been designated the mental health authority for the state of Washington. The Department of Institutions retained its official role as state mental hospital authority. At the time of this decision, the Department of Institutions was in no condition to administer a community program.

One result of the modernization of the 1950s was that requests were made to the Department of Institutions to establish mental health clinics in connection with the state mental hospitals. By 1961 the state hospitals were furnishing discharge summaries to the patient's family physician, and a statewide program had been established under which local medical societies would provide a doctor for discharged patients who had no regular family physician. A special nursing home placement program was begun in November 1960 in cooperation with the state Department of Public Assistance. In May 1962 the Division of Mental Health launched a new Hospital–Community Council Program. The division altered hospital treatment programs to shorten periods of hospitalization.

The new activities brought the state hospitals into contact with community agencies, particularly in the effort to return patients to active and productive lives. A statewide citizens' council was established to integrate the state hospital system with the community. The state hospitals also became "open staff," enabling physicians in the community to become members of attending staffs. The department set up child guidance centers to counsel in children's problems. The Mental Retardation Program also progressed rapidly in a short period of time. The Department of Institutions thus moved very close to the interests of the Department of Health. Common programs, but disparity of resources between the Departments of Institutions and Health, produced rivalry that influenced the shaping of policies in the mental health field.

The Department of Institutions operates the three state mental hospitals and the Mental Health Research Institute. Total professional staff in the division numbers about 400. An increasing admission rate and a decreasing patient population characterize these hospitals. In July 1964 the patient population stood at about 4,400—a reduction of more than 3,000 from its maximum figure several years previously, reflecting the shift to intensive therapy.

The division is concerned about its chronic population in state hospitals. The geriatric segment of the state population is increasing. It is hoped that the research program of the Mental Health Research Institute will be expanded, particularly in regard to the problems of children, geriatrics, and the chronically schizoid population.

The Division of Community Services of the Department of Institutions focuses on child guidance, and community and police consultation. Its primary concern is with maladjusted children and it is largely oriented to social work. It has a staff of about seventeen social workers and a number of part-time psychiatrists and psychological consultants distributed throughout twenty-three offices (seven regional and sixteen branch); its budget for the 1963–1965 biennium was nearly $750,000.

The major interest of the Department of Health in programing for mental illness is its community mental health clinic and consultation program. The community clinics are operated locally, though the state provides about 75 per cent of their support. Eleven communities in the state operate sixteen programs staffed by psychiatrists, psychologists, and social workers. For the most part they are demonstration projects to show what can be accomplished. Expenditures in 1964 for these programs ran to about $430,000 per annum, of which the state provided $190,000, the federal government $100,000, and the remaining $140,000 came from a variety of local sources.

The Public Health Nursing program is supervised by the Department of Health. An increasing proportion of the time of public health nurses is taken up with mental health problems.

The alcoholism treatment program is also supervised by the Health Department. About $147,000 per annum is spent for the treatment of alcoholism, of which $125,000 comes from direct legislative appropriation. The program includes case finding and treatment in three centers, educational activities, professional education, consultation services, and research. Local communities contribute to various parts of the program.

Personnel of the Department of Public Assistance bring cases up to the point of medical diagnosis and determination. The department also deals with nursing home facilities and care, which includes the mentally ill. Mentally retarded persons requiring (and eligible for) help through public assistance numbered 5,700 in January 1964. A study of 18,000 out of 130,000 cases involving disability and public assistance indicated that 50 per cent of the 18,000 included psychiatric problems.[2]

Of the 372 operating school districts in the state of Washington, 115 receive extra funds from the state Department of Public Instruction for working with handicapped children. The state appropriation for this program mushroomed from $25,000 in 1943 to $13,900,000 in the 1963–1965 biennial appropriation. As of July 1964 approximately 60,-000 children received such services, which was less than 10 per cent of the total school population. About 10,000 of this group were in special classes, two-thirds of whose members were regarded as mentally retarded.

Vocational rehabilitation is another activity of the Department of Public Instruction. A division in the department has been active in developing workshops and supervising work opportunity for the mentally retarded and severely disabled. Sheltered workshops provide the chief mechanism for the division's program in mental retardation. Expenditures for this program amounted to $595,000 for 1963–1965, of which a little more than half came from the federal government. The staff of the division is enthusiastic about the development of sheltered workshops by community agencies in a number of localities. The division supplies consultation, training, and funds for programs operated by organizations like Goodwill Industries and Occupational Rehabilitation, Inc. of Spokane.

Its very location in Seattle gives the University of Washington special significance as a metropolitan as well as a state resource. Under the direction of the Department of Psychiatry of the School of Medicine, the University operates four psychiatric in- and outpatient clinics for children and adults. Cases are accepted only by referral from physicians and the primary criterion for admission is the usefulness of the patient's condition to the teaching and research functions.[3] However, the clinics turn away very few persons whom the staff feels it could help. While the primary focus is on individual case studies, a broad orientation to treatment is emphasized for teaching purposes, including group therapy, drugs, and

[2] State of Washington Mental Health and Mental Retardation Planning Committee, *Minutes, Meeting,* July 13, 1964 (Olympia, Wash.: mimeographed), p. 10.
[3] In 1966 the University Hospital's policies were changed to permit self-referrals.

shock treatment. There is such a demand for treatment that a waiting period of six months is normal at the outpatient clinic. Both inpatient and outpatient children's services have long waiting lists.

Thus, four state departments (Institutions, Health, Public Assistance, and Public Instruction) attempt to cope with mental illness, though not to the same degree. The Department of Institutions, through its Division of Mental Health as well as programs concerned with child guidance and mental retardation, has by far the largest and most extensive treatment program. With the exception of the facilities and resources at the University of Washington, the Department of Institutions is the only state agency whose staff is actually engaged in treating mental illness and mental retardation. It has a virtual monopoly on resources and expertise.

In the past, evidence of joint planning among the departments, particularly between those of Health and Institutions, has been very slight indeed. The prevailing relationship between the two departments was more of competition and rivalry than cooperation. An attempt to develop a coordinated program involving both the Departments of Health and Institutions in the city of Everett and focusing on relating the treatment facilities and services of Northern State Hospital to the Everett community met with difficulties.

The majority of the state programs suffer from lack of financial support. Mental health activities have not enjoyed a high priority among legislators, with the exception of the improvement of the state mental hospital system. The initiative for such progress as was made came for the most part from the executive branch. By and large, the legislature has not recognized the importance of extensive outlays of money for mental health services. Attempts at coordination at the state level have been feeble affairs and have shown few results.

The Washington State Mental Health and Mental Retardation Planning Committee was appointed by Governor Albert D. Rossellini in October 1963. It originally served as a mental health committee but was enlarged early in 1964 to include mental retardation as well. Its membership grew from twelve to fifteen to twenty between October 1963 and April 1965.

It was composed of representatives of the state agencies, institutions of higher education, business, labor, and professional groups as well as the state legislature. Dr. Charles R. Strother, professor of psychology and psychiatry at the University of Washington, was chairman of the committee. He provided the primary guidance at the state level. The committee had a small staff to carry out its planning and organizing activities.

The role of the governor's committee loomed large because of the atomization and diffusion of programs, the special interests of the agencies working in mental health and mental retardation, the hostility between the Departments of Health and Institutions, and the absence of vigorous or unified support either from professional groups or voluntary agency representatives. The governor's committee did not attempt to impose an arbitrary scheme on the state but sought to build grassroot state and community support and thereby to increase chances for success and minimize conflicts. It reflected the divergent positions and interests of its membership, but at the same time it was committed to devising a unified plan for the development of community mental health centers that would also include a role for the state. The committee realized it had to gain the support of a majority of those working with mental illness and mental retardation. In 1964 it functioned gingerly at the state level and with great caution at the local level. In early 1965 it appeared that the committee might serve more as an arena for making decisions than as a decision-making mechanism itself. It was, for all practical purposes, the only symbol of policy and program unity in these fields in the state and its communities.

The breadth of representation on the committee produced problems as well as benefits. The fact that the directors of the Departments of Health and Institutions were present meant that the committee would inevitably provide a medium for the expression of their differences. As one monthly meeting of the committee followed another, it became apparent that the central problem of a statewide mental health authority would be among the most important to be faced.

The committee attempted to stimulate discussion and planning in the counties and combinations of sparsely populated counties by dividing the state into ten regions. Each was to prepare a plan for its area and all were to be integrated into a statewide plan. The local committees represented public and private organizations in the area; their task was to assess available services, identify deficiencies, and suggest priorities as well as ways and means of attaining their goals.[4]

[4] Mental Health and Mental Retardation Planning Committee, *Mental Health Planning* (Olympia, Wash.: State Printing Plant, 1964), p. 4.

The whole state program was inaugurated with a state Mental Health Congress, held on November 16, 1963, sponsored by the Washington State Medical Association in cooperation with the Department of Health. Over 300 professionals and laymen gathered to hear the governor and persons of national and state prominence discuss developments in the mental health field. The emphasis was on the value of community action.

The governor's committee was confronted with an impossible deadline of July 1, 1965. The state plan, with its county and regional components, as well as its recommendations for state organization, all were to be finished by that time. It became apparent early in 1965 that a plan could not be completed on time; the committee therefore extended its deadline to November 1965. Problems of data design, of getting county and regional committees to function, and of processing plans took more time and effort than was originally calculated.

The committee appointed twelve task forces, which were to provide expert advice and analyze data from a statewide perspective. The task forces brought together professional and lay persons knowledgeable in specific fields. Though the coverage and representation in the task forces were impressive, the degree and intensity of their work varied considerably.

The governor's committee emphasized the importance of local initiative and funding in the development and management of mental illness and retardation facilities and services. In one way this idea was tested by special legislation during 1965, authorizing the establishment of a community mental health and retardation facility in Kitsap county, to be operated by the Division of Mental Health of the Department of Institutions and to be financed wholly by state funds. The precedent of having a community facility fully supported and operated by the state could prove embarrassing to the principle of community-generated support. The governor's committee was concerned that the facility be as effectively constructed and serviced as possible. The Department of Institutions, for its part, took steps to involve the community in its operations.

In its relations with the 1965 legislature the committee recognized the need for continuity and coordination. Legislation was passed to authorize and empower the governor to take the necessary action to enable the state to participate in the federal program.[5] In the same act the legislature

[5] State of Washington, House Bill No. 647, 39th Regular Session.

reconstituted the mental health and mental retardation advisory council to be appointed by the governor. The Departments of Health, Institutions, Public Assistance, and Public Instruction were represented by their chiefs. The governor was empowered to add nongovernmental representatives for two- and three-year terms. The advisory council was to advise the governor on matters relating to development, standards of performance, and the review of plans.

Since the Governor did not act immediately to appoint the Advisory Council, the Planning Committee under Dr. Strother decided to recommend to the governor that the Health Department be designated as the construction-planning authority, without prejudice to its future role in the overall activity.[6] It further resolved that the Institutions Department be designated as the program-planning agency to work in full cooperation with the Advisory Council and without prejudice to the programs currently under the aegis of the Health Department. This was obviously a holding operation. The difficulty of coordination between the construction- and program-planning agencies was obviously known to the committee. Perhaps their resolution suggested a trial and shakedown period with the final decision to be made by the governor.

The committee was more a locus for the presentation of positions than a decision-making body in any *pro forma* sense. It did decide on county- or regional-based planning processes and provided task forces, but it did not, nor could it, resolve fundamental issues at the state level. Clearly it was difficult to make much progress without some resolution of the dispute between the Health and Institutions Departments. In relying on consensus and persuasion, the committee avoided strong direction. Whether its nondirective approach would offer a payoff in the form of a broadly based and approved scheme remained to be seen. Certainly the federal act itself pointed the way and perhaps the committee felt that sufficient direction had already been given by the statute.

To understand public mental health programing in Seattle, one must begin at the state level. The absence of locally supported and operated systems makes it necessary for the impetus for new programs to come from the state government. The principal state agencies, their major programs and commitments, influence the decisions made by local communities in the mental health field.

[6] Mental Health and Mental Retardation Planning Committee, *Minutes, Meeting of May 8, 1965* (Olympia, Wash.: mimeographed), p. 3.

The official attitudes that condition formal decisions can be drawn from statements of the director of the Department of Health and the supervisor of the Division of Mental Health of the Department of Institutions. Ordinarily the supervisor of a division in state administration is a level lower than the director of a department, but because of the strong support given the supervisor of the Division of Mental Health by the director of the Department of Institutions, the status differential is minimized.

At the inaugural Washington State Congress of Mental Health, held in Seattle on November 16, 1963, the state health director, Dr. Bernard Bucove, said he was aware that public health and mental health stemmed from different backgrounds "and still reflect some basic differences in orientation." [7] Public health, he argued, had long had a concern with the environment while mental health, based on psychiatry, had focused on individuals and particularly individuals in institutions. Later the mental health "program moved in the direction of the establishment of clinics, which at first were oriented toward treatment on a one-to-one basis, though sometimes group therapy has been added. Until recently, however, there has been little concern with the community, and relatively little with primary prevention or rehabilitation." [8] Recently, public health had become concerned with patient-oriented support, with the aged, with those suffering from chronic diseases. Problems of nursing homes and home care services had become increasingly pressing. Mental health, for its part, had become concerned with the relationship of the community to the mental hospital, rehabilitation, and similar environmentally focused issues. Thus, the philosophies, orientations, and perhaps even the techniques of public health and mental health were beginning to converge. This, he felt, was one of the most significant and positive current trends.[9]

Dr. Bucove stressed the importance of identifying "high risk groups" in mental illness, of noting the "susceptible host" within the community. He urged all those working in the mental health area to pull together, but nowhere in his address did he mention the work being done by his neighbors in the Department of Institutions.

---

[7] Bernard Bucove, M.D., *The Status of the Community Mental Health Program in the State of Washington* (Olympia, Wash.: State Department of Health, mimeographed, 1963).
[8] *Ibid.*
[9] *Ibid.*

The spokesman for the Department of Institutions, Dr. William R. Conte, pointed to the achievements of his agency with justifiable pride. He stressed the development of a large professional staff, implying that his agency had a monopoly on professional talent in the public mental health field. He emphasized the fact that the state psychiatric program operated by his department was community oriented. Study-planning groups were devoting their time and attention to geriatric problems, to the difficulties encountered with the care of the socially deprived child, to community participation and interrelatedness of mental health programs, to the psychiatric services in the general hospital, and to the evaluation and treatment of the offender.[10]

In discussing the growing importance of community psychiatric hospital service, Dr. Conte noted that many persons now being whisked away to state hospitals for treatment could be treated effectively in their communities, close to friends and families, if treatment facilities were available. The state mental hospital system, however, was legally prohibited from providing services directly to the community off hospital grounds. But the division was indeed looking ahead to the day when it could establish small psychiatric units within state hospitals that would serve a particular geographic area, county, or community.

Furthermore, Dr. Conte lost no time in telling this statewide audience who should adminster this community program. It should be the "agency with the highest level of competence in the hospital-community service field." He did not mention any contributions that had been or were being made by the Health Department. Evidently he did not feel that mental health programing belonged in any unit of the state government other than his own. His concluding sentence drove home the point in no uncertain terms: "In Washington we have been fighting the battle *alone* italics ours] for a long time and to see this organized interest in psychiatry is most gratifying."

A comparison of the bases for decisions in the two major departments would indicate that the Department of Health's goals and interests are focused on the traditional public health ideas of prevention and epidemiology as applied to psychiatry. Interest in treatment is secondary. The Department of Institutions is almost wholly concerned with treatment and has moved from custodial to intensive therapy methods. Research

[10] William R. Conte, M.D., *Psychiatric Hospitalization—A Look Into the Future* Olympia, Wash.: Department of Institutions, mimeographed, 1964).

is the cornerstone of its program, and the concept of prevention, particularly in relation to the community's environment, is strong.

The Department of Health in emphasizing community-centered and
-supported activities did not develop its own staff. There is little evidence
of any long-range planning. A limited professional staff indicates lack
of resources for effective planning and operation. This also gives credence
to the criticism offered by some that the Health Department tended to
treat mental health simply as another species of public health program.
On the other hand, the Department of Institutions in recent years has
made enormous strides and its staff has been actively engaged in planning procedures. It published plans for the future development of
comprehensive mental health services that advocated a combined mental
hospital and community mental health approach even before the establishment of the Strother's committee. It had expressed concern that
adequate aftercare programs, preadmission units, and other important
community-centered and community-located segments could not be established because of statutory restrictions.

The governor's Planning Committee held two conferences with the
departments of state government concerned with mental health and
mental retardation in the summer of 1964. The Departments of Health,
Institutions, Public Assistance, and Public Instruction and Vocational
Rehabilitation were represented. Professor Strother stated that the purpose of these meetings was to obtain "information from the various
departments about the nature and scope of the programs in each department which relate to mental health and mental retardation."

Nearly all of the second meeting of the state agencies with Professor
Strother on July 30, 1964, was devoted to mental retardation. The
Department of Institutions runs the schools for the retarded and the
Department of Health performs a variety of medical functions in communities throughout the state. The question of interagency cooperation
among all of the agencies involved did arise and problems concerning
the need for increased cooperation between the Departments of Institutions and Public Instruction as well as Public Assistance were aired.
On the whole, there appeared to be much more of a spirit of unity in
matters relating to mental retardation than in the mental health area.

In addition to the Departments of Health and Institutions, other
agencies of state government and groups functioning throughout the state

contribute to policy decisions in the mental health field. The Public Assistance Department sees itself as a user of mental health services and as a link for those who require services and the mental health and mental retardation facilities of the state. The department does not engage in mental health operations but provides housing, when necessary, for dischargees from state hospitals. It is concerned about the shortage of adequate outpatient clinics for those who are released from mental hospitals who need continuing treatment. It also maintains responsibility for finding foster homes for mentally retarded children, a task which has proved difficult. It further tries to find foster homes for a number of "extremely bad kids" for whom there is no room in institutions.

The Department of Public Instruction emphasizes the "total approach" to the whole child. Adult education, child guidance, in-service training for teachers and counselors are aspects of the task of coping with mental health and retardation problems in the schools. For example, the department in 1964 developed a mental health teaching unit as part of its health education course of study. Instruction is being provided to guidance personnel in the school districts, and the Special Education Section of the department holds workshops for teachers concerned with retarded children.

The perceptions of those responsible for administering the Vocational Rehabilitation program centered on the broad view of their field. Vocational rehabilitation is offered to physically and mentally disadvantaged persons, along with care and support, if necessary, for their dependents. The division operates the federal-state program of services to the physically and mentally handicapped. Efforts include studies on dropouts in the Tacoma school district, the functionally illiterate child, and sheltered workshops.

The pattern at the state level of professional groups was related to the roles that these groups performed in the Seattle metropolitan area. A few psychiatrists have been active at the state level. The former Committee of Psychiatrists for Community Action was instrumental in getting the Department of Institutions to hire Dr. Conte to run the Mental Health Division in that agency. The committee even lobbied for specific projects such as the establishment of a separate department of mental hygiene and acute treatment centers in the metropolitan area.

The Mental Health Committee of the Washington State Medical Association has been concerned primarily with educating physicians about mental health problems. To an extent its role was circumscribed by the attitudes of the association itself. The Mental Health Committee did, however, play an active part in convening the mental health congresses of 1963.

The Washington State Psychological Association evaluates the credentials of individual psychologists in private practice, school systems, hospitals, and institutions for the mentally retarded. It has a legislative committee to prevent what it regards as harmful legislation from being passed by the legislature.

The Washington Association for Mental Health has advocated more extensive programs of public information, aftercare, rehabilitation, referral services, and legislation. It has sought to play an active role in the planning process for mental health through the Governor's Committee on Mental Health and Mental Retardation Planning. The Washington Association for Social Welfare has been interested, but not really active, in mental health matters.

The State Council for Psychiatric Institutions lobbies on behalf of Department of Institution activities. Its purpose has been to foster the programs and activities of the Division of Mental Health. Its chairman lobbied with the governor and the legislature and has worked to achieve maximum program effectiveness and protection for its adopted agency. The Governor's Council on Aging functions through the Department of Public Assistance and focuses on the development of community concerns and action. The council meets annually and is subdivided into seven regional committees. It has pressed for more foster homes, better boarding homes, curriculum in the schools to prepare people more effectively for retirement; in this context it was concerned with the preservation of mental health.

Taken collectively, the professionally oriented groups have not been an effective force in fostering mental health and retardation programs at the state level. The professional groups were not motivated toward vigorous action, nor did their leaders feel that they should be. Some groups are primarily concerned with improving the competence of their members. They want to protect the level of services and to prevent the dilution of standards. Both the psychiatric and medical groups saw themselves as "paper organizations" in the mental health field until the last two or three years. The social workers' activities apparently emerged as an organized group only within the recent past and the psychologists have operated through their legislative committee only within the past eight years. On the other hand, the professional groups agree that their individual skills should be incorporated into whatever statewide programs are developed, although they are not clear how they should be fitted into whatever schemes are devised.

A marked difference in perception was evident between the major agencies concerned with mental health and those with partial interests in the field. The Health and Institutions Departments are more self-conscious on the matter of coordination and cooperation than the other less directly concerned agencies. Neither of the two giants in the state field find any cooperative scheme feasible for their purposes. Rather loose coordination devices have been used, such as the Governor's Inter-agency Council of Health, Education, and Welfare and the Hospital Community Council Program, as well as functional coordination in educational programs in which several departments participate. The Governor's Committee on Mental Health and Mental Retardation Planning is the first statewide attempt to bring the whole field into focus.

Nor were the leaders of the professional groups any more precise in their perceptions. The cochairman of the Mental Health Committee of the Washington State Medical Association suggested some sort of "forced cooperation" between the Departments of Health and Institutions. He also felt that the more groups concerned with mental health that could be brought together on a regional basis, along the lines of the November 1963 conference in Seattle, the better the chances for a general scheme of state cooperation. The chairman of the District Branch of the American Psychiatric Association declared simply that more state and community coordination was needed and suggested a separate department of mental health along with the establishment of acute treatment centers and aftercare clinics. The representatives of the Washington State Psychological Association were similarly aware of the need for coordination as well as the conflict between the Health and Institutions Departments. The psychologists appeared also to favor a separate Department of Mental Health if only because "when there are two kids fighting, you should bring in a bigger kid to stop it." The social workers perceived the need for the better utilization of existing resources, more involvement of all professions, and interagency co-ordination.

The voluntary agency representatives, one step further removed from the fray, suggested coordination with virtually no specifics. Little satisfaction was expressed, however, with the existing pattern.

A single Department of Mental Health may not be entirely unacceptable. There may be a predisposition to accept such a device for the stimulation, development, and supervision of mental health programs in the state, though approval would depend upon the organization and leadership of the agency. To put it bluntly, the Department of Health cannot see the Department of Institutions doing the job, and vice versa, yet each agency wants to have a part in any new mechanism that may be devised. Quite obviously the professional and voluntary groups have not organized with sufficient effectiveness to take the initiative in the planning and organizing process. Much depends upon the governor's Planning Committee and even more upon its ability to harness the antagonists and their supporters into an effective working force. Certainly, the governor himself has a role to play.

The governor's administrative right arm in many respects is the Central Budget Agency. The executive budget is relatively new to the state of Washington, it is the only executive management unit in the atomized and diffused administrative structure. In the matter of mental health, it tends to follow the governor's lead, which is to support and encourage the development of the Institutions Department's Division of Mental Health, without confronting the problem of the relationship between the Health and Institutions Departments.

The position of the Central Budget Agency is that custodial care is declining and new outpatient facilities are required. It recognizes the legal fact that the Department of Health is the mental health authority but feels that its staff is inadequate to carry out even programs supported by federal funds. It is also aware of the conflict between the Departments of Health and Institutions. In 1964, an election year, the governor was not willing to embroil himself in a controversy that might become a campaign issue.

Furthermore, the Central Budget Agency placed a good deal of faith in the capacity of the Governor's Planning Committee on Mental Health and Mental Retardation to cope with the problem of coordination. The committee further met the need for long-range planning, which no previous agency or coordinating body in the mental health field had been able to do. The Inter-Agency Committee on Health, Education, and

Welfare had not been oriented toward intensive, long-range planning. Insofar as its contribution to the making of any decisions is concerned, the Central Budget Agency is willing to follow the lead of expert policy advice and adhere to its criteria of financial and managerial efficiency within the policy commitments.

The role of Governor Rosselini was a passive one. He could have taken a positive role, even overriding the major conflicting state agencies. Such actions as the newly elected governor, Daniel J. Evans, took were designed to add prestige to the Planning Committee. At the same time there was little evidence of positive action from the governor's office. Mental health did not enjoy a high priority during the stormy first months of a new state administration preoccupied with the problems of legislative redistricting and major financial headaches.

The governor was loath to choose between the Departments of Health and Institutions. He hoped that these agencies could work out a solution to their problems, but the advent of federal legislation only intensified and crystallized their positions. While the Governor's Committee on Mental Health and Mental Retardation Planning did much to stimulate planning activity at the local levels, it is still faced with the problem of disposing of the underlying conflict at the state level. The subsequent establishment of the Advisory Council, in fact a metamorphosis of the Planning Committee, which has the potential to become a super-co-ordinating agency, could lead to a formal resolution of the problem by authority. The governor remains the central figure in that he has the power to decide, but it appears he wants consensus. On the other hand, the Planning Committee is reluctant to press for a decision imposed from above.

The state Committee on Mental Health and Retardation Planning is the only genuinely integrative force in mental health in the state. To be sure, in its attempts to move a large, amorphous complex of organizations, groups, and activities throughout the state toward a comprehensive view of mental health and mental retardation, the Planning Committee had its difficulties. It was not rejected, however; in the course of 1964 and 1965, one could detect activity on the part of a number of communities in the directions sought by the committee. Voluntary groups supported those integrative programs that did not threaten their program authority. For the state of Washington, the general activity in the direction of mental health programing cannot be dismissed lightly.

The Washington state legislature has in recent years been sympathetic to the development of sound (in the meaning accepted by those professionally engaged in the field) mental health programs. In a policy area generally considered low-pressure, the legislature has followed the lead of the executive in mental health legislation and budgetary support. Yet, for the most part, legislators were reluctant to respond to queries on mental health matters, perhaps because of the stigma attached to the field.[11] Even the few who were willing to answer questions for the most part were aware of their lack of expertness. Most of the lobbyists in the mental health field were "pro" mental health and retardation programs. The Washington state legislature had yet to be deluged with anti-mental health literature. Its members had a high regard for the directors of the Health and Institutions Departments and the judgment of the governor and the Central Budget Agency in this field. Most legislators concerned with mental health knew about the change in the field from caretaker functions to short-term therapy. They agreed it was desirable to return mentally ill persons to productive lives as soon as possible. The interested legislators by and large felt that community mental health centers were needed and that the legislature ought to provide at least some of the funds for these facilities. They also tended to support the establishment of psychiatric treatment centers in general hospitals. At the same time, the legislators who evidenced interest in mental health programs had reservations about the state's role in counseling, vocational, and recreational functions in the mental health field.

The limitation of available financial resources was most frequently cited by concerned legislators as the reason for the lack of more comprehensive programs. This would indicate that federal funds might lead to more favorable action by the legislature. Legislators were also aware of the lack of general public interest in mental health matters. Perhaps the absence of a vigorous mental health lobby also explains legislative lethargy. Furthermore, the very length of the legislative session works against measures that do not have tightly organized support. Sixty days each biennium are hardly sufficient to deal seriously with the array of high priority matters, let alone those with little support. Recent legis-

[11] Lawrence K. Lee, "Legislative Aspects of a Mental Health Policy in the State of Washington," unpublished report (Seattle: Department of Political Science, University of Washington, March, 1964). Mr. Lee's report (based on research under the author's supervision) is based on questionnaires he submitted to members of the 1963 legislature.

latures were preoccupied with major problems, at least superficially far removed from the mental health field. Legislative redistricting to meet the requirements of a court order took priority over other legislative functions.

Those legislators who were aware of mental health programs and problems understood the difficulties between the Departments of Health and Institutions. Very few wanted to maintain a status quo, though even those who expressed concern by and large were reluctant to propose solutions. Among those who did suggest specific changes, the idea of a Department of Mental Health was most often propounded, with the Department of Institutions assuming the full burden as a second choice. One member of the 1963 legislature proposed that the Department of Institutions be given the mental health program responsibility and, in the following legislative session, that a separate Department of Mental Health be established. He argued that the Institutions Department would thus have two years to orient itself to community service and support on a statewide scale.

On the matter of levels of governmental financial support, those legislators who were interested in mental health tended to divide along party lines, with the Democrats advocating greater federal participation in the funding. In this context it is worth reporting that among the interested legislators of the 1963 legislative session none of the mental health oriented legislators regarded continued state support as unacceptable. A number of the legislators with a realistic view of the capacity of local governments to sustain mental health programs felt that purely local funding was either undesirable or impossible.

An interesting note on partisan support is that in the Washington state legislature, among those evidencing public interest in mental health, the Republicans appeared to want a more comprehensive program but were less willing to pay for it while the Democrats, with more limited objectives, were willing to spend money.

Even this cursory examination of the views of a legislature's membership revealed a willingness to support mental health programs. This willingness must be qualified by noting that no prime movers have as yet emerged among the legislators to spark a full-fledged legislative commitment to mental health programs. Nor has outside pressure been strong enough to induce legislative action.

The mental health care that was available at no cost, or for a minimal fee, in Seattle was provided by the private sector. Not until 1963 did the Seattle–King County Health Department accord official recognition to mental illness; on November 1 of that year a physician was appointed to head its mental health unit. The first appointee to the post continued to act in his original capacity as director of maternal and child health services. His training was in public health, not in psychiatry. He was chosen to head the new unit because his work with child services and the visiting nurse program "is the closest thing we have to mental health services." The professional staff of the mental health unit consists of one part-time psychiatrist and one full-time psychiatric nurse. The funds for the mental health unit come from the state Department of Health and must be used specifically for mental health services. The city and county appropriate no money for mental health.

The mental health unit provides staff consultation to visiting nurses and other members of the Health Department. No direct therapy is offered; those who need psychiatric care are referred elsewhere. On a limited basis some attempt is made to follow up those who have been discharged from state mental institutions through the visiting nurse program.

Harbour View (King county) Hospital maintains a psychiatric outpatient unit. The clinic's director is a psychiatrist in private practice who holds an appointment as an assistant professor at the University of Washington hospital. The clinic has a dual role: providing short-term treatment to indigents or welfare recipients and offering clinical experience to medical students. The students see the patients and manage the cases, and the psychiatrist consults with the students. Approximately 1,500 patients are seen a year. No inpatient facility exists in the usual sense of the term.

The Seattle city school district is the most active local unit in the mental health field. It has two departments, Guidance Services and Special Education, whose activities deal with the psychological well-being of children in Seattle schools. The school system is not a treatment organization. The more seriously disturbed children are referred to community agencies.

The extent of governmentally sponsored and operated mental health programs in the Seattle metropolitan area is not impressive by any American standards. Nor, until recently, has there been any substantial pressure for local government to become actively concerned with mental health. No money is appropriated by the city of Seattle, King county, Snohomish county, or the smaller governmental units within the metropolitan area for mental health services. The school districts are an exception to a degree, but even they rely heavily for operating support on state grants-in-aid from the Department of Public Instruction.

Unless one can term the Seattle–King county consolidated Health Department a coordinator, virtually none exists among local units. What coordination one does find is vertical in that referrals are made from local units to state agencies. Thus the schools refer youngsters needing attention to the Department of Institutions, or to locally sponsored facilities such as the Community Psychiatric Clinic.

The state hospitals serve as primary governmental service units for mental health in the metropolitan area. Northern State and Western State Hospitals have divided the region among themselves. The Lake Washington Ship Canal that cuts through Seattle serves as an inexact dividing line. Northern State Hospital receives patients who reside north of the canal, and those whose homes lie south of the canal are served by Western State Hospital. Such administrative pie cutting reveals the lack of a metropolitanwide perspective of the problems of mental illness that need public action. The state facilities do enjoy a good reputation among psychiatrists. Good working relationships have developed between the medical community, public and private, and the hospitals.

The difficulties of working within a fragmented governmental and organizational pattern were at least tacitly accepted and did not stimulate metropolitanwide concerns in respect to mental hospital services. On the other hand, social workers, school administrators, public assistance officials, and the clergy most often have to cope with fragmentation, and some of the push for coordination and more effective local programs comes from these groups. Both the Institutions and Health Departments grew interested in developing local services in line with their interests and approaches. The Institutions Department had no desire to limit its services to state hospital facilities and wished to move its services and tie them more closely to population centers. It hoped to be a vigorous partner in the development and operation of local services. The state Health Department is committed to stimulating, supporting, and assisting in the growth of public and private local services. With the added impetus of the Governor's Planning Committee on Mental Health and Mental Retardation, the greatest push for effective local and community-oriented services would have to come from the state.

The majority of programs in the metropolitan area are conducted by community-supported agencies, some of which receive funds from the state Department of Health and the federal government. The territorial boundaries encompassed by these programs vary; a few are limited to Seattle, several to King county, and others to communities within the county. Such programs are fragmented in that no territorial, governmental pattern provides a geographical or rational boundary. Much as the agencies of the federal government have their own ways of designating districts and regions, local mental health programs had self-designated limits they regard as practical.

The community programs are locally generated, managed, and supported. Usually, a small group of highly motivated citizens and professional people give unstintingly of time and energy to establish a specific program and constitute its board and professional leadership. Money is sought, and often obtained, from United Good Neighbors, and for special purposes such as training, money is provided by the Health Department and the federal government (particularly the NIMH). The autonomous identification is intense. Those associated with many of these programs are proud of them and work hard for whatever small accomplishments they have achieved. Board members and professional persons involved in specific programs want increased support for their particular programs and are not greatly interested in coordinated, metropolitan-wide developments.

Evidence does exist that a growing group of persons who daily have to struggle with the crazy-quilt array of community agencies are more interested in effective coordination than are those involved in treatment programs within many of these agencies. School psychologists, consultants, and social workers confronted with an atomized collection of social service, welfare, and state agencies are as weary of the frustration of communicating with these units as they are aware of their own agency's inadequacies. The absence of effective coordinating units, particularly within local government, make the exchange of information, the transmittal of records, and referrals difficult. In point of fact, there is probably nothing to deter the Seattle–King County Health Department from serving in a coordinating capacity, though it does not do so.

On the other hand, fragmentation is not without its peculiar advantages. Variety could be discerned in the programs developed in the metropolitan area, no matter how inadequate they appear to their founders and administrators. The school systems in the region, for the most part, have their own programs, and some, such as the Shoreline and Seattle schools, do well in special fields. The scattering of autonomous units, therefore, provides a field in which experimental programs (though not necessarily regarded as such by their supporters) are begun and function in the chaotic welter of local government agencies. In a unified jurisdiction for governmental services, with required county or metrowide support for approval, funds, and supervision, some good programs might not survive the inevitable budgetary battles or the uniformity-seeking tendency of centralized administration.

It is not surprising that Seattle–King County Health Department offered no mental health treatment services at all in 1964 and only very limited education and consultative services. There is no reason to suppose that local units of government will have a rapid change of heart. Some members of the Seattle City Council seem interested in publicly supported mental health programs, as does one of the county commissioners. For the immediate future it can be anticipated that whatever mental health policy and action is made locally will be spearheaded by the private sector. If the existing pattern is continued, policy initiative and a major share of operating budgets will come from it.

INFORMAL STRUCTURE OF COMMUNITY RELATIONS IN THE MENTAL HEALTH FIELD

Mental health programs in the Seattle area, as in the state of Washington, are low-pressure, low-priority activities. Persons with professional interests or those directly or indirectly affected by the problems of mental illness and mental retardation provide the leadership. Small numbers of persons are involved in the mental health field. The prejudices and historically hostile attitudes toward mental illness and retardation have only recently undergone modification. The improvement of mental health services in the state government did not get underway until the mid-1950s, and most of the mental health and retardation programs in the Seattle area are recent.

Seattle's social structure, its power and decision-making components, have not been studied systematically, but one might suggest two differing though not unrelated hypotheses. One is a power elitist establishment picture of Seattle. The other emphasizes a "multi-nucleated" decision-making complex for the metropolitan area. The establishment idea holds that decisions are made in Seattle by certain civic, professional, and business leaders. The names of members of the establishment appear time and time again on the rosters of civic boards, as patrons of civic functions, and as entrepreneurial guides of civic enterprises. Its critics argue that the establishment is a power clique dedicated to the maintenance of a social and economic status quo. The Seattle establishment has its greater and lesser lights. It exhibits a strong defensive pride in the metropolitan region and a desire to maintain Seattle's control as the financial and social capital of the area. Its membership is large enough so that there is considerable dispersion in its actions and activities depending on individual interest and inclination. For example, those concerned with education serve on school boards and take part in related educational programs; those interested in transportation devote their energies to such problems as a second or third span over Lake Washington. Some overlapping in membership is evident. The ties are social and to an extent economic and financial. Large ventures such as the financially successful Seattle World's Fair of 1962 required the resources and cooperation of a substantial proportion of community leadership. Other civic activities may find the group fairly well dispersed. No evidence exists of a consciously organized formal structure, though unifying social associations exist in the Rainier Club and other exclusive organizations. If one accepts the power elitist concept, he would say that the Seattle establishment is a fluid, somewhat oligarchical leadership of long-time residents.

Multi-nucleation of the decision process in Seattle and other urban areas is defined as a system that exists when control over events within a metropolitan area is decentralized among a number of jurisdictions which are formally independent of each other.[12] In relating the establishment thesis to multi-nucleation one sees the former as a stimulus and instrument for implementing decisions arrived at, on occasion, through the bargaining process inherent in the latter. In encompassing mental health decision making in the multi-nucleated construct, one must bear

[12] Robert Warren, "A Theoretical Framework of Change: A Case Study of the Seattle Metropolitan Area," supplement, *The Western Political Quarterly*, XIV, No. 3 (Sept. 1961), 40.

in mind functional disjointedness as well. Most mental health programs are encased in autonomous organizations, and their leaders have not been motivated to view their relationship to the whole of either the community or the mental health complex. This helter-skelter pattern, if imposed on a multi-nucleated government structure, does not make for metropolitanwide solutions to the problems of mental health programing. The sense of suburban autonomy in the Seattle metropolitan area is strong. Within the mental health field, program autonomy is equally tenacious. Possibly, the mental health planning now underway may result in a network of interaction based upon common needs. Such a network could lead, in turn, to working out the relationships to meet that need without threatening the existing support structure in the community.

An array of agencies and organizations could be identified as interest groups that operate to support or oppose communitywide mental health measures. Interest groups in the mental health field in Seattle perform centripetal and centrifugal functions. An interest group is centripetally oriented when its contribution and/or support is necessary to establish and maintain a policy. A group is centrifugal in that it will tend to pull a policy commitment to its own orbit and interpret the policy and act in the light of its own needs and interests. An effective mental health policy for Seattle would have to bring about the confluence of the purposes of numerous groups and organizations that, up to this moment, have not had to be concerned with a common policy. The present mental health programs arose in the absence of an integrated or common policy.

The major mental health interest groups in Seattle fall into four categories: (1) organizations and groups professionally involved in the field, (2) program activities groups, (3) active state and local groups, and (4) community support groups.

The psychiatrists are critically important in the making of mental health decisions in the community. Their support is essential to the success of a program; their veto can prevent a program from achieving its purposes. As a group, however, the psychiatrists of Seattle are not particularly active. Most of them are in private practice. Their clientele, it is reasonable to assume, is almost wholly limited to middle- and upper middle-class groups. A Committee of Psychiatrists for Community Action of the American Psychiatric Association helped convene the first Congress on Mental Health in the state but does not appear to have accomplished much else. This committee was abolished and the Northwest Chapter of the American Psychiatric Association was formed. Its meetings are reportedly not very well attended and it has taken no positive action in the community mental health field. Psychiatrists are themselves divided as to the feasibility of community centers. The upshot of these differences, which on occasion were debated at professional meetings, is a reluctance to take strong policy action. However, a number of psychiatrists, acting as individuals, are actively engaged in the planning process.

Divisions of opinion among the psychiatrists practicing in the Seattle area further frustrated any development toward unified professional support. Seattle psychiatrists differ over the effectiveness of various methods of therapy. The local psychiatric community numbers about sixty, not small for an area of that size and population. But it is divided into analytic and nonanalytic camps. Most of those psychiatrists who are active in local mental health services lack knowledge of community developments and demonstrate only a limited concern. For the most part, the psychiatrists in private practice are extremely busy and, in some instances, have to turn away patients. Little time is left for community activity.

The state Medical Association has been strongly skeptical about community mental health centers, especially if the Department of Institutions was to run them. The director of the Division of Mental Health and the president of the Medical Association both expressed doubts about the centers' usefulness. The association tends to support the Department of Health as against the Department of Institutions in the rivalry between these agencies. It is not unlikely that the physicians of the state of Washington and the Seattle community, through their medical associations, will lobby against the establishment of direct community mental health units.

The clinical psychologists are another potentially important group in securing mental health services, but they are not organized for action in the public sphere. While the majority of clinical psychologists are employed in community and public agencies, they number only a total of twenty-seven persons. There was not more than an additional ten in private practice.

The Alcoholism Treatment Clinic in Seattle began operations in 1959. A good functional working relation exists between the Alcoholism Treatment Clinic and other agencies. For example, the Community Psychiatric Clinic refers those requiring such treatment to it almost as a matter of course. The alcoholism treatment program, while supported by state funds, regards its program as one apart from mental health. Supporters of the program in Seattle argued that it would suffer if it became identified with mental health. Mental health advocates have tried to persuade supporters of the alcoholism program that it belongs in the general mental health framework, but they have not been successful. Alcoholism treatment proponents agreed to take part in the King county mental health planning process, however, and this was considered by mental health planners as something of a moral victory.

The Atlantic Street Community Center, with its concern for problem children of junior high school age, is a specialized undertaking. The director of the center states that he participates only in those organizations of benefit to his organization; he feels that his agency serves a clientele group, lower-class minority groups, in which no one else has any real interest. As such, he and his charges are somewhat isolated.

The Crisis Clinic was formed in 1963 under the energetic leadership of a small group of professional, clergy, business, and academic people. The founders of this suicide prevention center sought state support at the outset and were, at one point, quite willing to have the state assume entire responsibility for its operations. Then its leaders ran into what they regarded as a barrier of sympathetic noninvolvement and decided to "go it alone." A board was founded, a telephone number was assigned even before the staff was readied, and the clinic, in effect, found itself in business. It did receive the half-time assistance, for a three-month period, of a Department of Institutions clinical psychologist. Conceivably, the Crisis Clinic could be counted upon to contribute to the development of overall publicly supported community mental health programs.

The Community Psychiatric Clinic has the advantage (and disadvantage) of being an "established" institution. It is something of a vested interest. It has been criticized by publicly oriented psychiatrists and psychologists for its long waiting lists, the slowness of its treatment, and its relatively meager (as perceived by its critics) contribution to community mental health. The director of the clinic is not a strong partisan of public support. In his judgment, federal pump priming, even state support, would not be as effective as private community commitment. Since the Community Psychiatric Clinic receives both United Good Neighbors support and an NIMH training grant, its leadership ostensibly is sensitive to these aspects of support. Whether or not it will become a positive force in moving toward metropolitanwide programs is difficult to decide. Its leadership has its hands full in maintaining the current program.

The Eastside Community Psychiatric Clinic (situated to serve the area on the eastern shore of Lake Washington) is relatively new. It receives some state support and occupies space provided by the Seattle–King County Health Department. Originally under some pressure to regard itself as a branch of the Community Psychiatric Clinic, its supporters decided to work independently. Its initial success makes it difficult to assess it as a contributor to any highly structured metropolitan organization or plan.

Taken as a whole, the degree of active leadership and support from the mental health organizations for a communitywide program is negligible. They are too busy and too poor. Those engaged in publicly and privately supported mental health activities sometimes are willing to take part in mental health planning, but they will not easily sacrifice their identification with programs for which they have labored long and hard.

The Mental Health Unit of the Seattle–King County Health Department is a relative newcomer. It does not provide direct psychiatric treatment, but its director feels a strong obligation to lead developing mental health community programs. The community, as he sees it, must be made to appreciate the problem of mental health. The director is active in King county's planning unit for mental health. Weak as it is, the Mental Health Unit is one of the few forces for the development of mental health services on a regional basis.

The Seattle–King County Mental Health Association has not been strong. After a period of travail that included being dropped from the United Good Neighbors rolls, it was reactivated in 1962 and hired a full-time director in April 1964. A new board of directors was appointed and the national office of the Mental Health Association provided a loan of $10,000. The leaders of the state and community interested in developing mental health programs made a conscious effort to activate the Mental Health Association, but it has not proven to be an effective spokesman for mental health.

In Seattle, as in many other parts of the country, there has been a tendency to separate concern for retarded persons from concern for mental illness. The Washington Association for Retarded Children is the most active group of its kind in the state. Its King county branch is no less vigorous. It emphasizes that four mentally retarded babies are born in Washington state every day. The Department of Institutions' waiting list of those who are totally dependent is increasing at the rate of one person a day. The association has been fighting for improved custodial care, research, and better educational facilities. The major interest of the association has been the establishment of a multiple-purpose center for the retarded in King county. Members of the association have worked with skill and vigor in this direction. They also played an active role in the state planning function on mental retardation.

There is no evidence, however, on the part either of mental health or mental retardation program supporters of a desire to merge. For planning purposes on a statewide basis, the two were brought together under the same roof. But separate budgets, professional staffs, and task force committees were maintained.

Ordinarily an agency such as the United Good Neighbors would not be considered an interest group. In Seattle its primary function is to provide support through planning, budgeting, and fund raising. A number of agencies engaged in mental health activities, including the Community Psychiatric Clinic, the Atlantic Street Center, and the Ryther Child Center, receive UGN assistance. The UGN's position on mental health programing has been important and its views carry considerable weight in the community.

The UGN is reluctant to take on additional mental health work. It is satisfied with its current support of agencies providing direct and indirect mental health services. Anxiety over declining UGN revenues undoubtedly have influenced this position. At the same time, the low pressure of mental health demands also has contributed to the organization's reluctance to support additional mental health services. UGN's position is one of a watchful observer and contributor to existing services. Several key members of its board and of its Council of Planning Affiliates have been active in mental health and retardation planning. The extent to which the UGN will participate in the implementation of the new community mental health program will depend upon how much financial support the federal and state governments will provide.

As with the UGN, the Seattle Area Hospital Council does not fall precisely within the category of a mental health interest group. Yet it clearly influences any community decision affecting the deployment or employment of hospital facilities. In fact, it has a veto over hospital utilization on a broad scale.

The Health Facilities Planning and Development Board of the council deals with such matters as long-range planning for mental health care in the hospitals in the area. The planning board engages in research and helps hospitals obtain federal grants. The view of the board is that a general hospital is the best place to locate mental health facilities regardless of the nature of the services to be rendered. Mental health is but one aspect of the total health picture. Hospitals have traditionally ministered to all health needs, hence the board feels it is only proper that hospitals be considered as the most rational facility for mental health purposes. It remains to be seen how the council would react to pressures for alternative solutions to mental health problems, including the establishment of centers removed from the physical facilities of a hospital.

There is no strong, well-organized mental health group in the informal group structure in the Seattle metropolitan area. The mental retardation program is in a better position since the Association for Retarded Children fulfills that role. But in the mental health field, there is only an amorphous array of groups, each advocating its own program and unwilling to sacrifice its independence for the good of the larger cause.

There is no fervent grassroots movement in favor of a strong community mental health program. Existing organizations are more interested in maintaining their own programs. Integrated community action does not appear to offer any resolution to their problems. Adjustment to a federally sponsored and state-stimulated concept would take time, adequate financing, and a guarantee of the maintenance of existing programs. Little likelihood appears that any attempt to integrate health services, more than in a loose confederation, would succeed.

The state government holds a key position in Seattle as well as in other communities in Washington. State leadership and support are critical if community-centered programs are to be launched at all. On the basis of experience, it appears that the conflict between the two major state agencies will prevent integrated action. It remains to be seen how much this situation can be changed by the Governor's Mental

Health and Mental Retardation Planning Committee, under the chairmanship of Professor Charles Strother of the University of Washington. The veto potential of the key groups appears greater than their ability to effect positive action. The professional groups, the agencies directly providing mental health services, the community support groups, the UGN, the Hospital Council can prevent mental health programs from being effective. Some, such as the professional associations, could withhold the legitimizing function of recognition and accreditation for practice, and the absence of such official cognizance could prove disastrous to the early nurturing of mental health centers. Others, especially those with influential boards and perhaps more broadly based popular support, could create so much hostility that a fledgling experimental program would be smothered. Even the absence of support from such a broadly based agency as the United Good Neighbors would in itself be disastrous.

The prospects for positive development are not as bleak as one might gather from these comments. Elements of change are in the air, if not clearly apparent. The governor's committee managed to interest a wider spectrum of leadership in mental health problems than one would have thought possible. Through its county committees substantial numbers of persons were invited to participate in gathering of data. This information-securing process helped to involve and educate people in the needs and requirements of mental health services to which the public sector might contribute funds, organization, and manpower.

This action must be placed alongside the fact of governmental fragmentation. Rapid population growth and the interest of suburban communities in facilities to treat mental disorders could lead to more territorial fragmentation. The generalized response to governmental fragmentation is to circumvent or manipulate it. Territorial boundaries tend to be set by the limits of a program rather than by any governmental pattern. Yet, the existence of widespread fragmentation or multi-nucleation does discourage a regionwide governmental approach to a problem of public concern. The impact of sewage on the pollution of Lake Washington has been the only issue to secure metropolitanwide support and to sustain metropolitanwide action.

The fragmented pattern of governments in the Seattle metropolitan area makes it difficult to construct programs tied to local units. A relevant exception to fragmentation was the Seattle–King County Health

Department, which however does not serve southern Snohomish county, which is part of the metropolitan area.

Leadership to promote improved services for the mentally ill in Seattle is not easy to find. Those who spearheaded mental health programs are usually devoted to a single program; therefore influential voices for community mental health movements have yet to be heard. The new concern for statewide and community planning could make a difference. It is possible to discern increased awareness and articulation of community needs. Opposition to mental health programs in the community is negligible and comes mainly from the crackpot fringe with no significant leadership locus.

Most of the professional groups in the field support some sort of mental health community program, as they indicated at the Regional Conference on Mental Health and Mental Retardation in 1964 at the University of Washington. The conclusions and report of the conference constituted a comprehensive set of demands for virtually all phases of mental health and mental retardation programing.[13] Generally, some sort of public response was prescribed.

It was clear that the professionals have a significant role to play. Any public program must rely upon the active support and broad cooperation of its practicing experts. For example, shortages of trained personnel would require sustained effort by those working in the field. Without the support and positive contributions of the majority of professional and technical personnel it would be impossible to build a strong community program. Yet, until the planning process was begun little had been done to bring about support from this crucial segment.

Active politicians in the maze of governmental units in the region have not been leaders in demanding mental health programs. Only one Seattle city councilman took part in the planning sessions, and only one city councilwoman could generally be counted upon to support such measures. The remainder of the Seattle City Council were not vitally concerned with mental health and many privately disapprove of a community-oriented program. One of the three county commissioners favored effective development of mental health programs. The mayor

[13] King County Medical Society *et al., Regional Conference on Mental Health and Mental Retardation* (Seattle: Governor's Mental Health and Mental Retardation Planning Committee, 1964).

of Seattle is not enthusiastic about mental health planning but could be expected to respond to strong community pressures.

In concluding this section one can only emphasize that the informal structure of mental health programs in the Seattle metropolitan area is loose, its peripheries not easily defined. The new element favoring effective programs was the Governor's Mental Health and Mental Retardation Planning Committee. Its actions in calling congresses and conferences, establishing county planning units, appointing task forces, and indicating the possibility of broad community and governmental support for mental health awakened interest and prompted involvement. The most important catalyst at the outset was Professor Charles R. Strother. He used involvement as a technique to bring together all groups of professionals in the work of his committee. His success in overcoming a high degree of professional and program isolation will be determined by his ability to activate the groups and organizations involved in the mental health field.

Decision Making in Mental Health

Decisions may be clear-cut or vague, consciously derived or accidental, directly germane to the issue at hand or subsidiary and supportive. The clustering of decisions affecting mental health policies may include decisions that are antithetical to the positive values held by proponents of mental health programs. This large and complex variety of commitments to act and react stems from the formal and informal group interaction, from formal commitments forged over a period of time, from informal self-perceptions, and from the inevitable ecological relationship of men, groups, and organizations to other men, groups, and organizations that constitute their environment.

The skills that are utilized in existing services taken together constitute a vital cadre of talent that is needed in any community program. The psychiatrists, psychologists, and psychiatric and other social workers are the core of professional leadership. Unless the community were to be inundated by incoming professional personnel to work in a greatly expanded community program, professional support is essential to a more integrated mental health activities scheme. To those professionally engaged in therapy must be added the professional and nonprofessional persons who serve as administrators of existing agencies. Not only would their knowledge be necessary to the installation and implementation of a larger scheme, but their active cooperation is essential as well.

The professional and lay leadership of the various boards that underpin the voluntary agencies serve as important links to the community. Most of the currently operating programs are a result of the considerable energy expended by the relatively small groups of people who perceive a need and utilize their talents and skills to structure a service to meet it. Obviously, such persons have a strong sense of identification and loyalty to their programs.

Planning in the metropolitan area was begun with the Regional Conference on Mental Health and Mental Retardation, convened in Seattle on June 27, 1964, at the University of Washington. The conference was called by the Governor's Mental Health and Mental Retardation Planning Committee and was cosponsored by the committee, the Washington State Medical Association, and the King County Medical Society. The 230 persons who attended represented the spectrum of interests and services in mental health and retardation.

Political leaders unfortunately were absent. General invitations had been sent by members of the governor's committee staff, which had made the conference arrangements, and it was assumed that city councilmen and county commissioners would not require a reminder. The omission was serious, for the conference would have provided an invaluable orientation for those persons from whom formal legislative sanction would have to be obtained.

In the context of framing policy decisions the conference was important. For the first time in the region a large group of persons were brought together to discuss their interests and needs in the field. The parameters of perceived needs were articulated and recorded. Second, the field was established for future operations. Third, the relationship of the Governor's Committee on Mental Health and Mental Retardation Planning to local planning was established. Chairman Strother of the governor's committee emphasized the committee's intent to have local committees organized on county lines (bi- or tri-county in the less populous regions of the state) and prepare plans under the general guidance of the governor's committee. The conference was a kick-off event, to inform the interested public, to have a variety of needs expressed, and to lead into the formation of the local King County Mental Health and Mental Retardation Planning Committee following the conference. The committee held its first formal meeting on July 9, 1964, and from that point much of the formal planning was in its hands.

With 33 per cent of the state's population, King county looms large in any statewide activity. It has most of the professional staff, particularly in private practice, most of the facilities, and the most impressive financial resources. Compared to the rest of the state its problems are of a different dimension. King county had its voluntary programs at the outset. While King county's progress has been slow, uneven, and not without internecine tensions; it did not have voluntary programs at the outset, and the majority of the regions outside the county had nothing.

The governor's Planning Committee had stressed the fact that regional committees should represent all segments of mental health programs as well as general community leadership. Fourteen categories of groups were represented in the King county committee, including churches, medical associations, schools, and local government. Fifty-four persons were invited to join the committee, but attendance at regular meetings varied from twenty-seven to sixty. In large measure the work was done by subcommittees.

At its first official meeting following the organization session, Seattle city councilman Wing Luke was elected chairman and Murray Meld, director of planning for the United Good Neighbors, secretary–vice president. Thus, two key persons whose support would be important to the implementation of any plan were placed in positions of formal leadership. The executive committee of nine members appointed by the chairman also was broadly representative.

The purpose of the county committee was prescribed by the governor's Planning Committee. It was to gather data and devise a program for the county that would be integrated into the state plan. Because the group was representative, it was hoped that a *modus operandi* could be negotiated for both the design and implementation of a countywide program.

One of the major difficulties encountered by the committee was the lack of staff, since the information to be gathered was very extensive. Furthermore, the sensitivities of those who were strongly committed to existing programs were obvious. After a few monthe of work, rivalries began to manifest themselves and some criticism of the data-gathering process was voiced.

The summary report of the state coordinating subcommittee on mental health contained few surprises. Its inventory of agencies revealed over-lap, conflict, duplication, and the absence of communications "in the schools particularly." [14] It was difficult to obtain records of what agencies were doing to assist particular cases. The committee found no central clearance mechanism. In the case of youngsters, parents would try to use every possible resource, which produced duplication of services. The question of distance from service facilities was noted. The subcommittee was not certain of the implications of its findings, but noted that the planning group would need to talk with knowledgeable people in outlying districts to assess how services are restricted by the distances that must be traveled by prospective recipients.

The range and capacities of services were found insufficient. It was difficult to find treatment for certain types of disorders and, equally important, for continuing services. Most children lacked preventive treatment, day-care, and residential care. The length of waiting lists was noted, as well as the fact that many agencies that had to turn away clients did not carry them on their lists.

In every way suggested by the governor's Planning Committee staff, the King county subcommittee on mental health felt that policy changes and methods were necessary to enable existing services to "cope more effectively with existing needs." It agreed on the need for better inter-agency cooperation, improved communication between agencies, better uses of available professional people, and for more and better trained staff. As for "new services" to be provided by existing agencies, the subcommittee suggested that a community council be established that would meet regularly to coordinate programs. New agencies were needed for diagnoses and evaluation, half-way houses for returned patients were required, as well as housekeeping services, local emergency psychiatric and expanded alcoholic care. In fact, the subcommittee asked for virtually the whole gamut of mental health programs.

The subcommittee agreed that an interagency mechanism would be helpful. The United Good Neighbors' Council on Planning Affiliates might provide an answer "as it represented central planning supported

[14] King County Mental Health and Mental Retardation Planning Committee, *Sub-Committee Report* (Seattle: mimeographed, 1964).

by voluntary funds and covered all agencies both public and private."
If it undertook this task, however, the council would have to be brought
into more direct and frequent contact with problems of cooperation,
communications, etc. on an "everyday operation" basis.

Unfortunately, the subcommittee did not consider itself competent
to discuss the matter of private insurance for mental health or the
financing of mental health, which it thought should be done by the
county planning group as a whole, nor did it attempt to deal with a
number of problems it felt had been adequately considered at the
regional conference the preceding June. The subcommittee recommended the committee seek expert advice upon special problems such
as determining the proportion of cost for mental health services which
could be carried by private insurance. In attempting to answer questions on community orientation toward mental illness, the subcommittee
thought that these questions should be answered by a panel of people
who carry a daily caseload as practitioners, not administrators.

The subcommittee on mental retardation was more specific in its
analysis and proposals than its mental health counterpart. In admirable
detail the subcommittee offered its proposals, agency-to-agency, serv-
ice-to-service, including budgetary recommendations, translating need
into financial terms. It found inadequacies everywhere. It reported that
the retarded of King county were estimated to number about 30,000,
or 3 per cent of the population. Existing services would be inadequate
even if the figure were only 2 per cent. The four state institutions for
the retarded served a total of 4,000, but they must serve the whole
state. They cared for a small percentage of the King county retarded.
The special education classes in King county would have a total enrollment of 2,764 for 1964–1965. The school-age retarded in King
county were estimated to number about 7,000, and adult retarded
were estimated at about 14,000. Known work opportunities in sheltered
workshops totaled about 150. Of the young adults graduating from Pacific School, only a fraction were able enough to take vocational training.

While the King county committee was still at work an important
event took place which presented new difficulties. The Department of
Institutions' Division of Mental Health received a hospital improvement program grant from the federal government to establish a King
county psychiatric unit in association with Western State Hospital but

located in King County General Hospital to evaluate potential admission to that facility and make recommendations to both the psychiatric staff and the committing court of courses of action that most clearly will meet patient needs. Furthermore, the staff of the King county unit would assist in establishing liaison with agencies, professional personnel, and others to facilitate the eventual transfer of the unit to the community. This was part of the Division of Mental Health's program to relate the isolated state hospitals to the rapidly growing urban communities.

King County Hospital was reluctant to provide space for the proposed new state unit. Its own psychiatric unit, which had been working under the handicap of inadequate support for a number of years, had a plan of its own for community involvement and it did not welcome a new state unit. Furthermore, the University of Washington School of Medicine's Department of Psychiatry had its own plans for becoming the regional center and at the same time providing an expanded training program in the mental health field for the entire state. Thus, the university's Department of Psychiatry was reluctant to endorse either the county or state proposal.

This battle of the giants presented the King county planning committee with a very real dilemma. It is reasonable to assume that local service agencies were confused by these conflicting proposals. On the other hand, one or all of the proposals, if they could have been integrated into a feasible plan and linked to existing services, might have provided an impressive beginning that the community as a whole could support. Furthermore, the establishment of a program under the auspices of any one or a combination of the agencies wanting to become involved would guarantee a professional standard of service otherwise difficult to attain. Nor was there any evidence of an emergent leadership other than that assumed by the university, Department of Institutions, and King County Hospital agencies. The major stimulus still came from outside the region.

The work of the county planning committee has been reviewed in some detail because it remains the central decision-making mechanism in the mental health and mental retardation fields. Programing for mental retardation did not pose as great a problem as in mental illness. Those supporting the development of effective programs in retardation were well organized, energetic, and successful. Within the mental health area there appeared to be little dynamism, but the activation of the state and county agencies might provide the spark out of which a program could be forged.

FINANCING MENTAL HEALTH ACTIVITIES

The pattern of financing mental health programs must be viewed from a number of perspectives. The community must make the basic value choice as to whether it wants to support expanded, publicly financed and operated mental health programs. This choice must be more articulate than it has been in the past, particularly in the Seattle metropolitan region and in the state. If the community so chooses, the resources are available, but other programs may be lowered in the priority scale as mental health is upgraded.

Once the choice to support public mental health programs is made, technical considerations become relevant. Any financial scheme must certainly be related to existing program objectives and systems of support. Additional legislation may be required to provide more adequate underpinnings. Constitutional limitations on financial patterns in the state of Washington are strict. Statutory authorization and amendments, however, could be sought if necessary to provide adequate structural support.

The restrictive nature of the Washington state revenue system has been referred to early in this study. Basically, three categories of funds are set up at the state level. The general fund is made up of a general account and a number of special fund components. The convenience of this arrangement can be seen in the fact that the general account deficit (overdraft) can be counterbalanced by surpluses in the special fund components and thus facilitate the overall administration and accounting of the fund. Thus, "while the general account showed an overdraft of $16.8 million at the end of the first year of the current biennium, the special accounts showed a total working balance of $35.7 million." [15] A second category includes special funds for ear-

[15] George A. Shipman, "A Projection of Washington's Financial Needs," *Washington Law Review*, Vol. 39, No. 5, p. 982, which has been used for the projections that follow.

marked revenues (motor vehicle, game, liquor excise), bond issues, bond retirement, and interest funds. In the third category are the local funds.

The three major programs supported by the general account fund of the general fund were public instruction, institutions, and public assistance. Together they accounted for approximately 92 per cent of appropriations in the general account fund. Professor G. A. Shipman has indicated that "the programs financed from the general account of the general funds are the ones most sensitive to the yield of the general revenue system." Thus, these three primary components are most visible and most subject to public and legislative scrutiny. The pattern of growth and need has been clearly discernible. Professor Shipman estimates that the appropriation for education for the 1963–1965 biennium, which was $598.8 million, may increase to $915–996.5 million for 1969–1971. His figure included public schools, higher education, and other educational programs tabulated in the general fund. In public assistance, Professor Shipman sees overall expenditures increasing, although less dramatically than in education. More significant, he sees the federal contribution as increasing in percentage terms and the state burden actually decreasing.

The Department of Institutions' demands on the general account, which includes juvenile rehabilitation, adult corrections, veterans' homes, and schools for the handicapped, as well as mental hospitals and mental retardation programs, showed a projected growth from $84.27 million appropriated in 1963–1965 to $101.9 million for the 1969–1971 biennium. The projection took into consideration the decline in patient years and the increase in admissions, revealing the shift in emphasis from custodial to intensive short-term therapy. It also included the increase in cost per patient-day expenditures as the quality of care improves, improvement that leads to shorter patient stays in the hospital.

Both cities and counties in Washington operate under millage limitations. Counties are restricted to a ceiling of eighteen mills, which includes from seven to ten mills designated for county roads. Cities are restricted generally to fifteen mills, which accounts, statewide, for about 40 per cent of their operating income, the remainder coming from utility collections, the business and occupation tax, property improvement assessments, fines, fees, and service charges. These limitaons have encouraged the utilization of service fee oriented enterprises, pecially funded and outside the pale of the local government general unds. With increasing costs and increasing demands for services the ressure for increased millage has been intensifying.

In King county in 1962, 38 per cent of its governmental revenues ame from the general property tax. This included the eight-mill maxinum permitted for general county government collected from incoriorated as well as unincorporated territories. An additional ten mills, vhich could be expended only on county roads, was collected in uninorporated areas. The remaining revenue sources included receipts rom the motor vehicle (and state gasoline) fund, restricted to roads, nd a portion of state liquor revenues that could be used for general und purposes. The state also contributed 82 per cent of the cost of he county hospital, which in 1962 amounted to $4.5 million, the renainder coming from service fees. Service revenues generally accounted or 12.6 per cent of the total in 1962, bond issues for 13.5 per cent; .6 per cent came from "other sources," including licensing, the issunce of permits, fines, penalties, the rental of equipment, and interest.[16]

In Seattle in 1963 the general property tax yielded 28 per cent of he "operating dollar." The business and occupations tax accounted or 20 per cent and included revenues from business, utilities, occupaion, loan companies, and admission taxes. The city's share of revenues rom state agencies and the counties (including liquor sales and excise, asoline, motor vehicle excise, and King county grants) came to 15 ier cent of the total. Use of money and property (general government eceipts, pension funds, parking meters, etc.) contributed 10 per cent. The remainder of the revenues came from a variety of sources, inluding fines and fees, departmental service, property improvements ssessments, garbage utility collections, sewer utility collections, and egulatory and other licenses.[17]

The financial picture within the metropolitan area is healthy. Both he county and Seattle, as well as the smaller cities in the metropolitan egion, are financially holding their own. One may question, however, he extent of services and their quality. In 1962 Seattle ranked four-

[16] League of Woman Voters of King County, Wash., *A Second Look at King County Government* (Seattle: League of Women Voters, 1964), pp. 14–16.
[17] City of Seattle, Wash., *Annual Financial Report of the Comptroller for the Fiscal Year Ended December 31, 1963* (Seattle: City of Seattle, 1964), pp. 20–21.

teenth among the sixteen cities of 500,000 to 1,000,000 population in total general expenditures. It was eleventh in the field of sixteen in total revenues.

The best available data on the costs of mental health services in relation to need, including projections of the economic gains of effective therapy, were prepared by the Task Force on Economics of the Governor's Committee on Mental Health and Mental Retardation Planning. The committee computed as best it could the direct costs (for therapy) and the indirect costs (losses to the economy of the state due to incapacitated earning power). It is understood that any designation and computation of indirect costs is very crude and inexact. The direct costs of mental illness in 1962 were estimated by the task force to be $35 million. This figure excluded federal expenditures and drugs. The indirect costs were about $20 million. Some specific evidence was provided by a recent study of economic costs of therapy in Washington state, which indicated that the average length of stay per patient had been reduced from twenty-four to eighteen months in the past decade. Intensive, short-term therapy was being used increasingly "at only very modest increases in direct expenditures." [18] Over the ten-year period this innovation in therapy and its consequent reduction in the length of stay might possibly have added $6 million annually to the state's income.

The estimated cost for outpatient service was found to be $115 per patient served per year. This figure was based on the information provided by clinics in the state reporting under the Uniform Reporting Program of the NIMH. The figure was an average, with costs ranging from $50 to slightly over $200 per patient. The median figure was about $100 per patient, but to this had to be added the increased, and thoroughly realistic, cost of having to rely more and more upon the private sector of psychiatry for services.

The best estimate was that approximately 37 per cent of the state's population would avail itself of such services if offered. The annual patient load would approximate 90,000 and the total cost for this outpatient service would therefore be about $10,350,000.

To outpatient and inpatient services had to be added the cost of

[18] Mental Health and Mental Retardation Planning Committee, *Report on Task Force on Economics, Kenneth McCaffree, Chairman* (Seattle: Mental Health and Mental Retardation Planning Office, 1965), p. 4.

partial hospitalization, which the task force estimated would be utilized by about 7,000 patients annually at a cost of $1,050,000.

The three figures cited total $12,840,000 per annum. If estimates for the other components of community services were added, including emergency services, expatient services, consultation, education, community planning, and similar important functions, the task force estimated an additional $2.5 million per annum would be added to the previous total. Thus, the cost for comprehensive community mental health care, in gross dollar terms, using current figures on mental health needs and costs, would be $15,340,000 per annum.

The task force assumed that the role of the state hospital would obviously change if community mental health programs were initiated. If the state hospital system did not move into the community, possibly as few as 20 per cent of the present hospital admissions would have to be cared for by state hospitals after a comprehensive community service had been established.

In fact, numerous alternatives for the support of a comprehensive community mental health scheme were offered by the task force. It was suggested that consideration might be given to having the individual pay a greater proportion of services than heretofore had been the case: "only about 15 per cent of the state hospital costs are now paid directly by patients, and this percentage has not changed for 15 years." Insurance programs were becoming increasingly available and, in view of short-term therapy and a great reliance on outpatient and partial hospitalization, it might be possible for the family to pay for a greater share. This possibility was unlikely in the near future, however, so the public would be asked to assume the burden.

Three alternatives thus remained: federal and state sources, local government sources, and volunteer community efforts. The voluntary community sources did not appear promising. The use of local government sources would really depend upon the willingness of the local communities, especially those in the Seattle metropolitan area, to divert money from other programs to mental health. The economics task force suggested that property tax funds being used for other programs might be diverted to mental health. For example, the decline of the tuberculosis program in recent years and the possibility that funds earmarked for its administration might be moved to mental health would no doubt receive careful consideration in the state.

One alternative raised by the task force was the division of costs among federal, state, local, voluntary, and service fee sources. The state, with federal support, might provide 60 per cent of the annual operating budget with the community providing the remaining 40 per cent "through local tax and voluntary funds and fees for service as paid by patients." The task force suggested that the state provide a total of $900,000 a year the first year and increase its contribution along with the local communities each year until, after ten years, a comprehensive scheme is achieved. Adjustments would obviously have to be made during this decennial period on the basis of the experience gained.

The task force estimates were, at best, informed conjectures. For the most part, the state had to bear virtually all the burden of operating the state mental hospitals and generally about 75 per cent of the cost of past and existing community-based programs. To provide 40 per cent of the cost for new services in the mental health field (new to the local units) would be to ask local units to assume responsibility for a program in which they had no past experience.

The SMSA 1960 total population for the Seattle area was 1,107,000. Using the 3 per cent utilization figure accepted by the economics task force, it could be estimated that 33,000 persons would have used such services if offered in the Seattle region at approximately $115 per patient per year, to total $3,795,000. For inpatient services, the estimated rate of utilization of 2 per 1,000 and the average number of days in the hospital projected at 8 days per patient provided a SMSA Seattle annual figure of 17,713 patient-days in hospitals (2,214 patients at 8 days per patient). At the cost figure of $30 per day for 17,713 days, the gross figure for inpatient service would have been $531,390 per annum. Again using task force reasoning, about 5/6 of the number of estimated inpatients would have required partial hospitalization, or 1,825, to which an additional ⅓, or 738, should be added, making the total partial hospitalization population 2,563 at a cost of $15 per day; the aggregate for partial hospitalization would be $384,450 per annum.

The sum of the estimates for the basic services for the SMSA Seattle region in 1960 would then have been:

Outpatient care	$3,795,000
Inpatient care	531,390
Partial hospitalization	384,450
	$4,710,840

If one added ⅙ of $4,710,840 (the approximate proportion of the present state total used by the task force) to represent emergency, expatient, consultation services, and educational and community planning functions, the addition would be $785,140.

The total estimate for mental health services in the metropolitan area (excluding mental retardation, for which comparable data was unavailable at the time of this study) amounted to an annual figure of $5,495,980. This sum was based on current population, so that any decennial projection would have to take into account population increments and increased costs of services. It is also possible that the estimate was conservative. Furthermore, the figures were based on gross population and cost; in all probability they could have been as much as ¼ over or under true experience data. Interestingly enough, however, the per capita expenditure for the metropolitan region was $4.96, which was below the overall state average for 1961.

The Seattle metropolitan area then would account for about ⅓ of the total state expenditures in the foreseeable future. This concentration could effect a certain economy of scale which, if realized on a statewide basis, would reduce the total cost of services to the state. On the other hand, the very concept of community mental health centers limits the amount of large-scale specialization, making the program rather more expensive. Only the experience of several years of a comprehensive network throughout the state or in a number of communities could provide the basis for judging the full social and economic impact of such a program.

As of the date of this study, the local governments spend little or nothing for direct costs in mental health services in the metropolitan region. The County Hospital support comes largely from the state; its mental health program is not adequate. School district programs are specialized and uneven. The bulk of the money spent in the metropolitan region for mental health and mental retardation services comes from federal or state funds and voluntary contributions. The funding does not approach the sums projected for comprehensive services, and voluntary funds are limited and certainly offer no prospect of backing for a comprehensive scheme.

One can only conclude that funds are insufficient now in the Seattle metropolitan area for mental health needs. They are not likely to become available in the future unless mental health can be given a much higher priority in the minds of political decision makers. If that can be done by rallying wide community support, funds no doubt can be made available, but even then it will not be easy.

MENTAL HEALTH MANPOWER

The overriding fact about mental health manpower in the state and metropolitan region is that, no matter how viewed, there are not enough people to staff publicly oriented programs, nor are there likely to be in the near future. A shortage exists in every category of the mental health field except patients. Thus, serious questions are raised about the capacity of the "best laid plans" to fulfill the desires of the mental health program enthusiasts, even if sufficient funding were available. Can current concepts of therapy be modified to compensate for the shortage of professional and subprofessional personnel currently regarded as essential? Can educational and professional programs be redesigned to provide greater output of trained personnel? These queries are basic to mental health planning and programing. No easy answers seem to be on anyone's horizon.

A recent survey by the American Psychiatric Association indicated there were 238 psychiatrists known to be residents of Washington, of whom 213 were in practice.[19] Approximately half of the number in practice were in the Seattle metropolitan area, although total population of the area is only one-third that of the state. If community centers were established in the metropolitan region, it is reasonable to assume that the majority of the psychiatrists in private practice or associated with the University of Washington would not take full-time employment with the centers. Thus, there might well be a need for twice the number of practicing psychiatrists as are now in the state.

While the psychiatrists in the state came from various schools and communities in the country, the resources of the state itself were important in the supply of additional professional personnel. The University of Washington School of Medicine was the sole supplier in this field. The School of Medicine sent 15 per cent of its graduates into psychiatry, 8 per cent above the national average. The task force on manpower and

[19] Mental Health and Mental Retardation Planning Committee, *Task Force Report on Manpower and Training; Dr. Thomas H. Holmes, Chairman* (Seattle: mimeographed, 1965), p. 3.

training conjectured that the reason for this was a "strong" department and the concentration of psychiatrists in the community.[20] The residency program in psychiatry at the University of Washington is the only fully accredited program in the state and includes child psychiatry as well as regular inpatient and outpatient services. The Department of Institutions maintains residency programs of a more limited sort at its Northern and Western State Hospitals. In 1964 the total output of psychiatrists in the state was about twelve to sixteen annually. This figure is not expected to increase significantly in the near future.

Both the University of Washington and Washington State University train clinical psychologists at the rate of ten to fifteen Ph.D.'s per year from each institution, regarded by the task force on manpower and training as "entirely inadequate to meet the needs of the state." The task force felt that the two major state universities were strongly oriented toward the production of research Ph.D.'s rather than therapists. As a professional degree the M.S. in psychology has been seriously downgraded. Both institutions of higher learning evidently use the degree for training junior-level researchers and junior college teachers. Most of the students are people who for one reason or another cannot go on to the Ph.D.

In 1952 the state of Washington required all nurses to have psychiatric training and practice in order to be registered. While the preparation in the past had varied and had been for the most part inadequate, those responsible for the preparation of nurses were in 1967 giving greater attention to more sophisticated approaches to mental health. Nursing curricula today emphasize integration of mental health aspects throughout the entire program.

The best estimate the task force could find for the number of nurses actively employed was 8,528 (a 1957 figure), 4,597 of whom were practical nurses. The task force also noted a potential resource of about 5,000 registered nurses who were inactive, but who kept their licenses current. The task force conjectured that a number of nurses on the inactive list might be sufficiently challenged by properly established

---

[20] *Ibid.* Unfortunately, figures were not available for the number of clinical psychologists and other psychologists practicing and/or employed by organizations and agencies for the state as a whole. The number of psychologists in private practice in King county was estimated by the Planning Committee staff to be ten full-time and fifteen part-time. No figures are available on the number of psychologists employed in public institutions or community organizations.

mental health programs to want to take an active part in them. No evidence was cited to support this contention.

The state's educational resources for nursing care will provide approximately 400 nurses annually. The University of Washington is the only institution offering graduate work in the nursing and allied fields. In 1963–1964 only eight of the fifty-one master's degrees in nursing were awarded for psychiatric nursing. Child psychiatric nursing was instituted in 1963, however, and plans are underway for post-master's work in mental retardation.

In view of the demands and turnover in the nursing profession, plus the chronic shortage of nurses, particularly those trained in the mental health fields, and more especially those who are oriented toward mental health with some training and background in public health, the situation in the state is serious.

No special survey was made of the number of social workers actively employed in the state or metropolitan region. The Graduate School of Social Work estimated the number to be about 1,000, of which one-third to one-half were employed in the Seattle region. The output of the Graduate School of Social Work, the only educational and training resource for social workers in the state, was from 65 to 70 each year with a planned increase to 125 in the next five years. All told, the demand for social workers will continue to exceed the supply that can be provided by the state's educational resource. In addition to its regular two-year graduate curriculum, the School of Social Work offered workshops for personnel of children's institutions and public welfare agencies.

Some attention was given in the state to providing training for the clergy. In 1964 the Department of Psychiatry at the University of Washington offered its first course exclusively for ministers. The Greater Seattle Council of Churches conducted a seminar for understanding the mentally retarded. While the preparation of individuals varied considerably, numerous clergymen in the region sought additional training in the mental health field.

Some mention should be made of preparation for teaching in the public schools. The various teacher education curricula include units on mental health and mental retardation. In counseling, guidance, and other forms of educational reinforcement activities, mental health training plays an increasingly significant role. The use of clinical psychologists and psychiatrists is more and more prevalent in school districts. However, school teachers in the state are in short supply and there are many vacancies. Indeed, the task force on manpower and training reported shortages in all classes and categories of mental health personnel.

The staffing problem for mental health is especially difficult because the field is so ill-defined. The skills necessary for manning community mental health centers demand a breadth of knowledge and creativity that is difficult to attain. The difficulty is that it is impossible to meet current staffing needs using traditional means, not to mention the requirements of a greatly expanded program. Where is the staff for the mental health centers to come from? Certainly the resources in the state of Washington would not provide them. Supplier states such as California, Massachusetts, and New York will themselves be hard-pressed for personnel. Furthermore, if the mobility of professional groups in other fields provides any index at all, such skilled persons are not likely to move to Washington.

It is also possible that current concepts of staffing will prove inadequate once the centers are established. Indeed, even if the broadest and most permissive concept of a center is used, the types of skills required to provide effective services might significantly alter with experience. Perhaps less formally trained, but no less competent, subprofessional categories might be devised to step up the output of qualified personnel. In-service training might be used more intensively than has been the case. Some of the traditional service components might be merged to share scarce manpower resources.

In a world of accelerating scientific knowledge and discovery, the very techniques and theories of diagnosis and therapy may change. Different skills, perhaps more specialized, perhaps more general, may be required to operate the centers. In this context, it might be wise at the outset to tie the centers to larger units, such as departments of mental health and universities.

One should keep in mind, too, the traditional intraprofessional rivalries. Relationships between the medical profession and the psychiatric community leave a great deal to be desired, to say nothing of problems within the psychiatric group itself. The roles of nurses, social workers, psychologists, and others have to be worked out, if possible, in such a way as to provide a maximum degree of effectiveness in the program of the centers.

In regard to good management, one of the psychiatrists interviewed for this study emphasized the need for skilled administrators to run the centers. He doubted whether there were enough trained people available to administer the number of centers projected for Seattle. He felt that the success of these enterprises might well hinge on the skills of a professionally trained psychiatric administrator. Therefore, he felt, it would be wiser to have one well-run center than four or five poorly run. He defined an administrator as one who could coordinate the resources and skills of the facility, and who could get the components working together smoothly.

SUMMARY AND FINDINGS

Governmental fragmentation reflects historical patterns of growth in which the political values of the society were assumed to be constant irrespective of its political organization. All the pieces of a fragmented metropolitan area are in form and theory democratically oriented. Popular controls through some system of representation, whether used or not, are invariably structured into the system.

Seattle is no exception to the prevalence of fragmentation. It is replete with governments, districts, and authorities of a variety of sorts, multi-purpose and special, each reflecting a public response to a demand for services. Governmental fragmentation in Seattle is the accepted way of life. Advocates of new programs accept it and attempt to manipulate its system.

Fragmentation is no serious deterrent to the development of new programs. It could even assist program development by providing the mechanisms for diverse, experimental attempts, as in the case of school districts whose programs are varied. It could also help to provide multi-based support for a program, and it could provide a jurisdictional sharing of the cost burden through contractual relations.

On the other hand, fragmentation can become fracture. Fragmentation does not necessarily inhibit the formation of regional organizations. Seattle's experience with metropolitan government is a case in point. When the dangers of water pollution were made clear and its regional implications became evident, a metropolitan unit was established. The same may prove true of metropolitan transportation, air pollution, and mental health.

Fragmentation does not preclude social homogeneity, or the existence of an amorphous, relatively open elite. Seattle is not without its activists and influentials, though their influence has yet to be empirically determined. Obviously it would help to have the establishment on one's side, but the amount of support necessary to start a program in mental health is an open question. Nor is it known whether the activist leaders can veto a broadly based popular program.

The mental health policy field in the state of Washington and in the Seattle metropolitan region is a relatively low-pressure area, quasi-private in the local sector, in the process of being upgraded under national stimulation. The provision of an outside catalyst, in this case the federal government, has had an impact on an atomized pattern of organizations and services. But, if there had not been a dispersion of local programs, each with its own enclave of support, the conflict between the two major agencies at the state level would have had a disastrous effect on mental health programs.

In Washington, as in other states, the proper perspective for analyzing mental health is to begin with the state and proceed to the community. Jurisdiction for mental health programs is divided between the Department of Institutions and the Department of Health. The state mental hospitals are under the control of the former and responsibility for the development of mental health community facilities (prior to the current federal legislation) rests with the Department of Health. In the 1950s the Department of Institutions was reformed; its Division of Mental Health was staffed with able and competent professional personnel. The state mental hospitals were overhauled and they, too, were staffed with the best available talent. As a consequence, the Division of Mental Health became in fact the mainspring of competence and program initiative in the state. Custodial care in the state hospitals was replaced by short-term, intensive therapy, and research became an important adjunct of the division's program. Inevitably, the division's professional personnel and leadership became increasingly interested in relating the state hospitals' functions to the community. Equally inevitably, this movement brought the Division of Mental Health into rivalry with the Health Department.

The Health Department, with a minimal staff in the mental health field, was oriented toward the traditional public health view and sought to build support in the communities for the design and development of programs. It was concerned with an epidemiological, preventive view toward mental health rather than the therapeutic focus that it attributed to the Institutions Department. Other state agencies involved in mental health were either interested in special programs, as was the Public Instruction Department, or were engaged in a service relationship with one or both departments, as was the Public Assistance Department. Their role in the formation of mental health policies for the state was secondary.

The rivalry between the Health and Institutions Department for jurisdiction in the mental health field became one of the facts of life in state administration. When federal money became available for planning purposes and for construction of community mental health centers, both agencies felt they warranted designation as the single mental health authority for the state. The resolution of the rivalry remains a major difficulty.

The governor's Committee on Mental Health and Mental Retardation Planning was established independently of either agency to develop a comprehensive plan for the state. It chose a path of representativeness and local participation, following the obvious requirements of federal legislation and the ideas of its leadership. It established its own staff and stimulated the development of local (county and multi-county) planning committees to draw up plans for community-oriented centers. Task forces of experts in the substantive fields of mental health and mental retardation were established to advise the Planning Committee and the local committees, and also to integrate their materials and help with the development of the state plan. To be sure, the various state departments, including those of Health and Institutions, were represented on the Planning Committee, and the Department of Health contributed the services of its leading mental health authority to the planning staff of the committee. Considerable energy and enthusiasm were generated in many local committees and positive programs were initiated in several communities. Some of the Planning Committee and its staff became concerned lest the enthusiasm fade at the time when positive community support might be required in the future.

If one views the state level in the context of decision making, it would appear that the field is congested. Numerous loci for decisions are discernible. The governor's Planning Committee has been the most active, if not the most powerful, and has built up a wellspring of community support for mental health programs. But it did not do much about the central problem of conflict between the Health and Institutions Departments at the state level. The legislature, meeting biennially, and preoccupied with other problems, including legislative reapportionment, has not taken a forceful position.

Also in the Seattle metropolitan region, the mental health field is atomized. With the exception of limited services offered by the county health department and the county hospital, local government services did not exist. Most services for citizens unable to afford help from the private sector are provided by voluntarily supported community agencies, and these are in short supply in the region. Two of the state mental hospitals serve the region but are not located in it. There is no integrating mechanism for screening and referring patients who need help.

Those agencies that do render mental health services are governed by private boards, many of them financially buttressed by UGN aid and by grants from state agencies and the federal government. For the most part, these agencies had been established only after considerable effort, usually by a small group of concerned citizens and an ardent professional staff. As a consequence, these people are identified strongly with their missions. This identity is an important element in understanding the response of such agencies' leadership toward any move in the establishment of community centers that requires the integration of a number of programs into a center.

Financing mental health programs could prove to be a serious problem. The question is basically one of choice and of the selection of mental health over other programs. If the community is willing to make the choice, the money can be diverted to support mental health. Money for existing programs is scarce and the costs for these programs are rising. But effective mental health programing is not beyond the reach of the community with initial support from the federal government and the state.

The financial challenge pales in the face of staffing needs. The supply of professionals needed for effective services in mental health and mental retardation is inadequate to meet even current needs. The expansion of community mental health centers will make the staffing picture impossible. Existing educational resources in the state will be quite unable to meet the demand. A new concept of staffing for community mental health services is needed.

The underlying difficulty faced by the proponents of mental health lies in the conceptualization of the field itself. Mental retardation has a distinct advantage in that its parameters are more readily ascertained and it has a relatively clear-cut range of programs to propose. In Washington and in the Seattle region, the proponents of programs for the mentally retarded are vigorous and purposeful in defining their needs and programs. They have been more successful than their mental health counterparts.

Mental health activities in Seattle are characterized by a number of disconnected programs for the most part independently governed and operated. Mental health decisions in the metropolitan area are on an individual program basis. The impetus came from the strongly motivated professional and lay persons intensely interested in given programs. Neither the state nor the county Mental Health Associations have exhibited strength or vigor in providing professional or program leadership. The professional psychiatric community in Seattle is not socially motivated to take an active part in the community mental health field. Physicians and psychiatrists have been at loggerheads; psychiatrists differ among themselves, clinical psychologists differ with psychiatrists, and other professional groups have had their disagreements as well. The differences within the professional mental health field as to the definition of mental health and therapy make many elements of mental health programing difficult to justify in the quantitatively oriented world of governmental policy making and management. Attempts to measure the effectiveness of various forms of therapy have not been carried out to the extent of empirical validation. Some of the more sophisticated types of short-term therapy in which, as one therapist explained, all that could be done was to "shore up the defenses of the patient" to cope with everyday problems and life, might in fact be all that mental health proponents could claim for a broad public approach to the field.

No flocking to the banners of mental health in Seattle is discernible. A slow, tedious campaign to secure effective support at the community level is possible, provided a segment of the community leadership is willing to assert itself. Strong support could be achieved rapidly in the metropolitan area. In light of the sensitive relationships of mental health and mental retardation organizations and personnel, any system that is devised would have to be carefully structured to secure the positive support of the professionals and interested lay community. Manpower, finance, and a host of professional and technical problems remain to be resolved even with strong support. Perhaps in a decade the objectives of the Mental Health Act could be achieved.

VII: NEW ORLEANS

DAVID R. DEENER

FOUNDED IN 1718, New Orleans is one of North America's older major cities. Though a century younger than Boston or New York, the city has seen a fulsome life. Its span of history has witnessed events as varied and exciting as any struck off by the will of man and the whim of fortune. The twentieth-century metropolitan area reflects its past. It lives with its memories of fever and floods, pirates and pirogues, quadroon balls and the code duello, but the city enjoys its present as well. It partakes of jazz and jambalaya, midwinter sports, Mardi Gras and Carnival balls. New Orleans looks to the future. It seeks answers to the problems of racial tensions, culture contrasts, religious differences, bitter politics, and economic growth in the space age.

ECOLOGY

As defined in the 1960 census, the New Orleans standard metropolitan statistical area embraced three parishes or counties: Orleans, Jefferson, and St. Bernard. These three parishes form a cluster at the lower delta reaches of the Mississippi in the southeast corner of Louisiana. The surface extent of the three-parish area is 2,900 square miles, or about 6 per cent of the total area of the state. In 1960 the area's population was 868,480, or somewhat less than 27 per cent of the state total. New Orleans is the most populous of the five metropolitan areas in Louisiana, ranking well above Shreveport, Baton Rouge, Lake Charles, and Monroe.

A change has occurred since 1960 in the boundaries of the New Orleans standard metropolitan statistical area. In 1962 the Bureau of the Census added the parish of St. Tammany, which in 1960 had a population of 38,643. The addition of St. Tammany materially changes the geographic configuration of the New Orleans metropolitan area. Future expansion of the New Orleans metropolitan area may involve two additional parishes, St. Charles and Plaquemines.

Geography determines many of New Orleans' characteristics. Set on the Mississippi River some 90 miles from the Gulf of Mexico, New Orleans is primarily a port city. If water is one of the area's greatest resources, it also presents one of its greatest problems. The New Orleans metropolitan area is waterlogged. Of the approximately 4,040 square miles in Orleans, Jefferson, St. Bernard, and St. Tammany parishes, only a little more than 50 per cent (some 2,030 square miles) is land. The major portion of the area's surface is lake, river, bayou, and coastal bay.

Of the surface waters, Lake Pontchartrain and the Mississippi River are especially important. Pontchartrain has presented a barrier to northward expansion of population, but one lessened considerably by the completion in the late 1950s of the "world's longest bridge," a 23-mile concrete causeway across the lake. The Mississippi River has operated as a barrier to the south. Until the 1930s there was no bridge across the lower Mississippi. The first bridge, built by the Huey Long administration, was located several miles up the river from the city of New Orleans. A second bridge opened in 1958, running through the heart of the city. Additional spans across both the lake and the river are in the making.

Open surface water is only a part of the area's water problems. The New Orleans metropolitan area lies on delta land, built on the silt of the centuries, sucked from the heart of America by the Mississippi and spewed into the Gulf of Mexico. Land is therefore surprisingly low; some spots in downtown New Orleans are two feet below sea level. Land must be protected by extensive levee works against flood waters, the fresh waters of the Mississippi, and the tidal waters of the Gulf. Delta lowland is also swamp land. To be made usable, land usually requires drainage and levee installations. Even after land is drained and leveed, it must be filled and protected by pumping systems. And even this is not the end. Subterranean New Orleans is largely mud. Underground construction is virtually nonexistent. Furthermore, building foundations tend to settle, and until very recently tall "skyscraper" buildings were simply not erected. On the whole, readily usable space has been scarce and costly.

The overall effect of both surface and subsurface water has been to constrict the great bulk of the area's population within a relatively small area. Beginning as a small dot on the bend of the Mississippi in 1718, the city spread slowly, following the highest land along the river edge and two high ridges between the river and Lake Pontchartrain. But land was drained very slowly, and even by the 1930s the city had not reached Lake Pontchartrain, only 7 miles from the Mississippi. Better pumping systems, extensive levees, and a seawall on the south shore of the lake facilitated expansion during the first half of the twentieth century. Even so, the settled area remained only a small fraction of the total land area, as figures for Orleans parish will illustrate. In 1950, of some 127,000 acres of land area in the parish, only 26,000 were fully developed with another 20,000 acres ready for development, and most of this developed area was in the westernmost corner of the parish. Since 1950, bridge construction across the lake and the river has hastened land development outside the settled portion of the central city. Extensive land reclamation and development in Orleans "East" are announced goals for the decades of the 1960s and 1970s, as the impact of population growth is felt in Orleans and other parishes of the metropolitan area.

Water also has its advantages, however; it is the Mississippi which makes New Orleans the second busiest port of the United States. The lakes, bayous, and the Gulf provide ample recreation. Commercial fishing and shrimping are economically important and provide succulent contributions to New Orleans' celebrated cuisine. Perhaps more important is the attraction of an abundant water supply to many types of industry, which have begun to locate in the New Orleans metropolis and thus provide a more varied economic base for the area and its growing population.

In Orleans parish the rate of population growth since the beginning of the Civil War has been fairly constant as the city increased from 168,675 in 1860 to 627,525 in 1960. The rate of growth outside of the city has been quite different. Until 1920 the population outside the city remained roughly 10 per cent of that within Orleans parish. In the decade from 1920 to 1930 the population spurted in Jefferson parish, and then leveled off in the 1930s. After World War II it skyrocketed, quadrupling from 50,427 in 1940 to 208,769 in 1960. St. Bernard and St. Tammany parishes contribute only in a minor way to the total population of the metropolitan area. In both of these parishes, the significant population growth has occurred since World War II, as indicated in Table 1.

Table 1: New Orleans Metropolitan Area, Population Growth, 1940–1960

Parish	1940	1950	1960	% Increase 1940–1960
Orleans	494,537	570,445	627,525	27
Jefferson	50,427	103,873	208,769	316
St. Bernard	7,280	11,087	32,186	346
St. Tammany	23,624	26,988	38,643	55

Yet, since World War II, the New Orleans area has not grown as fast as many other Southern metropolitan areas. It ranked first in the South in 1940, but only fifth in 1960. The area's rate of growth from 1950 to 1960 was 27 per cent, only slightly above the national average (25 per cent) for metropolitan areas; but it was lower than any of the other four metropolitan areas in Louisiana. The area reached the million mark in the mid-1960s and population estimates for the future suggest that the rate of growth in the New Orleans area will show an increase and exceed the national average by about 7 per cent, with the overall population reaching between 1.4 and 1.5 million in 1980. During this period Jefferson parish is expected to grow three times as rapidly as Orleans and consequently to provide an increasingly larger share of the area's people.

The New Orleans metropolitan area presents a spectrum of diverse social and cultural groups. The first settlers of New Orleans were the French and their Negro slaves. Spanish rule did not result in much Spanish colonization. After the Louisiana Purchase came the first Yankee invasion. The clash between the culture of the Creole and that of the Yankee was severe and produced a segregated residential pattern based on nationality, overtones of which still persist a century and a half later. In the mid-nineteenth century Irish immigration became significant, to be followed in the latter part of the century by an Italian influx. Germans settled in the 1700s and again in the period before the Civil War. In the twentieth century, and particularly since World War II, another Yankee infiltration has come, partly in connection with the movement of industry southward. Too, New Orleans' close ties with Latin America attract increasing numbers of Spanish-speaking peoples, especially from the Caribbean and Central America. All of these groups contribute to the cultural complex of the area, but the French Catholic and the Negro play particularly distinct roles.

In Louisiana the term "French Catholic" conjures up two different images. One is of the Creole, a representative of a sophisticated culture, accustomed to the arts, of discriminating taste, of old and high social status. The other is of the Cajun, a denizen of the bayou, master of the pirogue, close to nature, of lusty tastes and little pretensions to elegant society.

Creole and Cajun have contributed much to the culture of southern Louisiana. But the society for which they stood—paternalistic, class-bound, mercantile and rentier minded, as well as family-focused—is vanishing. The French Catholic is being overshadowed, especially in the New Orleans area, and his ways of doing things are being displaced as new men, new ideas, and new economic enterprise enter the region.[1]

The Negro appears to be on the rise, both in numbers and influence. In 1920 the Negro constituted about 27 per cent of the metropolitan area's population, a proportion that rose to 31 per cent in 1960. Within the area, the Negro is heavily concentrated in Orleans parish, which contains approximately 90 per cent of the area's Negro population. Moreover, in recent years, the proportion of Negroes to whites has risen sharply in the city of New Orleans, from 32 per cent in 1950 to an estimated 40 per cent in 1965, while falling drastically in the surrounding parishes. Since World War II, political participation on the part of Negroes has increased in Orleans parish and will certainly gain in impetus.[2]

The rural-urban population cleavage varies markedly within the metropolitan area. Orleans parish was classed 100 per cent urban in 1960 and Jefferson parish as 94 per cent urban. The proportion of urban population dropped sharply in St. Bernard to 66 per cent. St. Tammany parish is predominantly rural, with only 34 per cent of its population classed as urban. However, for the metropolitan area as a whole, about 95 per cent of the population falls into the urban classification.

[1] The Archdiocese of New Orleans estimate as of 1966 was that 47 per cent of Orleans parish should be classed as Catholic, and that the percentage for the state as a whole was just under 50.

[2] In 1940 there were less than 1,000 Negroes registered in the state; this figure had risen to over 150,000 in 1960. In Orleans parish, Negro registrants numbered 37,000 in 1960 out of about a 200,000 total.

There is also variation, particularly between the two principal parishes, Orleans and Jefferson, with respect to age groups within the population. Orleans parish represents an aging population cluster. In 1960 only 32 per cent of the parish population was eighteen years of age or younger, while 7.5 per cent was sixty-five or over. In Jefferson parish, however, the youth group made up over 40 per cent of the population and the aged only 4 per cent. Population projections suggest that the age differential between the two parishes will continue. Estimates for 1980 indicate that Jefferson will have a significantly larger proportion of young people (37 per cent) than Orleans (29 per cent), and a smaller proportion of aged (6 per cent as compared with 10 per cent for Orleans). The above figures may be read another way. They also indicate that there will be no significant percentage changes in the economically active age group (eighteen to sixty-five). This group will continue to be around 60 per cent of the population in Orleans parish and 57 per cent in Jefferson, although changes in the area's economy will affect the economic tasks of this group in many ways.

Shipping, inland transport, warehousing, wharfing, importing, and exporting—these and other port activities constitute the core of New Orleans economic life. Naturally the retail, wholesale, real estate, banking, utility, educational, and service enterprises necessary for a population approaching the million mark are by no means insignificant. In addition, tourism in Orleans and the extraction of gas and oil, especially in Plaquemines parish, are important. There has also been some movement to the region of light manufacturing and chemical, particularly petro-chemical, industries.

But what is clear is that the New Orleans area is not primarily an industrial and manufacturing center. Of approximately 350,000 workers employed in the area, something more than 20 per cent are engaged in manufacturing. Of this number, almost one-third have come into the labor picture since the early 1960s as a result of the expansion of shipbuilding works and the opening of the NASA Michoud plant.

In New Orleans, the cost of living is relatively high and the median income low. The middle-income class has been relatively small, although growing in recent decades. The area has a relatively large upper-income class but few families with great wealth. The lower economic class has been relatively large, and the Negro falls into this class in disproportionate share as data for the New Orleans area illustrates. In 1960 the median family income was $5,195 in the area, but for nonwhites it was only $2,977.

Another index of the area's general economic posture is the quality of its housing. The 1960 census revealed 58,357 of the metropolitan area's 271,642 units to be substandard. This represented 22 per cent, a figure higher than the national average of 19.6 per cent and the Southern average of 17.4 per cent.[3]

The future for economic growth in the New Orleans area appears cautiously optimistic. Since 1962, trade and investment, particularly in building construction, have increased. On the other hand, to take personal income as a gage, the area ranks well below the national average in median urban family income, the New Orleans figure being 81 per cent of the national median in 1959. As the national economy grows, indications are that the area's economy will grow at about the same rate. But the likelihood of faster growth, of closing the 19 per cent gap, depends not only upon greater investment but also upon an altered pattern that will emphasize industrial growth.

Unlike many large metropolitan areas, New Orleans is not beset by an excessively large number of separate local units of government. In Louisiana the basic unit of local government, the parish (county), is not subdivided into unincorporated townships. Furthermore, school districts are organized on a parishwide basis. More important, the parish of Orleans is consolidated with the city of New Orleans; there is no separate parish government. There are a number of incorporated towns and cities, but these are located in only two of the four parishes comprising the metropolitan area. The picture of fragmentation becomes more complex when lesser units such as special districts and independent boards and commissions are taken into account.

As of 1962 the total number of governmental units in the New Orleans area was thirty-one. Of these, thirty exercised a taxing power. Table 2 provides a breakdown by parish of these governmental units.

To the thirty-one governmental units listed in Table 2 should be added twenty-three "special taxing areas," which are clearly subordinate to parish governing bodies. Such "special taxing areas" (which may be water districts, road districts, recreation districts, mosquito districts, and the like) are found in all but Orleans parish.

---

[3] Louisiana is the only state not authorizing its cities to participate in the federal urban renewal program. New Orleans leaders were unsuccessful during the spring 1967 legislative session in an attempt to obtain authorizing legislation.

Table 2: New Orleans Metropolitan Area, Governmental Units, 1962

Parish	Municipalities	School Districts	Special Districts	Separate Parish Gov't.	Total
Jefferson	5	1	1	1	8
Orleans	1	1	2	. . .	4
St. Bernard	. . .	1	6	1	8
St. Tammany	8	1	1	1	11
	14	4	10	3	31

The low ranking of the New Orleans area in fragmentation is offset by two factors. The first is the existence of a wide variety of boards and commissions, such as the New Orleans City Board of Welfare, the Dock (Port) Board, the Mississippi River Bridge Authority, the Sewerage and Water Board, and the French Market Corporation. Some of these boards and commissions are authorized to charge tolls and fees for services; others may have particular tax revenues dedicated to them. Their total number runs between fifty and seventy, depending on definition.

The second factor offsetting the area's low index of fragmentation is the nature of population growth. What is developing is a metropolitan area containing two great power clusters—New Orleans city and Jefferson parish. The resulting bipolar situation may affect attainment of uniform metropolitan policy as much as the existence of all the other fragments of government put together, especially in view of the political structure of local government in the area.

The governing authorities of all the major governmental units in the New Orleans area are popularly elected. The city of New Orleans operates under a home-rule charter effective in 1954 that provides for a strong mayor-council form of government. The mayor and seven councilmen serve four-year terms. Jefferson parish adopted a president-council (seven members) system in 1958, to replace the traditional police jury (counterpart of a board of supervisors or commissioners) parish government found in Louisiana. In St. Bernard and St. Tammany parishes the old elective police jury system continues, although St. Bernard now has a home-rule charter. The municipalities in the area are governed by an elective mayor and board of aldermen, usually five in number. While the mayor has some supervisory authority, individual aldermen or committees are also active in administration. The school boards in each parish are also popularly elected. The remaining units, special districts as well as boards and commissions, are constituted in various ways. Some are appointed by the governor, directly or together with local authorities, and others by the parishes or the city of New Orleans. In some instances, the parish authority or a part thereof serves as the special unit.[4]

State control of local units varies, of course. Perhaps the most important control is financial. Local taxing powers, millage rates, and borrowing capacities are limited by legislation and, in some cases, by constitutional provisions.

Formal coordination and cooperation among governments in the area have been almost nonexistent. Contractual arrangements for furnishing certain services have occasionally been made, as, for example, between New Orleans and Jefferson parish. Recently a Metropolitan Planning Commission has been established, with representatives from New Orleans, Jefferson, and St. Bernard. Also, an areawide transport planning authority may be constituted.

Informal cooperation has been complicated by the political party structure. While nominally a one-party Democratic state, Louisiana is in fact rent by factions, both at the state and local levels. Indeed, political power at the local level centers heavily in elective local officials—the sheriff, district attorney, and tax assessor—who are not really part of the local governing authority structure. No local Republican Party exists, except in a formal legal sense.[5] Hence, in the past, local coalitions within the Democratic Party formed and dissolved, with tax assessors and

---

[4] For descriptions of governments in the area, see L. Vaughan Howard and Robert S. Friedman, *Government in Metropolitan New Orleans* (Tulane Studies in Political Science, Vol. VI: New Orleans: Tulane University, 1959); Bureau of Governmental Research, *The Government of St. Bernard Parish* (New Orleans: Bureau of Governmental Research, 1960); and Robert J. Richardson, *Orleans Parish Offices* (New Orleans: New Orleans Bureau of Publications, 1961). The standard history of New Orleans is John Smith Kendall, *History of New Orleans* (3 vols.; Chicago and New York: Lewis Publishing Co., 1922).

[5] There were 20,471 registered Republicans in the state in 1966 (as against 1,254,405 registered Democrats); this compares with 5,290 registered Republicans in 1952 and 2,850 in 1948. In Orleans parish, there were 3,563 registered Republicans in 1966 (and 204,996 registered Democrats); this compares with 1,133 in 1948. The Republican vote, especially in presidential elections, is all out of proportion to registration. In 1964, Goldwater received 509,000 votes in the state; this was 56.8 per cent of the votes cast. A few Republicans have won in state and local elections in recent years. Republicanism is a significant ideological force in Louisiana, but not an effective organization within the state.

sheriffs remaining more or less constant, while government leaders and would-be leaders contended for their and the electorate's favors. Since World War II, however, some local government figures such as the mayor of New Orleans have tended to gain in prestige, and within parish limits, local tickets advocating policy positions have begun to appear. Perhaps of greater portent, citizen and citizen group participation in politics is on the increase.

A major source of common policy in the area is the state government. In certain fields, such as public welfare, public health, and education, the state sets basic policy and even provides some of the administration. In other areas, and mental health for instance, there is virtually no local policy or service; it is almost wholly a state function. But even the state is being supplanted by the federal government in certain fields, notably education, public housing, and highways.

Given the increasing impact of the state and federal government on the New Orleans metropolitan area, perhaps the pattern for common action to envisage in the future will not emphasize cooperation between local units and local officials, but will rather put a premium on efforts of state and federal legislators in assuring that the area shares in the benefits of programs authored in Washington and siphoned through Baton Rouge.

MENTAL HEALTH ORGANIZATION AND FACILITIES

Elements of New Orleans' mental health structure trace far back into the area's history. Charity Hospital in New Orleans dates from 1735. Originally founded privately, Charity was taken over jointly by the state and the city in 1811. A few years later, in 1814, the hospital became wholly state administered.

Charity Hospital began caring for mental patients in 1820. In the early 1840s the hospital constructed a separate building for the mentally ill, designed to serve the whole state as well as New Orleans. Following a siege of epidemics in 1847, the state legislature provided for an "Insane Asylum of the State of Louisiana," located upstate at Jackson, and for the transfer of mental patients at Charity to the new institution. At the time the act of 1847 was passed, New Orleans was the state capital (state laws, incidentally, were still being published in both French and English texts). The location of the new asylum was closer to Baton Rouge, where the

state capital was moved in 1849, a move indicative of the upstate legislators' distrust of New Orleans as a "modern city of Sodom."

The closing down of Charity Hospital's service for the mentally ill after
passage of the act of 1847 stripped New Orleans of its facilities for mental patients, and the new upstate asylum really did not fill the area's needs,
since it did not have the capacity to take in all the persons committed to
it. Municipal authorities began using local jails and prisons to house mental patients, a practice that continued well into the twentieth century. This
situation left its mark on relations between New Orleans and the state.
The legislation of 1847 had made the care of the mentally ill a state
function, but at the same time the only state mental health facility in New
Orleans, the Charity Hospital service, was eliminated. Insofar as New
Orleans was concerned, therefore, mental health became in fact a local
problem, a point that the city came to resent and did not forget.

In the latter half of the nineteenth century, some private mental health
facilities were established in New Orleans, most notably the La Retreat
in 1861, the forerunner of De Paul Hospital. In the early 1900s the state
opened a mental hospital and colony for the feebleminded at Pineville,
but these were even farther upstate from New Orleans than the East State
Hospital at Jackson.

In 1909 the New Orleans city council created the post of City Alienist
to provide some treatment for the mentally ill who continued to be placed
in the city jail and the house of detention. Then, in 1911, the City Hospital for Mental Diseases was established. The hospital was not greeted
with universal enthusiasm. In fact, a municipal commission, reporting
in 1912, urged that the city hospital be closed and that the state carry out
its responsibility for caring for the insane by, among other things, opening up again at Charity Hospital a psychiatric ward and outpatient department. The commission's recommendations came to naught.

Late in the 1920s further stirrings in the New Orleans community
began to produce some action. A child guidance demonstration clinic was
established in 1929 through the combined efforts of the Orleans Parish
School Board, the Tulane School of Social Work, and the Commonwealth
Fund. It foundered in 1932 due to lack of finances, to be later revived
for a short period through support from Samuel Zemurray. Then, in
1937, an endowment from Mr. Zemurray enabled the city of New Orleans to establish an Institute of Mental Hygiene, which opened a guidance center in 1938.

It was in the mid-1930s, however, that developments on the state level began that eventually made the state the dominant figure in mental health in the New Orleans area as well as throughout Louisiana. In 1936 an attempt was made to set up a centralized administrative system for state health facilities. In that year, a state Hospital Board was set up, with a mandate to appoint a state hospital director and an assistant director. Then, in 1942, the board was abolished, and all state general (except Charity of New Orleans) and mental hospitals, along with state penal and correctional institutions, were brought together under the state Department of Institutions. Also, in 1942, the state legislature, mainly as a result of the importunings of the Louisiana Association for Mental Health, made appropriations for the opening of a psychiatric unit at Charity Hospital. Thus, after almost a century, Charity was back in the mental health business.

In 1948, following the National Mental Health Act of 1946 and the Hill-Burton Act of the same year, the Louisiana legislature repealed the legislation of 1942 and reestablished the state Hospital Board. While the 1948 act returned many of the state hospitals to the control of their own separate boards, it did provide the basic impetus for the development of mental health organization and planning in the state. The state board was designated the sole agency for carrying out the purposes of the Hill-Burton Act and the state mental health authority. It was further empowered to adopt a state mental health plan, to submit to the Surgeon General a budget for implementing the plan, and to administer funds provided for that purpose. The state board itself was composed of ten members appointed by the governor, who was a member ex officio. The board appointed a state hospital director and an assistant. The 1948 legislature also established a state Advisory Council, appointed by the governor, who served as chairman. One member of the Advisory Council was required to be "a person of recognized ability and interested in programs designed to improve the facilities for the care and treatment of the mentally ill."

Following the legislation of 1948, several basic features of mental health organization and planning in Louisiana appeared. A separate mental health unit was created, at first termed the Mental Hygiene Division, operating under the state hospital director and the state Hospital Board. The state Hospital Board began to formulate annual state plans, which typically devoted separate sections to each major kind of health installation coming under the board. For example, the 1951 plan contained sections on general hospitals, chronic-disease hospitals, tuberculosis hospitals, mental hospitals, and public health centers. For each type of health installation the state was divided into geographical areas, with the idea that a minimum standard of services would be planned for each area. The size and number of the geographical areas varied with respect to type of installation. To take the 1951 plan as an example, for general hospitals, the state was divided into eight hospital regions and fifty-seven hospital service areas. For mental hospitals, there were six areas. The standard to be attained in each geographical area was usually measured in beds per one thousand population, the precise number being related to nationally suggested ratios and varying with type of facility. Each area was then rated according to the degree to which the desired standard ratio was attained in the area, and the priority in planning for future facilities was assigned to those areas rating lowest. One particular feature deserves special note. The plan encompassed not only state public facilities, but local and private facilities as well.

Other mental health developments occurred in the early 1950s. The Louisiana Commission on Alcoholism and the Louisiana Youth Commission were both established in 1950. But the most notable development was legislation of 1952, which again abolished the state Board of Hospitals and returned almost all state general, mental, mental retardation, and tuberculosis facilities to the Department of Institutions, along with the state's penal and correctional institutions. This legislation was short-lived.

In 1956 the Louisiana legislature created the state Department of Hospitals, headed by a director appointed by the governor. The Hospital Board was reestablished, but as an advisory and policy-framing body. The legislation of 1956 also attached the Commission on Alcoholism to the Hospitals Department. A separate act of 1956 created the Commission on Aging, but did not attach it to the department.

Developments since 1956 have continued to emphasize the principal features of mental health organization in Louisiana. With the Department of Hospitals at Baton Rouge, there was established an assistant director for mental health, who was responsible for (a) state mental hospitals, (b) mental health community clinics, (c) mental health educational activities, and (d) alcoholism programs. In 1960 the Department of Hospitals was designated as the agency responsible for developing a residential care program for the mentally retarded and to participate in the development of a comprehensive program for the mentally retarded. For a few years, mental retardation (headed by an administrator for mental retardation services) was organizationally placed under the assistant director for mental health. After enactment of the national legislation of 1963, mental health and mental retardation were formally separated within the department. The offices of commissioner of mental health and commissioner of mental retardation were created under the overall control of the director of the department. The two commissioners are stipulated to be of equal status within the department.

Accompanying the growth in central mental health organization in Baton Rouge has been a continual development of the geographical mental health area system, which dates from the late 1940s. By the early 1960s the number of mental health regions had increased to nine, and by 1967 to twelve. After 1963 the mental health district was established and the state was divided into three districts, each embracing several regions.

The district-region system is also utilized to attempt a decentralization in administration of mental health services. The departmental mental health subdivisions in Baton Rouge are designed essentially as coordinating units, while the districts are viewed as the effective administrative units each under a district director.

It is perhaps a little too early to say how well this decentralized district-region system will work out. There are obvious areas for tension. One is between the coordinators at Baton Rouge and the district directors. Another is within the districts, between the mental hospitals and the community-oriented mental health services. A further factor may enter the picture. The overall organization of Louisiana's health programs has begun to evoke calls for broad-scale reform. A substantial reform proposal issued in 1967 by the Public Affairs Research Council suggests a merger of the present Department of Health and Department of Hospitals into one state Department of Health and Hospitals. Within the proposed single department, however, there would still be separate divisions of mental health and of mental retardation, along with divisions for sanitation and environmental health, patient services (nonmental), planning and federal programs, and administrative services. Bringing mental health, mental retardation, and public health together in one administrative structure might yield some catalytic heat.

Mental health facilities in New Orleans and Louisiana have increased markedly since adoption of the regional planning system in the late 1940s. The early plans focused almost entirely on mental hospital beds located in state mental hospitals, state general hospitals, and private hospitals, as the state plan for 1951 will illustrate. This plan, on the basis of 5 beds per 1,000 population, allowed 13,350 beds for the whole state, of which 10 per cent were planned for psychiatric units of private general hospitals. As against the optimum total of 13,350 beds, there were 5,805 acceptable beds existing in 1951, leaving 7,545 additional beds needed. The mental hospital patient population at that time was around 8,000. Two of the six areas into which the state was divided had no mental health hospital facilities within their borders.

Later plans reflect the impact of newer approaches to mental health as well as growth in mental health facilities. Mental health outpatient clinics, day-care centers, alcoholism clinics, guidance centers, and evaluation centers began to appear in the state in the 1950s. In 1957 state facilities included twelve guidance and outpatient clinics, one mental health clinic, and one evaluation center, in addition to the usual array of mental hospital beds. By 1957 a decline in the mental hospital population (which had risen steadily in the decade 1947–1956) was noted. This decline was due, so it was supposed, to increased staff, better facilities, and the use of new drugs and method of treatment. During the same year, outpatient clinics provided over 20,000 consultations to some 3,363 patients. Another development of 1957 was the institution of a state program to train mental health personnel, particularly students of psychiatry, psychology, social work, psychiatric nursing, and other forms of therapy. In addition to training, the importance of research in mental health had become clearly recognized at the state level.

During the decade ending in 1957 over a dozen outpatient mental health installations providing services of various kinds were added to the state's stock of mental health facilities. A comparable increase in outpatient facilities occurred in the next decade. By 1967, twenty-five outpatient facilities were in operation, with seven more definitely planned.

The mental health districts are roughly equal in population (a little over one million each, on 1960 data), although not in area. Each district contains a state mental hospital, and these along with bed-spaces in the state general hospitals constitute the public inpatient long-term mental health facilities. Total public hospital beds available in 1967 numbered slightly over 8,000 with 7,800 of these in the three state mental hospitals. The average daily total of inpatients at the three mental hospitals has run about 6,500 during the past two or three years. Southeast Hospital at Mandeville (498 beds) emphasizes intensive, short-term treatment; Central at Pineville (3,368), and East at Jackson (3,943) provide long-term and custodial care. In addition to the 8,000 mental hospital beds in state institutions, there are some 360 beds in private hospitals and 130 in federal hospitals.

Unlike the district, the mental health regions are by no means equal in population. They range from Region XII (New Orleans) with 700,000 persons to Region VI (Crowley) with 117,000. For each region, there is envisaged a mental health center plus satellite mental health and alcoholism clinics, depending upon population. The centers offer a more comprehensive range of services than the clinics, and the centers have the responsibility for coordinating the outpatient services available in the region. During 1964–1965, some 10,200 persons were admitted to the state's outpatient mental health services, a threefold increase over 1957. In addition to regions, the state is marked off into thirty-five catchment areas, or roughly one to every 100,000 of population.

Whether a separate state outpatient facility is to be located within each catchment area is not clear. In this respect, admissions data strongly suggests that physical location is a factor determining use of outpatient services. Those parishes in which outpatient facilities are situated provide the great bulk of admissions thereto, and there is some evidence that this may result in prevention of later, more severe mental illness. At any rate, a surprisingly large number of young persons use the outpatient services of the mental health centers and clinics; in 1964–1965, for example, persons seventeen years old and under accounted for about 41 per cent of outpatient admissions.

Whatever advantages the state district-region system for mental health may have, it does add another element of fragmentation to the New Orleans scene. The system trifurcates the metropolitan area, which consists of Jefferson, Orleans, St. Bernard, and St. Tammany parishes. Jefferson, however, is in Region XI, St. Tammany in Region X, and Orleans and St. Bernard are in Region XII.

As to mental health facilities located within the New Orleans metropolitan area, a survey of public and private facilities was conducted in 1964. This survey was part of the state's long-range comprehensive mental health planning in connection with the federal Community Mental

Health Centers Act of 1963. For the New Orleans area, a total of 101 mental health facilities were inventoried. This total broke down into 19 "psychiatric" facilities (meaning that a psychiatrist had responsibility for its operations), 18 "other" facilities (meaning that some psychiatric services were offered but a psychiatrist was not in charge), and 64 "auxiliary" facilities (meaning that psychiatric patients were accepted, but no psychiatric services were offered). The figures of the inventory probably understated the number of mental health facilities and services in the New Orleans metropolitan area. The special teachers programs conducted by parish school boards were omitted, as were a number of facilities which certainly would fall in the auxiliary category. And, of course, there have been developments since 1964.

Three of the New Orleans metropolitan area's psychiatric facilities are operated by the federal government. The largest of the federal facilities is the Veterans Administration Hospital, for outpatients and inpatients. The third federal installation, the United States Public Health Service Hospital, maintains a Psychiatric Service and a Social Service Department. Until the early 1960s, the Public Health Service Hospital was named the Marine Hospital, and the men who go to sea remain its major clientele.

Nine of the psychiatric facilities located in the New Orleans metropolitan area are state or state/local agencies. One of these is the Southeast Louisiana Mental Hospital at Mandeville. When built in the early 1950s this was designed as a regional mental hospital. It still functions as such but will not admit bedridden patients nor usually accept patients with chronic brain syndromes or mental deficiency that will not respond to treatment. It is an "open" installation, with a basic bed capacity of 498. The hospital has special programs and facilities for alcoholics, young children, and adolescents.

Three mental health centers are located in the metropolitan area. The largest of these is the New Orleans Mental Health Center, which also operates two mental health clinics in the suburbs. The New Orleans center provides diagnostic, precare and aftercare, and training services. The Metairie Mental Health Center (Jefferson parish) and the Covington Mental Health Center (St. Tammany parish) offer a similar wide range of services.

The Southeast Aftercare Clinic, a state facility located in New Orleans, provides aftercare mainly for persons who have been inpatients at the Southeast Louisiana Hospital, Mandeville, and the East Louisiana Hospital, Jackson. The Clinic for the Diagnosis and Treatment of Alcoholism, another state facility situated in New Orleans, is an outpatient unit. There is also the Psychiatry Department of Charity Hospital, a 160-bed inpatient facility. The Charity unit is closely associated with the Tulane and Louisiana State University Medical Schools and their teaching and training programs. The Louisiana State University Medical School through its Department of Psychiatry also provides the inpatient and outpatient mental health services at Charity Hospital. In addition to engaging in the usual range of psychiatric services, the LSU unit has projected a day-care service, a child clinic, a rehabilitation service for handicapped children, and a day school for handicapped children.

The third group of psychiatric facilities in the New Orleans area consists of those operated on a private basis. There are nine of these in operation with two more in the planning stages. De Paul Hospital is a 195-bed facility, operated by the Daughters of Charity of St. Vincent De Paul. An outpatient clinic is planned to be attached to the hospital. Four psychiatric facilities in the area are attached to private hospitals. Southern Baptist Hospital provides inpatient services only and does not accept chronic or emergency cases. Only mild, acute, nondangerous patients are admitted. The main service provided is diagnostic, although Southern Baptist does participate in a Clinical-Pastoral Training Program. Ochsner Foundation Hospital's Psychiatric Unit and Clinic provide services both on an inpatient and outpatient basis. Touro Infirmary through its Division of Neurology and Psychiatry provides a fairly comprehensive range of services to both inpatients and outpatients.

Four psychiatric services operated on a private basis in the area are attached to Tulane University, but as with most university-operated units admission of patients is highly selective. As might be expected, the facilities of the Department of Counseling and Psychiatry of the Student Health Service are open only to Tulane students and faculty. Plans were underway for a top-priority, $2 million community mental health center to be added to the Tulane complex, but the university may have to withdraw because of financial factors.

Some idea of the quantity of service rendered by the psychiatric facilities in the New Orleans area may be gleaned from the admissions and separations records during 1964. Figures available indicate that there were 11,421 admissions and 9,117 separations during the year. Federal facilities accounted for 6 per cent of the admissions, state facilities for

61 per cent, and private for 33 per cent. At the end of the year there were 5,757 cases on the rolls; of these, federal facilities accounted for 19 per cent, state for 58 per cent, and private facilities for 23 per cent.

The precise number of "other" mental health facilities in the New Orleans area is not easy to determine. Much depends on the definition of "other" facilities, and not a little on who does the counting and when. The eighteen such facilities listed in the 1964 survey are certainly a minimum.

One group of "other" facilities includes several day-care centers for retarded children, which began operations in 1964. These are cooperative ventures, involving the state Department of Hospitals, the state Department of Education, and the Louisiana Association for Retarded Children. The New Orleans Regional Mental Health Center provides administrative support and consultation for the day-care centers. There are also five privately operated schools for the mentally retarded in the area.

Within the New Orleans area are three large family service organizations, the Family and Children Service of Jewish Welfare Federation, the Associated Catholic Charities, and the Family Service Society. Each provides for a regularly scheduled psychiatric consultant.

Several court and prison installations in the New Orleans area provide some mental health services for those taken into custody. For the juvenile offender, the Youth Study Center, which opened in 1959, serves as a detention home and makes use of a regularly scheduled psychiatric consultant. The Orleans Parish Juvenile Court has also utilized the regular services of a psychiatric consultant. The state Department of Public Welfare maintains a Juvenile Probation and Parole Service in its Orleans area office.

For the adult offender, both the Orleans Parish Prison and the House of Detention afford some psychiatric services, and in an appropriate case a person may be transferred from these to the mental ward of Charity Hospital. It seems, however, that security arrangements for such tranfers are far from adequate, as rashes of prisoners break out of Charity's mental ward from time to time. It may be mentioned that the Louisiana Association for Mental Health has become interested in mental health aspects of police work and conducts an educational program designed to alert arresting and other officers to the possibilities of mental health factors affecting persons taken into custody. The mental health services provided in connection with police and prison operations are generally regarded as minimal, however. In particular, the probation and parole services are felt to be most inadequately staffed.

To the above categories of agencies may be added a miscellaneous group providing in one way or another some mental health services. This group includes the Lighthouse for the Blind; McKinney House, a halfway house; the Milne Municipal Boys' Home; and the Division of Vocational Rehabilitation of the state Department of Education. This last agency has evidenced concern with job handicaps resulting from mental disability. In all four of the metropolitan area's parishes, there are visiting teacher programs, with that in Orleans the largest in scale. Although the visiting teacher program is designed to serve students in both public and parochial schools, the Catholic schools make almost no use of it.

According to the 1964 inventory, sixty-four auxiliary facilities are located in the New Orleans area. Of this total, forty-four are classed as nursing homes or homes for the aged with a bed capacity of about 2,200. The next largest group consists of foster homes. There are four sheltered workshops in the area, and, to fill out the list of auxiliary facilities, an Information Center on Alcoholism.

In terms of numbers of mental health facilities alone, the New Orleans metropolitan area is the most heavily endowed in the state. Indeed, in the planning under the federal legislation of 1963, the New Orleans area ranked construction of new mental health facilities last in priority among the area's mental health needs. Still, vociferous complaints about the situation in the area continue to be voiced. The existence of waiting lists suggests that capacities are not always sufficient to serve needs, although the absence of hard criteria by which to measure needs makes assessment and planning difficult. Perhaps more significant is the criticism of interagency coordination, or rather the lack of it. As it has been put, mental health agencies in the New Orleans area go about their daily tasks "hermetically sealed off from each other."

MENTAL HEALTH INFRASTRUCTURE

Since the beginning of World War II, the infrastructure of mental health in the New Orleans metropolitan area and throughout Louisiana as well has burgeoned markedly. Interest and informal groups concerned with mental health have increased in size and organization, as well as in numbers. Some of these groups are properly termed mental health interest groups, for their concern with mental health problems is major and direct, if not exclusive. In addition, many other groups have become at least peripherally involved with mental health problems, although their major interests lie elsewhere. A number of the groups comprising the infrastructure of mental health have a statewide organization, as well as units operative within the New Orleans area. Other groups are local in character. In some instances statewide and local bodies may have national affiliations. Thus, the informal structure of mental health in the New Orleans area is at once a distinct cluster roughly coinciding with the area's bounds, and at the same time part of a larger statewide, and even national, pattern.

Among the mental health interest groups, the Louisiana Association for Mental Health stands out. The New Orleans area was the birthplace of the Louisiana association. The first meeting of the group which eventually incorporated as the association in 1942 was called by Miss Eva Smill, director of the New Orleans Family Service Society, on October 30, 1939. This meeting served to bring together a variety of New Orleans civic leaders who had become concerned with mental health problems. Among the founders of the Louisiana Association for Mental Health were persons from the business sector, such as Joseph M. Jones and Walter Barnett; members of the medical profession, as represented by Dr. C. H. Holbrook and Dr. T. A. Watters; religious leaders, such as Rabbi Julian Beck Feibelman; and society personages, particularly Carmelite Janvier and Mrs. J. W. Reilly. Insofar as prestige and status are concerned, the founders placed the association on a solid basis. To take a few examples, Joseph M. Jones was one of New Orleans' acknowledged business leaders and president of the Tulane University board of administrators at the time of his tragic death a few years ago. Miss Janvier symbolized the interest in community problems of one of the area's oldest families, a family synonymous with high Mardi Gras festivities. And Rabbi Feibelman is eminent in New Orleans Jewish religious circles.

The Louisiana Mental Health Association maintains a permanent central office in New Orleans under an executive director. The first executive director was Mr. Felix Gentile, who served until 1945, when he took a position with UNRRA. In 1945 the Louisiana Mental Health Association obtained as director Dr. Loyd W. Rowland, who previously had been chairman of the Department of Psychology at Baylor University in Texas. He served as director until 1963, when the present director,

George L. Saporito, took office. Dr. Rowland has continued his contacts with the association as director of education and research.

Its governing body consists of a board of forty members, drawn from throughout the state. In addition, the association has formed chapters to operate in each of the mental health regions of the state. Of the forty-member governing body, twenty were from the New Orleans area in 1965–1966. The New Orleans contingent also included the president of the association as well as four of the five remaining officers. The governing board, it may be mentioned, also doubles as the association's chapter for the New Orleans mental health region. Thirty-five of the board members came from Louisiana's metropolitan areas.

About a third of the association's board in 1965–1966 were women. There were a half dozen doctors, including some psychiatrists, and there was a small Negro representation. Several lawyers, a New Orleans city councilman, an officer of the AFL-CIO, several persons attached to universities, a minister or two, and at least one person connected with the daily press also appeared on the roster. A few of the names on the board would be recognized as among the more socially prominent in New Orleans, and one or two had high financial connections. Generally speaking, however, on an elite scale, the 1965–1966 board fell in the second, perhaps even third, rank. Certainly, with respect to the New Orleans contingent, it was not drawn from the area's top-most business, financial, political, or social strata.

Two years later, in 1967, the board had undergone a considerable changeover in personnel, with only eighteen of those serving in 1965 still remaining. In other respects, the changes were not so great. Members from the state's metropolitan areas continued to dominate, with thirty-four of the forty members, and the New Orleans contingent numbered nineteen. The number of women members remained the same, at thirteen. There were still a half-dozen doctors, a representative of labor, some lawyers, and one or two people connected with universities. The status of the group had not changed much, either; the board could hardly be said to be drawn from the highest business and social circles.

The Louisiana Association for Mental Health has not attempted to engage in large-scale membership drives. In the mid-1960s, however, the association did form a ladies' Auxiliary, which attracts members from Junior League circles and the social strata the League represents. The Auxiliary sponsors benefit shows, Christmas sales, and other activities designed to raise money for various mental health causes. The financial support of the association comes almost entirely from United Fund and Community Chest sources. It is, of course, affiliated with the National Mental Health Association.

The Louisiana Association for Mental Health is not a mass-type, high-pressure organization. Its tactics in furthering mental health have not been of the militant, bare-knuckle variety. Not that the association has refrained from entering the political decision-making arena, however, as will be detailed in the discussion below of mental health decision making. But it has preferred to use the more subtle arts of political influence, private persuasion, and sometimes just plain perseverance to achieve specific mental health goals. In addition, the association engages in a number of public education efforts. One of these is "Pierre the Pelican," the creation of Dr. Rowland, which consists of a series of pamphlets designed to reach expectant parents and all parents of first-born children. "Pierre the Pelican" has been translated into German and is in full-scale use in Berlin and Munich. In another effort, the association produced a manual and several training films for use in educating police officials in the handling of suspects who might in fact be mentally disturbed. The association has become increasingly concerned with the problems of persons returning to the community from mental hospitals and has developed a manual dealing with social clubs for such persons. The national association has undertaken distribution of this manual. The Louisiana association has also played its part in popularizing the notion that "after all, mental illness is illness."

A second interest group important to mental health is the Association of Retarded Children of Greater New Orleans, a local affiliate of the Louisiana Association for Retarded Children. In fact, New Orleans served as the birthplace for the Louisiana Mental Retardation Association. The Louisiana Association for Mental Health hosted meetings of the American Association on Mental Deficiency in 1949 and 1950. From these meetings came the impetus for the Greater New Orleans Association, founded in 1953, and the statewide association, established in 1954.

The New Orleans Mental Retardation Association has a board consisting of five officers and some twenty directors. The directors as of 1967 included two New Orleans city councilmen, three doctors, a couple of lawyers, nine women, and several business people. Many of those active in the association have a personal interest in mental retardation. It is fair to say, however, that the directorate of the association is not representative of the higher echelons of the area's elite structure.

The mental retardation associations have been more militant than the Mental Health Association, in part, certainly, because of intense personal participation by parents of mentally retarded children. The associations have successfully pressed for new facilities, such as the Belle Chasse school and several day-care centers in the New Orleans area. They have also been successful in getting mental retardation concerns separated administratively from mental health within the state Department of Hospitals. It appears, however, that the state association has not been as active as the Greater New Orleans Association, which seems to be a sore point insofar as some members of the metropolitan association are concerned.

Another active mental health group in the area is the Committee on Alcoholism for Greater New Orleans, Inc. It was founded in 1960 and has a twenty-four-member board of directors. On the board as of 1967 are representatives of New Orleans Public Service, Inc. (light, gas, and public transport), Southern Bell Telephone, Jackson Brewing Co., two large department stores, two shipping companies, an insurance company, as well as some attorneys and other business people. Also included are a minister, a psychiatrist, a local judge, a dean of one of the local universities, and two women. The composition of the board probably reflects a growing concern on the part of business establishments with alcoholism and its effects on their operations. The board also contains some names that would be recognized as belonging to the area's elite. The committee engages in a publicity campaign of considerable dimensions, including television. Through the Clinic for Alcoholism, the committee cooperates in offering services such as guidance, counseling, and referral for treatment.

There are other interest groups, some of which come and go, that become exercised over problems of juvenile delinquency, aging, crime, drug addiction, and sundry health-related ills of society. In some instances these problems have occasioned the creation of state bodies such as the Louisiana Commission on Aging. Crime has become of increasing concern in the New Orleans area, as the formation of the Metropolitan Crime Commission attests.

A second category of groups making up the infrastructure of mental health consists of a number of professional associations. Among these is the Louisiana Psychiatric Association, whose direct concern with mental health is patent. The Louisiana association was founded in the early 1950s as a branch of the American Psychiatric Association. The membership of the Louisiana Psychiatric Association stood at 131 in 1964 and had risen to 163 in 1967. Most of the members, about three-fourths, are located in the New Orleans area. The Louisiana Psychiatric Association was largely nonfunctional until the early 1960s. Since then it has undertaken a number of activities. It raises issues of statewide significance in psychiatry and mental health. It checks on activities of the state Department of Hospitals in psychiatry and mental health; in particular, it "watchdogs" (as one member has described it) the fees charged and services offered by state mental health agencies. The association has backed a few pieces of legislation and publishes a newsletter, which has taken a political stance in editorials. Some recent officers of the association have viewed the organization as quasi-political, at least.

The Louisiana Psychiatric Association exhibits some problems within itself. One involves a conflict between the Tulane University group and the Louisiana State University group of psychiatrists. This may be something more than the long-standing competition between these two institutions of higher learning and their two medical schools. Involved also is the question of private psychiatric practice versus the public practice presumed by the federal legislation of 1963. Further, there is the trade union question of whether psychiatrists should be in administrative control of mental health facilities or whether other professionals should be responsible for administration. To return to the Tulane-LSU conflict, the Tulane psychiatric program has been more community- and public-oriented than the LSU one. Also, under the leadership of Dr. Robert G. Heath, the Tulane Medical School's Psychiatry Department has pushed itself and its ideas vigorously into many phases of mental health in the metropolitan area and the state. Its very success is calculated to breed a measure of resentment. Needless to say, the issue of public versus private services follows the Louisiana psychiatrist into his basic medical organization, the Louisiana State Medical Society.

The Louisiana State Medical Society is the state chapter of the American Medical Association. Both the national organization and the state society have a long history as political interest groups. The state society has at least two committees of importance to mental health. One is the Legislative Committee and the other is the Mental Health Committee.

The chairmen of both of these committees as well as other officers of the state society have been involved in mental health decision making in Louisiana.

Two additional professional groups, psychologists and social workers, have an immediate interest in community mental health. The Louisiana Psychological Association has a membership of approximately 100. The association sponsored state legislation in 1964 for licensing psychologists. The Louisiana chapter of the National Association of Social Workers has about 325 members. Both of these professional groups have a "trade union" interest in the job ramifications of the community mental health program. Perhaps more important, they along with the psychiatrists have a special concern with the bureaucratic problem of who controls whom and to what degree in the administration of mental health centers and clinics. At another level, that of leadership in the development and assessment of the scientific concepts underlying the community mental health program, psychologists and social workers share with psychiatrists a major professional responsibility.

There is another circle of professional groups within the infrastructure of mental health. The interests of these groups in mental health are particular and narrow, although they may broaden as the community health program itself expands. Nurses, practical nurses, teachers, and therapists all have at least a "trade union" concern with the job ramifications of the community mental health effort. Such organizations as the Louisiana State Nurses Association and the Louisiana Teachers Association have already become involved in the mental health planning for New Orleans and the state. Lawyers and the State Bar Association have an obvious interest in the legal requirements surrounding commitment. The Louisiana Hospital Association also has an obvious concern with certain of the institutional aspects of mental health, hospital accreditation, for example.

A third category of mental health groups are those voluntary organizations active in the private and public social welfare programs of the New Orleans metropolitan area. One of the most important of these is the United Fund. Through the annual United Fund campaigns, substantial funds are raised and a number of mental health facilities in the area receive United Fund allocations. To head up the United Fund, there is usually selected one of New Orleans' most prominent business and social leaders, and the chairmanships of the working committees of the campaign are often similarly staffed.

Working closely with the United Fund is the Social Welfare Planning Council. The council was founded in 1921, largely through the efforts of the New Orleans Chamber of Commerce. It predates the Community Chest, the predecessor of the United Fund. It had ninety-four agency members in 1967. The Council has a board of directors numbering in excess of thirty, plus a representative of the United Fund and a representative of Total Community Action serving ex officio. As of 1967 the board included ten women, three clergymen, the judge of the juvenile court, a couple of doctors, several attorneys, the superintendent of the Orleans parish public school system, the director of the Port of New Orleans, as well as some businessmen. A few names on the board would be recognized as prominent in the area. The council's most important function is the planning and coordination of social welfare services; in this respect, its liaison with the United Fund is important in the allocation of Fund monies among some seventy-five of the area's social welfare and mental health agencies. The council also provides four central services: community information, community volunteer, Christmas bureau, and research consultation. In addition, it has undertaken with funds supplied by Total Community Action some specific tasks in the area's war on poverty.

Beyond the mental health interest groups, the professional associations with mental health concerns, and the array of community social welfare agencies, there is a widely diverse agglomeration of area groups whose activities impinge in one way or another upon mental health. Within the New Orleans area, there are several citizen "good government" groups which have an interest in public policy and its making. These include the Bureau of Governmental Research, the Metropolitan Area Committee, the Citizens' Crime Commission, the League of Women Voters, and the Chamber of Commerce and its related organizations. Moreover, the New Orleans area is studded with small political organizations, some devoted to a particular person, others to the well-being of a particular locality, and still others to a particular cause. These can be motivated to take a stand on a particular mental health issue.

Operating on a statewide basis are several bodies dedicated to "good government." Prominent among these are the Citizens for a Better Louisiana (a high prestige group concerned with the economic future of the state) and the Public Affairs Research Council of Louisiana, Inc., which is located in Baton Rouge and produces analyses and reports on political problems and issues. Organized labor, too, has taken an interest in mental health, as attested by the service of Victor Bussie, president of Louisiana's A.F. of L. organization, on the State Council on the Construction of Community Mental Health Centers and as president of the Louisiana Association for Mental Health in 1966.

One further point about the infrastructure of mental health in New Orleans deserves especial mention. It concerns the Negro. The Negro constitutes about a third of the metropolitan area's population and is an important consumer of mental health services. But the Negro was virtually unrepresented in the area's mental health infrastructure until the mid-1960s, when a few Negroes began to appear on directorates here and there. There is a growing awareness in New Orleans, especially in the top circles, that community groups can no longer function as real "community" groups unless the Negro plays an appropriate role therein. Yet there is a dilemma here. Participation of Negro leadership in community groups may not be as easy as it seems, for it may spell the end of existing Negro political organizations. But if participation does not occur (and perhaps even if it does), the possibility of the rise of Negro groups which reject a community orientation is very real.

The main locus of strength of much of the mental health infrastructure in Louisiana is really in the New Orleans metropolitan area. There are various reasons for this. In some instances, as with the Mental Health Association, organized concern first appeared in New Orleans and then spread to the rest of the state. In the case of some professional associations, like the Lousiana Psychiatric Association, the bulk of the practicing professionals are located in the area. Concentration of certain kinds of professional talent in the New Orleans area is partially due to the area's population, but other factors are important, too. The state's two medical schools, its only dental school, and two of the state's three law schools are located in the New Orleans area. Also, the New Orleans area has seven institutions of higher education within its bounds, including Tulane University, one of the state's two major doctorate-granting universities.

Times and circumstances are changing, however. Other metropolitan areas are fast developing in the state. New Orleans is no longer the sole source of urban problems in the state and the sole seedbed of groups and organizations concerned with their solution. The burgeoning of the mental health infrastructure both within and well beyond the New Orleans metropolitan area's boundaries adds a critical twentieth-century dimension to the mental health decision-making process.

MENTAL HEALTH DECISION MAKING

Mental health decision making in the New Orleans area is not an autonomous process. Mental health is a state function in Louisiana. Decision making in New Orleans is not organically separate from decision making at Baton Rouge. The metropolitan area is a part, albeit a very distinct part, of the overall, statewide mental health decision-making and planning field.

The statewide mental health decision-making field may be likened to a set of Cartesian coordinates with the office of commissioner of mental health at the center. On the vertical axis, the commissioner meets forces pressing down from above, emanating mainly from the state director of hospitals, the governor, the state legislature, and the federal government. From below come the pressures generated by the mental health regions and the various interest and pressure groups concerned with mental health. Along the horizontal lie the competing state services, ranging from those akin to mental health like mental retardation and vocational rehabilitation to those farther afield like education and highways. Any given policy movement in mental health is in the nature of a resultant of the forces and counter pressures operative in the decision-making field.

In the vertical axis and operating above the commissioner of mental health is the director of the state Department of Hospitals. Major policy decisions naturally require the formal approval of the director; occasionally, a matter is taken to the governor. Informally, the commissioner has a great deal of say-so, perhaps a little more than a strict hierarchical view of things would suggest. On the "big decisions," there will likely be a meeting of minds of the commissioner, the director, and the chairman of the Hospital Board (even though the Hospital Board is, strictly speaking, a purely advisory body). By and large, the state directors of hospitals have been sympathetic toward mental health and the community program.

Beyond question, the single most important political decision-making office in the state is that of governor. Louisiana's governor emerges from the state's Democratic Party primary system, often only after two bitter primary races. In the first, the field of candidates is narrowed from as many as half a dozen to two. In the second or run-off primary, Democratic Party factions and candidates for the legislature and a host of other elective offices in the state tend to line up with one or the other of the two gubernatorial aspirants, thereby forming competing "tickets." Since Republican opposition for state offices in the general election has been virtually negligible, the victorious Democratic gubernatorial candidate has in effect "whupped" the field. He comes into the governor's mansion in position to dominate the state legislature, the state Democratic Party Executive Committee, and the state administration. Moreover, a constitutional amendment adopted in 1966 that permits a governor to succeed himself for a second term may well enhance his position.

The powers and prerogatives that contribute to the political stature of the Louisiana governor are varied. He may call special sessions of the legislature and set the agenda therefor. Indeed, it is not unusual for the Louisiana governor to go on the floor of the house or senate to argue for his measures. He has the item veto. He exercises wide authority in the areas of job appointments and removals and in letting state contracts. He controls the budget, both getting and spending.

Within the state bureaucracy the governor's agency, the Division of Administration, controls the budget-making process. In presenting the budget to the legislature, the Legislative Budget Committee plays a dominant role. This is a seventeen-member joint House and Senate committee, but the governor appoints (and can dismiss) thirteen of the seventeen members. Moreover, the Division of Administration furnishes the staff for the Legislative Budget Committee. Thus, the budget comes to the legislature with a significant segment of both houses feeling ties of commitment to it.

With respect to mental health, the governor's office has played a positive role, at least since World War II. The evolution of mental health organization in the state, the emergence of a separate "commissionership" for mental health and the overall regional and district system, has been on the whole an orderly, albeit slow, process. It did not encounter political hostility from the governor's office, with all that such hostility would have meant in view of the powers of the Louisiana governor. Actually, some governors have taken an active interest in certain particular mental health programs, alcoholism and youth services being good examples. Also, the legislation of 1948 that reestablished the state Hospital Board and the act of 1956 that established the state Department of Hospitals were due largely to the desire of Governor Earl Long to maintain the state's hospitals and hospital-type services in a separate administrative division apart from other institutions, a pattern of separation that had been developed in the Long era of the 1930s.

Political relationships of the New Orleans area to the governor's office exhibit constant as well as variable aspects. Louisiana governors tend to come from the north of the state, which is thought of as Protestant, white, and "redneck," in contrast to southern Louisiana with its Catholic, Negro, and Cajun elements. It is a virtual axiom of Louisiana politics that a candidate from New Orleans has little chance to occupy the governor's mansion, an axiom demonstrated as recently as 1956 and 1960 in the unsuccessful attempts by New Orleans mayor de Lesseps Morrison. At times, relations between New Orleans and the state administration are strained, to say the least, as when the Huey Long regime brought the city to its knees and forced its mayor to resign. On the other hand, Governor John McKeithen proved instrumental in getting a constitutional amendment adopted so that the New Orleans area could proceed with plans for a covered "superdome" sports stadium. If in New Orleans the feeling persists that it does not get a fair shake in the state capital, this is counterbalanced by a sentiment in Baton Rouge that New Orleans often acts as if it were a separate little political world all its own.

A third force above the commissioner on the vertical axis is the state legislature. The legislature, like the governor, has played a positive role in mental health generally. The development of mental health organization and services in the state has, of course, required legislative support and action. Within the state legislature, the Legislative Budget Committee is the most important single committee for mental health as, indeed, it is for most state activities. Certainly this is the committee with which the commissioner has most dealings.

In a more specific vein, some individual legislators appear to understand mental health, but others do not. Legislators have been invited to visit mental health facilities, particularly newer installations like Mandeville, if for no other reason than to dispel the notion that all mental health involves is locking people up in padded cells. While several legislators have shown more than the normal run of interest in mental health, no legislator as yet has made it a personal cause. Mental health has no champion in the legislature comparable to Mrs. Lilian Walker, recognized as a spokesman for mental retardation causes. It may well happen that a legislator or two will develop a specialty in mental health; this would probably not be frowned upon by the Mental Health Division. In the state legislature the New Orleans area is well represented. Lawmakers from the area, or at least from the city of New Orleans, act at times as a delegation to press for area or city goals as the case may be. Legislators from the metropolitan area have taken more interest in mental health in recent years and have, on the whole, supported the mental health program, as has perhaps to a greater degree the Baton Rouge legislative delegation. One element of the mental health program has traditionally excited the concern of legislators: the geographic location of mental health facilities. Legislative preferences as to the exact geographic location of state facilities are still important, despite the development of statewide comprehensive mental health planning.

Exerting pressures on the commissioner's office from below are the forces emanating from the local units of government, the mental health regions and districts, and the various interest groups concerned with mental health issues. By and large the concern of local governmental units with mental health has not been high. This is especially true of the city of New Orleans in recent years. From Baton Rouge's standpoint, New Orleans seems to look to the state rather than exert local effort to obtain mental health services. Indeed, it has been exclaimed (without, perhaps, too much exaggeration) that the city of New Orleans is the only city of its size not spending a cent on mental health. Among other parishes in the metropolitan area, St. Bernard has likewise shown little interest in mental health. With St. Tammany and Jefferson parishes, the situation has been somewhat different. In the former, the local police jury cooperated with a local private group to obtain land for the installation in Covington, and in Jefferson Parish the local council has agreed to finance in part the new Metairie Mental Health Center.

The picture of local government involvement throughout the state is not markedly different. A number of parishes and other local units have taken some action in the area of mental health, usually by providing modest financial support for state installations (occasionally by means of a millage tax). But the tendency has been for this financial support to dry up as the years go by. Other parishes have shown little interest. It should be pointed out, however, that state representatives and senators are sometimes more active in mental health than local officials. The reasons for low interest at the local government level are not difficult to discern. The tight financial pinch of all local units is an important one, as is the effect of the now historic "pegging" of mental health as a state function.

Along the horizontal axis of pressures operating against the commissioner's office lies first of all the state mental retardation program. A separate commissioner of mental retardation was established, it will be recalled, after enactment of the federal legislation of 1963. Officially, the view is expressed that mental health has not suffered as a result of the formal separation of mental retardation services. But mental retardation is still regarded in some quarters as really a mental health program, and the impression is given that the division is more uneasy than appears on the surface. Perhaps the situation is well summed up in the remarks sometimes heard that mental retardation people do not want to get mixed up with "crazy" people, and mental health people do not want to get mixed up with "defective" people.

Nor does the Division of Mental Health and the state Department of Hospitals provide all of the state mental health services, despite the designation of the department as the state mental health agency. The Department of Education and the local school boards operate the special teachers programs, and in the same department is located the Office of Vocational Rehabilitation, which assigns rehabilitation counselors to state mental health centers and hospitals. The state Department of Health engages in activities of a mental health character in the area of prenatal care. There are also arrangements with the Department of Institutions for provision of mental health services within the state's correctional establishments. With the Welfare Department there are obvious problems of mutual concern since persons having basic contact with that department also may require mental health services. As indicated, in many instances contracted-type arrangements with other state agencies make possible the provision of mental health services, but the basic problem remains. Regardless of the logic of functional division of state operations, it is difficult to carve up the individual human recipient just to make that logic work.

And there is the last horizontal set of pressures. Certain social services, education and welfare in particular, seem likely to carry a higher priority than mental health, possibly even health in general, when it comes time to allocate the state's financial and other resources. And the competition of nonsocial services such as highways, of course, is yet another source of pressure.

Forces such as the legislature, the governor's office, the competing state services and the interest groups associated with them, and local governments represent in the Louisiana context inertial factors in the mental health decision-making field. That is, they tend to depress or at least to keep the political priority of mental health low, unless they are overcome or neutralized by forces of momentum. The forces of momentum in the mental health decision-making field consist mainly of the commissioner of mental health and the bureaucracy under him, certain of the mental health interest groups, and the federal government, more particularly NIMH.

The momentum provided by the state mental health bureaucracy has been steady and quietly innovative rather than noisy and demanding. The basic concept of dividing the state into mental health regions and the use of planning to ascertain regional needs and ways to meet them is largely the product of the state Mental Health Division, although seeds of this approach appear in the Hill-Burton program. Closely associated with the development of the regional concept and comprehensive mental health planning is the name of Mr. H. J. "Blue" Walters, long-time official in the Mental Health Division and serving currently as assistant to the commissioner of mental health. Mr. Winborn Davis, who served some twenty years in a variety of mental health capacities, was chief of the mental hygiene division in 1948–1951, when the regional system had its beginnings. He also played an instrumental role in establishing in the mid-1950s the state's mental health training and research program, and served as the mental health program director at the critical period of the impact of the federal legislation of 1963. As previously noted, the state hospital directors have been sympathetic toward mental health. For example, Mr. Jesse Bankston, a strong proponent of the separate department of hospitals administrative structure, was helpful in the initiation of the alcoholism program and the psychiatric internship training program.

The regional and comprehensive planning approach of the Mental Health Division has proved readily adaptable to the changing emphases and developments in the mental health field. The transition from emphasis on the mental hospital to the use of outpatient facilities was made without great incident in the mid-1950s. The guidance clinic movement of the early 1950s flourished under the regional concept, and later these same clinics became transformed into elements of Louisiana's comprehensive community mental health centers program. And the planning approach of the Mental Health Division virtually anticipated the planning emphasis touched off by the federal Community Mental Health Centers Act of 1963.

The Division of Mental Health has not used strident, demanding tactics in the decision-making arena. Its plan for action has not been to determine that a particular region needs certain mental health facilities and then to insist before the governor and legislature upon the wherewithal to provide them. Instead it has preferred to wait until groups within a region have recognized the need for facilities and then to assist in obtaining them. It is true that the division has on occasion taken the lead in suggesting to local groups that they might request facilities. But, on the whole, the philosophy followed projected mental health goals through planning and the regional systems, and premised action upon local awareness of needs.

The degree to which community awareness of mental health needs develops is in part, perhaps in large part, dependent upon the activities of the interest and action groups comprising the mental health infrastructure. The prime infrastructure group in this respect is the Louisiana Association for Mental Health. From its very inception, the association, in addition to its educational efforts, has followed the tactic of zeroing in on selected mental health targets. Thus, in 1942, the target was the opening of a psychiatric ward at Charity Hospital in New Orleans. Later, the association sponsored a U.S. Public Health Service survey, which recommended a third mental hospital in Louisiana. The association and the Louisiana State Medical Society in 1946 then sponsored legislation that, after a period of haggling in the legislature, was reduced to provide modest funds, $200,000, for survey plans of a hospital. Although the reduced measure passed, it was vetoed by the governor. Members of the association's board then approached the state Board of Liquidation, which provided the initial sum for the survey. Later legislative appropriations authorized construction of the Southeast Hospital, but north of Lake Pontchartrain rather than south, a location which at the time limited its usefulness to New Orleans. By a curious twist of history, however, the revision of the New Orleans SMSA in 1962 to include St.

Tammany parish brought the Mandeville Hospital within the confines of the New Orleans metropolitan area.

In 1950, through association efforts, the George S. Farnsworth contracting organization agreed to provide funds for nine psychiatric internships in the state's mental hospitals, and Joseph M. Jones gave funds for one. The experience of the Farnsworth Fellowship program led to legislative action in 1956 that placed the mental health training and internship program on a statutory basis. Other specific mental health objectives pursued by the association include the establishment of a mental health center in Shreveport, the opening of an aftercare clinic in New Orleans, and legislation of 1966 creating the Advisory Council on Mental Health.

As noted earlier, the Louisiana Association for Mental Health has not been a mass, high-pressure organization. It has instead utilized its board members who had access to those holding power, usually in the legislature or governor's mansion, to plead its causes. Such a member may be a prominent New Orleans citizen, like the late Joseph M. Jones, or a labor leader, like Victor Bussie, president of the Louisiana AFL-CIO. Indeed, Mr. Bussie, whose lobbying organization in Baton Rouge is said by capital observers to be one of the best anywhere, served as president of the association's board in 1966 and has worked effectively for mental health aims in the state capital and elsewhere.

Possibly because of the successes of the mental retardation associations, whose organizations have been more popularly based and whose tactics more militant, the Mental Health Association has received criticism from some quarters. It has been argued that the association should have been more active in developing grassroots demands for mental health services in communities throughout the state. The decision of the association to form chapters in all mental health regions may reflect, in part, such criticism.

Other groups within the mental health infrastructure have entered the decision-making field from time to time. Some, like the retardation groups, have in effect competed with mental health for the state dollar. Others, like the alcoholism committees, have helped advance mental health goals. As to the decision-making roles of the major professional groups, doctors, psychiatrists, psychologists, and social workers, these have not led public crusades in New Orleans or throughout the state, either for or against mental health. In some instances they have assisted in the attainment of specific aims. The cosponsorship by the State Medical Society of the initial legislation looking toward the Southeast Hospital is one example. The work of Dr. Robert Heath of the Tulane Medical School in placing psychiatric interns in the state hospitals is another. It may well be that the significant decision-making roles of the professional groups lie in the future, as they react to the implications of President Kennedy's "bold, new" program and the impact of the federal legislation of 1963.

The entrance of the federal government into the Louisiana mental health arena actually predates the federal mental health act of 1946, as the Public Health Service survey of 1945 illustrates. Under federal stimulus, the state Hospital Board was designated the state mental health agency in 1948 and was authorized to formulate state mental health plans. Through the Dallas regional office, NIMH maintained close contacts with mental health developments in the state. Federal demonstration grants and research and training grants contributed to mental health activities. Research and training grants have been especially important in New Orleans, since the universities and medical schools of the area have been the major recipients.

As indicated earlier, statewide comprehensive mental health planning in Louisiana anticipated in many respects the emphasis on planning generated by the federal Community Mental Health Centers Act of 1963. Annual state plans date from the state legislation of 1948. In 1961 the state Department of Hospitals began the formulation of a long-range comprehensive mental health program. This process merged into the planning undertaken in 1963–1965 in connection with the federal act of 1963 and with the assistance of grants from the Department of Health, Education, and Welfare.

Planning got underway with the creation of the Division of Planning in the state Department of Hospitals on July 1, 1963. Mr. H. J. Walters, a long-time official in the Mental Health Division, was appointed mental health planning coordinator. The next step was to appoint the state Advisory Council on Mental Health Planning, a step taken in August 1963. In September 1963 regional planning councils and coordinators were appointed in each of the then nine mental health regions. The planning edifice was completed in 1964 when the state Council on Construction of Community Mental Health Centers was established by statute.

The flow of the planning process went something like this. The regional planning council had the basic task of developing a plan to meet the mental health needs of the people of the region. The council did not go about this task untutored, however. State planning officials supplied the council with detailed instructions and statistical data; state consultants were also made available. A standard planning report outline drawn up by NIMH was required to be filed by each regional council around June 1, 1965. This report set forth the mental health needs and priorities for the region. The state coordinator and the state Advisory Council on Mental Health Planning then reviewed the regional plans. The regional plans were also reviewed by the state Council on Construction of Community Mental Health Centers. As a result of these reviews, the regions themselves were ranked for priority with respect to unmet needs.

Over a thousand persons were engaged in one way or another in the planning of 1963–1965. Who these people were and what interests they represented may be seen in the composition of the various planning councils.

The state Advisory Council on Mental Health Planning consisted of twenty-four persons, of which eleven were from Baton Rouge and eight from New Orleans. Wide geographic distribution was not, so it appears, an important factor in determining appointments to the council. On the other hand, there was wide representation of interest groups. Four psychiatrists were on the council. Other professions represented were social work, sociology, nursing, and the clergy. The executive director of the Louisiana Association for Mental Health and the president of the Louisiana Association for Retarded Children also sat on the council. Legislators included two state representatives and one senator. There was a rather large contingent of state officials. No member of the state Department of Hospitals sat on the planning council, but several departmental officials served as consultants.

The regional planning councils varied in size. Originally set at twelve to fifteen members, they ultimately ranged from sixteen to over thirty members. Appointments to the planning councils were made upon the recommendations of a variety of mental health interest groups. Recommendations also came from the state Departments of Education, Institutions, and Public Welfare and the state Board of Health. Civic groups, labor unions, business firms, police juries, and the like were also consulted.

For each region, a planning coordinator was appointed upon the recommendation and approval of the state Council on Mental Health Planning and the state coordinator of mental health planning. The regional coordinators, who also served on the regional councils (in several instances, the coordinator also was chairman of the regional council), were drawn from professionals working in the mental health field. Six of them, it may be noted, were administrators of mental health centers.

Since the planning councils generally proceeded along similar lines, the workings of the New Orleans regional council will illustrate the manner in which the mental health and construction plans of 1965 evolved. The New Orleans council was the largest in the state; ultimately some fifty persons participated in one way or another. Medical doctors made up the largest single contingent, numbering twenty-three, of which fifteen were psychiatrists or doctors engaged in mental health activities. The medical contingent included the deans of the Tulane and the Louisiana State University Medical Schools, the chairman of Tulane Medical School's Department of Psychiatry, plus four additional members of the Tulane medical faculty.

As did the other regional councils, the New Orleans council established subcommittees or task forces. The particular subcommittees of the New Orleans council dealt with (1) education, training, and research; (2) facilities and treatment of adults; (3) facilities and treatment of children; (4) mental retardation; (5) prevention; (6) geriatrics population; and (7) buildings.

The subcommittees were responsible for amassing factual data in their areas and preparing recommendations. The reports of the subcommittees were reviewed by the steering committee, which then made recommendations to the council as a whole. The council proved too big, really, for efficient working; it attempted to meet about every two months, while the steering committee met more frequently.

As the initial step, the regional council was organized as a working body in September 1963. During the next several months the task forces collected data by means of surveys and site visits and made interim reports. At the state level, data and guidelines for planning were collected and prepared and furnished the regional council. In the middle of 1964 a statewide effort was made to encourage community interest and participation in the planning process. Regional and statewide conferences to which professional, business, labor, civic, and social group representatives were invited discussed the problems of mental health planning and preliminary recommendations for a comprehensive state plan. Following these conferences, the regional councils directed attention to the acquisition of ecological and epidemiological data for each parish within the region. During the latter months of 1964 considerable emphasis was placed on the development of a statewide construction plan.

The planning process entered its final phase in early 1965. The Department of Hospitals transmitted an "Outline for Submitting a Report on the Regional Plan for a Comprehensive Mental Health Program," prepared by NIMH, to the regional coordinators. The outline indicated that the regional council would be required to file a comprehensive report on or before June 1, 1965. The outline called for a detailed reporting and analysis of various characteristics of the mental health region.

The outline placed before the regional councils five "Goals of Mental Health Planning" and requested the councils to state whether they concurred therein. Briefly stated, these goals were (1) to develop a continuum of mental health services in the local community, (2) to find successful approaches and programs for the prevention of mental illness, (3) to increase manpower and research in the mental health field, (4) to develop a coordinated plan for financing regional mental health services, and (5) to transfer responsibility to the local community for administering mental health programs.

The outline specified a series of thirteen mental health needs. The regional councils were required to rank these needs as to the degree to which they were unmet by existing services and facilities. Also the regional council was required to give its findings, with respect to the population receiving and needing mental health services, the continuity of mental health services, recent changes in services offered in the region, remaining mental health services problems, interagency coordination, and to make a concrete set of recommendations of what should be done during the period 1965–1970 to meet the region's needs.

What were the results of the planning process in the New Orleans mental health region? As to the five goals of mental health planning, the New Orleans council agreed with the first four but did not agree with the last, which proposed a transfer of responsibility to the local community for administering comprehensive mental health programs. The New Orleans council recommended that this goal be restated in the following terms: "To encourage the involvement of the local community in the financing and operation of local mental health programs."

As to the ranking of mental health needs, the New Orleans council arrived at the following priorities: (1) prevention, (2) budgetary needs, (3) in-service training, (4) manpower, (5) education and information, (6) treatment, (7) early detection, (8) research, (9) consultation, (10) auxiliary services (rehabilitation), (11) renovations and additions (buildings), and (12) new construction.

The New Orleans council concluded that neither new construction nor renovations or additions to buildings were primary needs. Indeed, it concluded that the "greatest need" of the region was "better and fuller use of existing physical plants." Nonetheless, the council proceeded to recommend the construction of six new community health centers, three new auxiliary facilities, and a new alcoholic facility during 1965–1970. The first recommended new community mental health center was to be at Tulane University at an estimated cost of $1,950,000. The reason for the recommendation for a new center at Tulane appears to be simple: Tulane was the only group to bring a concrete proposal before the council. The council noted that DePaul Hospital, Touro Hospital, and the Louisiana State University School of Medicine were developing plans for mental health facilities and indicated that these should be given top priority when funds became available.

The New Orleans council made a strong recommendation for continuous mental health planning in the region. It proposed the formation of a "Citizens' Committee for Mental Health Planning," which would run about forty to fifty in size. The citizens' committee would have an executive committee of about twelve to fifteen. The council emphasized the importance of having "community leaders not primarily identified with mental health efforts" on the citizens' committee. It also recommended that the governing body of each parish in the region be represented. Another point emphasized was the necessity of a staff with experience in community planning for mental health and money for continuous planning. The council felt that several organizations, and not the Department of Hospitals alone, should participate in the financing.

The council's recommendation for a continuous planning body reflects several points concerning the relationships of the New Orleans area to mental health. The call for involvement of community leaders not primarily identified with mental health suggests what has already been noted, namely, that the mental health influentials are not in the same class really with the community elite. The suggestion that parish governing bodies be involved certainly touches upon the factor that local governments, especially the city of New Orleans, contribute very little in the way of money to the mental health program. The council did not feel that the planning project of 1963–1965 had had an impact on the community that would help "materially" in future planning. It is not surprising, then, that the council argued that continuous planning might "strengthen the public image" of mental health. Finally, the council strongly endorsed the active participation of private practitioners in community mental health programs and felt it essential that "organized medicine" be involved in continuous mental health planning.

As might be expected, the results of planning in the New Orleans area differed in many respects from results elsewhere in the state. As to the five goals of a comprehensive mental health program, most regional councils were in concurrence with them. New Orleans, however, expressed apprehension over the particular goal of transferring responsibility to the local community for administering the mental health program; the New Orleans council was joined by the Baton Rouge council in this sentiment.

With respect to the priority rankings of mental health needs, New Orleans ranked "prevention" first. Over the state, however, "prevention" was placed midway in priority among the twelve specific mental health needs ranked. The situation was reversed in the case of "new construction," which the New Orleans council ranked last in priority. Statewide, "new construction" was given a middle-range priority ranking. The number one priority need on a statewide basis was "manpower," but in New Orleans it was only fourth. There was general concurrence as to "budgetary needs"; the need for money was number two in priority both in the New Orleans area and on the average throughout the state.

Finally, the New Orleans council expressed doubts as to whether the planning process of 1963–1965 had materially helped future mental health planning in the area. This was contrary to the conclusions of the other regional councils, all but one of which felt that future planning had been helped. The New Orleans council also made a strong plea for development of a mechanism for continuous planning. In this it was joined by the other regional councils, although usually in a milder way.

At the conclusion of the planning of 1963–1965, the state's mental health regions were given priority rankings. The New Orleans region received the top priority, followed by the Monroe, Houma, Shreveport, and Baton Rouge regions. Lowest priority went to the Lafayette region and the next to lowest to the Alexandria-Pineville region.

The planning process of 1963–1965 represented the first federal effort under the Community Mental Health Centers Act of 1963 to make a massive impact upon the mental health decision-making field in the New Orleans area and throughout the state as well. In line with the philosophy of President Kennedy's "bold, new" program, the process also represented an attempt to reverse the historic balance that had placed mental health on the state level and to return the mental health function to the "grassroots" local community. How successful was the initial federal effort?

In terms of number of persons involved, the mental health infrastructure groups participating, the formal planning structures created, and the data and documentation amassed, the results of the process of 1963–1965 indeed appear impressive. But the immediate results in terms of decision making and planning were not so impressive. For example, despite the overall modest priority ranking of "new construction," the regional councils called for quite a few new facilities for 1965–1970. These included at least four comprehensive mental health centers, five community centers, twenty-one "satellite" centers or clinics, seven alcoholism facilities, and approximately seventeen assorted day-care centers, half-way houses, youth study centers, emergency psychiatric facilities, geriatric units, and acutely ill units. The totality of new facilities proposed would have easily tripled the number of facilities existing as of 1963 when planning commenced. But, for the first years of the period 1965–1970, the Advisory Council on Construction of Community Mental Health Centers gave priority to only six new centers or clinics, one of which was to be located in New Orleans. Five of these six were state (or state-local) facilities that had already been "planned" by the state Mental Health Division before the exercise of 1963–1965 began. The sixth was the center proposed by the Tulane Medical School. While the Tulane center traces its immediate origins to the federal legislation of 1963, its inclusion in the plan is due to the initiative of the university's

Department of Psychiatry, not that of the New Orleans regional council.

Further developments have occurred, at both the state and metropolitan area levels, since the comprehensive mental health planning of 1965.[6] At the state level, Governor McKeithen, acting in response to the federal Comprehensive Health Planning and Public Health Services Amendments of 1966, established the Louisiana Interdepartmental Health Policy Commission in June 1967 to coordinate all planning and policy matters relating to health, including mental health, in the state.

Within the New Orleans area and led by the Mental Health Association, plans are in progress to incorporate the Metropolitan New Orleans Mental Health Council. Membership is to consist of two representatives from each of the mental health centers, clinics, and other organizations involved in the mental health field in the Greater New Orleans area. Functions of the proposed Council include the coordination of the activities of the member agencies, the standardization of procedures, the promotion of the highest quality and efficiency in mental health operations, and the discussion of problems of a medical administrative nature. Further purposes of the Council are to increase public participation and support, to obtain community involvement, and to secure funds for mental health services, projects, and research. Also at the local level, a group of private citizens, sparked in part by the 1966 federal comprehensive health planning legislation, have formed the New Orleans Area Health Planning Council. Playing instrumental roles in its establishment were Tulane University, the Chamber of Commerce, and the Bureau of Governmental Research, and its leadership is drawn in part from the area's top business and medical circles.

Insofar as mental health decision making and programing are concerned, these post-1965 developments may have an impact on problems resulting from splintering and fragmentation. The Interdepartmental Health Policy Commission and the proposed State Health Planning

[6] Basic documents relating to the planning under the federal legislation of 1963 are *The Louisiana Plan for a Comprehensive Mental Health Program* (Louisiana State Department of Hospitals, Baton Rouge: Sept. 1, 1965); *Louisiana State Construction Plan for Community Mental Health Centers, Fiscal Year 1965 and Fiscal Year 1966* (Louisiana State Department of Hospitals, Baton Rouge: June 1, 1965). For later developments, see *Louisiana's New Plan . . . Mental Health Services* (Louisiana State Department of Hospitals, Baton Rouge: July 1, 1967) and *The 1967 Modification of the Louisiana State Construction Plan for Community Mental Health Centers, July 1, 1966–June 30, 1967* (Louisiana State Department of Hospitals, Baton Rouge: April 1, 1967).

Council may alleviate some of the effects of splintering at the state level, although the price may be a greater merging, perhaps submerging, of mental health interests with those of health and welfare generally. On the metropolitan area scene, the proposed Mental Health Council appears as a possible antidote to local fragmentation, which, curiously enough, the 1963 federal legislation and developments thereunder compounded by adding several catchment areas to the checkered mosaic of the New Orleans area.

MENTAL HEALTH MANPOWER

Mortar, men, and money—these are the basic elements of any social services program. More mortar, as represented by new physical facilities, did not emerge among the highest priority needs in Louisiana's mental health planning of the mid-1960s. But with manpower, it was different. Indeed, manpower achieved the top priority ranking for the mental health needs of the state as a whole. For the New Orleans metropolitan area, however, manpower needs did not obtain a critical rating.

Of the manpower engaged in mental health programs, certainly the psychiatrist is in the top category. As a state, Louisiana ranks relatively low in terms of the number of psychiatrists practicing within its borders. In 1964, according to the roster of the Louisiana Psychiatric Association, there were 131 psychiatrists in the state. The geographical distribution of psychiatrists throughout the state is very uneven. As might be expected, they are concentrated in the metropolitan areas. In fact, in 1964, only 13 of the state's 131 psychiatrists were not located in a metropolitan area, and 11 of those 13 were in the Alexandria-Pineville complex. The New Orleans area alone accounted for almost three-fourths of Louisiana's psychiatrists. Since 1964, the number of psychiatrists in the state has increased. There has also been some tendency for psychiatrists to locate outside of New Orleans, but the large majority remain in the metropolitan area.

The figures above do not distinguish between private practitioners and those psychiatrists engaged on a full-time or part-time basis in those facilities embraced in the state's mental health program. These, it will be recalled, consist of both public and private facilities. Actually, only a little more than half (68) of Louisiana's 131 psychiatrists in 1964 were attached either full- or part-time to a mental health facility in the state program. All but two or three of these were located in the state's metropolitan areas or the Alexandria-Pineville area, with New Orleans accounting for 53 per cent (36) of the total.

The psychiatrist, though the key person, represents only one of several professional components of mental health manpower. Some idea of the total professional manpower problems facing the state as it continues expansion of community mental health services is indicated by data from a statewide survey of mental health resources conducted in 1964. The survey estimated that by 1970 the number of psychiatrists must be increased by 25 per cent over the 1964 figure, psychologists by 16 per cent, social workers by 31 per cent, psychiatric aides by 20 per cent, and all types of mental health professionals together by 18 per cent.

The geographical distribution of professional mental health manpower in general is similar to that of psychiatrists in particular. It, too, is concentrated in the metropolitan areas, with one aberration arising from the location of the state's mental hospitals. Because the survey includes personnel of state mental hospitals, it gives a distorted picture of the personnel actually engaged in Louisiana's community mental health program. To illustrate, the Baton Rouge Mental Health Region in 1964 claimed ten psychiatrists engaged in mental health, but eight of these were with the East State Hospital at Jackson, and only two were associated with the community program.

One further point concerning the state's mental health personnel involves the problem of the outlying parishes. For the private practitioner in psychiatric and mental health services, it is a sound principle to go where the people are, to the larger urban and metropolitan areas. But Louisiana's district-region plan for mental health services is based in part on the theory of geographical distribution of services. The two principles need not necessarily conflict. In fact, they may reinforce each other, as when facilities were placed in urban centers like Monroe and Lake Charles. What happens, however, when facilities are located in the smaller towns and cities like Bogalusa and Houma, which on their own are not likely to attract a psychiatrist or a similar professional? The answer is mixed; full-time personnel may not be available, but part-time personnel are obtainable.

On almost every count, the New Orleans metropolitan area fares well with respect to manpower involved in the state's mental health program when compared with the rest of Louisiana. The mental health personnel located within the metropolitan area numbered 691 in 1964. These included half of the psychiatrists in the entire state who were engaged in state programs, a fourth of the psychologists, and a third of the social workers.

In 1964, the present New Orleans metropolitan area comprised about 28 per cent of the state's total population. The percentage of the state's mental health personnel in the area was 30. Thus, it appears that the availability of personnel in New Orleans placed the metropolitan area in a favorable situation relative to the state as a whole.

For the metropolitan area, as for the state overall, personnel directly engaged in community type activities represents the minor portion of the total mental health manpower pool. In the case of New Orleans, three large mental hospitals take a goodly share of the area's personnel. De Paul Hospital, the Veterans Administration Hospital, and Southeast Louisiana Hospital (Mandeville), plus a Veterans Clinic and a USPHS Hospital, accounted for 13 of the area's 36 psychiatrists involved in the state's mental health program. An additional 22 psychiatrists were attached to Charity Hospital, Ochsner Hospital and Clinic, and Tulane University and Louisiana State University Medical Schools. This left but one full-time psychiatrist employed in a community mental health institution, the Southeast Aftercare Clinic in downtown New Orleans. This meant that the area's two community health centers, the New Orleans Center and the East Jefferson Center, and the one community clinic, the St. Tammany Clinic, had no full-time psychiatrists on their staffs as of 1964.

The situation with respect to other professional personnel serving in community mental health units was not much different from that of the psychiatrists; they, too, were largely on a part-time basis. The New Orleans Mental Health Center had the greatest number of full-time professionals.

In addition to the mental hospitals and the community units, the New Orleans mental health services contain a third element, not found in other areas of the state. This element consists of the psychiatric services attached to the medical schools in New Orleans, Tulane University and Louisiana State University, and to Charity Hospital, which is used as the teaching hospital by both. These account for a significant portion of the metropolitan area's mental health manpower.

The manpower differences between these psychiatric units and the community units became even more marked when gauged by the total man hours provided per week. In relative terms, psychiatric manpower in the community centers loomed less than half as large as the proportion in the psychiatric units. On the other hand, social workers provided the greater part of the manpower hours in the centers, while their role in the psychiatric units was barely minimal.

There are probably several reasons for the different allocations of manpower among the types of mental health facilities. One factor may relate to inpatient versus outpatient services. The centers are wholly outpatient and make extensive use of social workers, but very little use of nurses and psychiatric aides. The Charity Hospital service, on the other hand, is basically inpatient; its utilization of social workers is minimal, but very heavy for nurses and aides. The Tulane and L.S.U. Medical School units make the greatest use of psychiatrists. Undoubtedly, the teaching, training, and research functions of the medical school units are important, if for no other reason than that these give greater access to funds. If psychiatric manpower must be increased in the community centers, one device would be a greater linking of the centers with the Tulane and L.S.U. training and research programs. Otherwise, the financial burdens on the centers necessary to permit any significant increase in psychiatric manpower may prove virtually insurmountable.

To what extent does the New Orleans mental health manpower situation meet current and projected needs? This question may be approached by comparison with the staffing pattern for a community mental health center proposed during passage of the federal staffing legislation of 1965. The proposed staffing pattern indicated that a community mental health center would provide a total of 2,030 professional man hours per week to serve a population of 100,000. None of the mental health centers in the New Orleans area came even close to offering the magnitude of services contemplated at the time the 1965 Act was passed. The largest unit, the New Orleans Center, was providing only 681 man hours per week, or about one-third the total envisaged for a 100,000 population scale center. The smallest center, St. Tammany, was providing an abysmally low total of 96 man hours per week.

The mental health manpower attached to the area's community health centers in 1964–1965 represented only a drop in the bucket insofar as needs were projected under the federal staffing legislation of 1965. When the full range of area community type facilities was taken into account, the area manpower situation brightened. Sufficient psychiatric manpower seemed present to meet needs as set forth in the federal staffing pattern. The situation with respect to social workers was not dark. Thus, if all the manpower, full- and part-time, available in all of the area's mental health facilities could be utilized in community mental health programs, the presumed needs of New Orleans might be substantially met. Such utilization would require extensive reallocation of manpower, which in turn would be dependent upon (1) redefinition of clienteles, (2) reorientation of state program goals, and (3) restatement of standards by which needs are ascertained.

For the manpower of the State Mental Hospital at Mandeville and of the federal installations to be reallocated fully to area community type programs would necessitate two kinds of redefinition of clientele, including a geographic redefinition. The Mandeville Hospital serves the entire state of Louisiana, the Southeastern District particularly, and the federal units are not restricted to service in the New Orleans area. Whether it would be either wise or possible to redefine geographically are separate questions, but unless it occurs, the New Orleans area will share these mental health resources with other geographic areas. With respect to geographic redefinition, the fact that the New Orleans Mental Health Region ranks among the best endowed in the state is an additional factor. In the case of the federal installations, another kind of redefinition would be necessary, in particular one which would open these up to nonveterans. Redefinition of this type would quickly involve, among others, the veterans' interest groups. Finally, there is a clientele problem that hinges on personal finances. The low-income groups generally have ready access to public units; the well-to-do presumably can afford to purchase mental health services without much financial juggling. The middle-income groups seem to be the worst off, not qualifying for public facilities and not readily able to commit family resources to large outlays for mental health services. Perhaps expanded insurance plans, both private and public, are the answer for the middle-income classes.

A second prerequisite for substantial reallocation of manpower to community type services involves a reorientation of mental health program goals. So long as a goodly portion of mental health manpower is allotted to large custodial mental hospitals, it cannot contribute fully to community type programs. The 1963 federal Act presumes a de-emphasis of the custodial hospital. Even if this occurred in Louisiana (and this does not appear likely), it might not release much manpower because Louisiana is already far below the standard ratio of 5 hospital beds per 1,000. The New Orleans area illustrates another problem of reallocation. Since the Tulane and L.S.U. medical schools are primarily interested in teaching and research, their professional staff may not serve the general stream of clinical patients.

Finally, there is the question of standards. What should be the proportion of professional categories in relation to population served? New Orleans manpower figures suggest that the ratio of psychologists presumed in the federal staffing pattern might well be reexamined. Either psychologists are not so important, or their functions are being performed by psychiatrists or social workers, or the programs are suffering severely. There is also the matter of full-time versus part-time personnel. On a full-time basis only, New Orleans area mental health facilities are lacking in manpower. But, by adding part-time personnel, the area begins to approach the man-hours-week standard. Does this mean that the manpower demands of community programs are attainable in the immediate and middle future only through heavy reliance upon part-time personnel? And if so, will the services afforded suffer in comparison to those rendered by facilities manned by full-time staff?

If the federal mental health center staffing pattern of 1965 is taken as a guide, the mental health manpower needs throughout Louisiana are of a greater magnitude than in the New Orleans area. The federal pattern calls for six full-time psychiatrists per center, providing a total of 210 man hours per week of services. In 1964–1965, no community mental health center in the state came close to this standard. The best in the state was the Baton Rouge Center, providing 96 man hours per week of services. Most of the centers and clinics were providing 20 to 32 man hours per week.

The question is whether federal staffing grants have helped the manpower situation in New Orleans and Louisiana. The short answer is: so far, not much. Insofar as state mental health facilities are concerned, no staffing grants have been applied for. One reason for this is an apprehension that the commitments involved in a federal staffing grant would put the state in over its head when the grant expired. Instead, the state Mental Health Division has developed its own staffing pattern and has largely succeeded in getting the legislature to appropriate the necessary funds. In fact, some funded positions in state facilities remain unfilled and it is not felt that this is especially due to inability to offer competitive salaries.

In the New Orleans area two private community centers, Touro and De Paul, have applied for federal staffing grants. As of spring, 1968, De Paul had received a grant, but Touro had not.

A particular point in the Louisiana mental health scene that deserves special note is the development of the concept of the mental health center administrator, a position now officially designated. To qualify as a center administrator, training in social work is required.

In sum, Louisiana's mental health planners of the mid-1960s did not anticipate reaching the federal staffing standard in all categories of manpower by 1970. Indeed, it is doubtful whether that standard played any role at all in the planning process. The contrasts between manpower planning goals reached at the state and local level and those concocted in Washington are very great in some instances. The feasibility of either set of goals, moreover, involves consideration of mental health money and financing.

FINANCING MENTAL HEALTH

Taxes and tithes, alms and fees—these are the sources of mental health money in New Orleans and Louisiana. The state and federal governments are the chief provenders of tax monies for mental health; local governments on the whole contribute little. Alms in the form of charitable and religious efforts help support a variety of mental health activities. Fees play a minor role in public mental health financing, but loom larger in the economics of mental health in the private sector. Mental health financing in the New Orleans area is heavily dependent, as it is everywhere in Louisiana, upon state funds.

Indices of mental health expenditures indicate that Louisiana, like Southern states generally, ranks nationally in the lowest fourth of the states with respect to expenditures for public mental hospitals. Among Southern states, however, Louisiana ranks in the upper half on most counts. For community mental health programs, on the other hand, Louisiana expenditures run better than the national average, and the state emerges as leader among Southern states in this field. It should be noted that the state ranks forty-sixth nationally and seventh regionally with respect to per capita personal income. On the national scale, Louisiana's financial effort on behalf of mental health ranks higher than might be expected on the basis of the state's personal income situation.

State expenditures for mental health have increased considerably since World War II, but only in part as a result of the development of the community oriented program. In 1956–1957, state expenditures were $7,872,000, of which a mere $97,000 was allotted for community outpatient services. By 1966–1967, this had increased to $18,520,000, of which $2,519,000 went for community outpatient services. Thus it would appear that expenditures for mental hospitals increased 106 per cent over the decade, while those for community services increased 2,487 per cent.

The expenditure increases over the decade 1956–1966 are somewhat deceptive. In 1956 there were about a dozen mental health outpatient and alcoholism clinics in operation, but they were not financed through the budget of the State Department of Hospitals. Thus, the fantastic percentage increase for community mental health services over the decade is largely due to a change in bookkeeping. On the other hand, the figures do not show state expenditures for mental health facilities which are part of Charity Hospital in New Orleans and of Confederate Memorial Hospital in Shreveport. Nor do the figures reflect spending for training and research or for mental retardation. All in all, it seems that state mental health expenditures in 1966–1967 easily topped the $20,000,000 mark; total expenditures through the Department of Hospitals for mental health and mental retardation certainly topped the $30,000,000 mark.

Funds spent through the Department of Hospitals do not represent the full total of state money spent on mental health. The entire picture would include the costs of mental health related services provided by other state agencies, such as the State Departments of Education, Health, Institutions, and Welfare.

A further point concerning mental health expenditures is in regard to the relative costs of the mental hospital versus the community approach. For the year 1962–1963, the cost per patient per year in a mental hospital was $1,596, while the same cost in community clinics was $79. The cost per patient per year in mental hospitals appears to be rising steadily, from $1,300 in 1959–1960, to $2,317 in 1965–1966. The relative newness of community type services may render existing data for this type somewhat inconclusive, but the cost per year seems to be decreasing as yearly admissions and the total cared for rise sharply.

As mentioned earlier, the bulk of the finances for community mental health services in Louisiana comes from state funds. In 1964–1965, the total of the budgets of the 21 community centers and clinics was in excess of $1,400,000. Of this total, over 90 per cent represented state appropriations. About 4 per cent (around $50,000) came from fees, and about 6 per cent (around $80,000) came from local alms, tithes, and tax funds. The police juries in St. Tammany parish provided some support to centers and clinics. A number of towns and cities also made small appropriations. It may also be noted that in appropriate cases state welfare funds can be used to purchase drugs used in mental health treatment.

Although providing but a small proportion of state mental health funds, fees do raise some important policy questions. Both indigent and paying patients are eligible to use state mental hospitals and mental health centers and clinics. Louisiana law, however, requires that the patient or his legally responsible relative be charged for services in accordance with ability to pay.

The State Department of Hospitals has adopted a uniform schedule of fees. For treatment in mental hospitals, fees usually are not charged persons with an annual income of less than $3,000 (with prospects that the ceiling may be raised). For visits to outpatient clinics and centers, the fees range from 25 cents to $7.00 a visit. As the law now stands, all fees collected are placed in a special research and training account and are used to support research and the training of medical and other health personnel.

The primary source of mental health money in the New Orleans area is taxes. Whether state or federal taxes take the lead is a difficult question, in view of the variety of federal grants coming into the area for research and training. But one point is crystal clear: Local tax support has been negligible. Secular tithing through the United Fund is an important source of mental health money. Indeed, secular tithing seems to have been substituted for local taxing. Nor can fees as a source of mental health funds be dismissed. True, in the public mental health facilities, fees do not appear to be a substantial source. But New Orleans has several private psychiatric facilities (not counting private psychiatric practice), and these require more than modest sums to support their activities. Figures with respect to alms (as distinct from secular tithing) are not easy to come by. However, the New Orleans area had a goodly number of charitable and religious auxiliary facilities, and these derive some support from alms.

Is the New Orleans mental health money situation much different from that in the state at large? In recent mental health planning (1963–1965), the New Orleans area planners did not consider budgetary needs as a high priority item, while throughout the state budgetary needs received the second highest priority among unmet needs. Probably the statewide ranking is more realistic than the New Orleans ranking, if Louisiana's mental health program is to approach the dimensions envisaged in the federal legislation of 1963 and 1965. It would probably take a tenfold increase in the state's appropriations for community mental health programs in 1964–1965 to bring the state and the New Orleans area's programs close to the federal pattern, and this would mean more than doubling the total state 1966–1967 expenditures for mental health.

How well do health in general and mental health in particular fare in Louisiana's state capital decision-making arena? For 1966–1967, the state's overall health program was budgeted for $123.1 million (including federal and local funds), a figure which placed it fourth in rank of state program expenditures. Health expenditures fell behind education ($461.8 million), public welfare ($200.3 million), and highways ($187.6 million). However, when state money alone is considered, health programs rose one step in rank. State funds for health amounted to $87.3 million, a figure above the $61.5 million in state funds spent on public welfare, but still less than for education ($391.8 million) and for highways ($96.8 million). Federal funds for health accounted for $32.5 million (26 per cent of the total) and local funds for $3.4 million (only 3 per cent of the total).

The above expenditures relate to the overall health program of the state. What share of these go to mental health? If the estimate arrived at earlier of $20 million for mental health in 1966–1967 were used, it would account for 16 per cent of the total $123.1 million allocated to health. This proportion for mental health compares with $37.9 million (30.8 per cent) for general hospitals, $37.2 million (30.2 per cent) for medical assistance provided through the Welfare Department, and $9.7 million (7.9 per cent) for mental retardation.

The real property tax, long the backbone of local governmental revenue, operates under severe limitations in Louisiana. There is a constitutional limitation on the millage rate that a local authority may levy. To raise its millage rate, the city of New Orleans, for example, must obtain a constitutional amendment and this, in turn, involves a statewide vote on the issue. In addition, there is a problem of assessment. The constitutional requirement is that property be assessed at its real value. But what is the real value? Assessors in Louisiana are popularly elected and have shown little disposition to assess property at its market value. On the contrary, assessments are usually low. Much to the chagrin of the buyer, about the only time there is an increase in assessment is when property is sold. Estimates suggest that real property in the New Orleans area is assessed at perhaps 25 to 30 per cent of the market value.

The sales tax is another important source of local revenue. Any local sales tax must be levied on top of state sales tax and, furthermore, requires legislative authority.

In 1967 the city of New Orleans was prepared to propose to the state legislature that it impose an income tax. However, in part through the efforts of the legislators from the adjoining parish of Jefferson, the state legislature passed a law which forbids one parish to levy an income tax on residents of another parish.

Finally, there is the matter of local bonds. In New Orleans, the Board of Liquidation of City Debt must approve city bond issues. The Board will not approve a bond issue unless the yield from the real property tax will be adequate to service the new debt. Thus, the city of New Orleans is limited in any given year by the rise in assessments of real property during the year as to any new bonds it may issue. Here again, the fact that the tax assessors are popularly elected is an important consideration.

Given the financial limits on local units, it is not surprising that mental health has not received much local tax support. Indeed, both the state and the metropolitan area might well be regarded as underdeveloped areas, in that the basic governmental services such as education, paved highways, police protection, adequate sewage, etc. are below par. Until these basic needs are adequately met, it is not likely that mental health, which in the popular mind is likely viewed more as a luxury item, will receive high fiscal priority.

VIII: SYRACUSE

JULIAN R. FRIEDMAN

ONCE THE CENTER of a powerful federation of Indian tribes, today the Syracuse metropolitan area, comprising Onondaga, Madison, and Oswego counties, is a "prime industrial region, an important distribution point and a financial center" bolstered by a comprehensive retailing setup, a major university complex, expanding cultural facilities, and attractive recreational opportunities. Once "a fever-stricken swamp," "dark, gloomy, and impenetrable, a favorite resort for wolves, bears, wildcats, mud turtles, and rattlesnakes," today the area is a thriving theater of human endeavors.[1]

In area the Syracuse SMSA ranks second in the state. Extending from the Adirondack Mountains to the Finger Lakes, it covers approximately 2,420 square miles. Cities occupy 58.5 square miles, or 100 square miles with their urbanized fringe and suburbs. The remaining area, 96 per cent of the total, is rural. Of the three counties, Oswego is the largest and Madison the smallest, ranging in size from 970 square miles to 660 square miles.

The terrain of the metropolitan area varies moderately. Geography has allowed growth in transportation in line with both technological and economic revolutions. Except during the occasional blizzards no portion is totally isolated from the city of Syracuse and the Upstate Medical Center. An expanding highway system has brought all mental illness and retardation facilities within direct, though not always convenient, reach of all the inhabitants of the area.

I wish to acknowledge with appreciation the help of Robert Lee and Thomas Wolfe, research assistants, in preparing this chapter.

[1] C. E. A. Winslow, *A City Set on a Hill* (Garden City: Doubleday Doran & Co., 1934), p. 20. This account fails to do justice to the more felicitous conditions to the south and east of the city of Syracuse.

ECOLOGY

With an estimated population of 619,367,[2] the Syracuse metropolitan area stands fifth among the seven Standard Metropolitan Statistical Areas in New York state. Seventy-six per cent of the population (468,154) is concentrated in Onondaga county, 15 per cent (92,244) in Oswego, and the remainder (58,969) in Madison county. Onondaga county has a population density of 591 persons per square mile, Oswego 98, and Madison 89. Of the total population approximately 42 per cent reside within the limits of the cities, though the city of Syracuse and its suburbs contain more than 65 per cent of the Onondaga county inhabitants. With the cities declining in population, the metropolitan area is undergoing a suburban explosion.

The Syracuse SMSA shares honors with the Rochester area for population growth since the 1960 census, 9.9 per cent for the six-year period. But Onondaga county expanded 10.7 per cent during these years, although its rate of growth has declined since 1963. Moreover, Syracuse suburban development is occurring beyond the county line into the neighboring counties.

The population of the Syracuse SMSA is younger than that in New York state as a whole. For the Syracuse area the median age at the time of the 1960 census was 29.5 years; for the state it was 33.1 years. The cities here as elsewhere in the United States attract those over fifty-five and the elderly. The higher the age group being considered, the relatively greater number of females will be found in the cities. By contrast, newer families with young children are drawn for obvious reasons to the suburbs.

As for ethnicity and the ethnic pattern, according to the 1960 census one in every four inhabitants of the Syracuse SMSA was of foreign stock, and one in every three in the city of Syracuse. Countries represented in the national origins of the foreign born and the parentage of first generation Americans included, in order of importance of contribution, Italy, Canada, Germany, Great Britain, Poland, and Ireland. Italians have gravitated to Syracuse, Fulton, Oswego, and Oneida, while

[2] New York State, Department of Commerce, *Business Fact Book New York State 1966 Supplement* (Albany: Department of Commerce, 1966), p. 9. This figure is a July 1, 1966, estimate.

the Canadians tend to settle in nonurban parts of Oswego county. Ethnic neighborhoods are noticeable in Syracuse and ethnic politics are one overt consequence of their existence.

Voluntary family service organizations and other social services have maintained close ties with religious bodies, and thus the religious composition of the SMSA is pertinent. In the city of Syracuse approximately 51 per cent of the population is Roman Catholic, 40 per cent Protestant, and 7 per cent Jewish. In the metropolitan area, Roman Catholic and Protestant churches predominate, with the former well represented in Oswego county and the latter in Madison county. The Jewish community is found concentrated in the cities and certain suburbs.

Caucasians constitute the vast majority of the population of the SMSA, but the minorities include Negroes and Indians. Eleven out of twelve Negroes reported in the 1960 census lived in Syracuse, eight out of the eleven in three census tracts, with 26 per cent residing in a single tract. Beyond the city limits the Negro is a rarity except as a house servant or a seasonal migrant laborer.

According to recent estimates, the Negro population has increased but is still confined to the city of Syracuse. Intracity mobility is now high as a consequence of urban renewal projects that hastened the relocation of the Negro inhabitants from the properties selected for redevelopment. As a result, in 1967 the Negro was residing in other census tracts, but he still finds himself in ghettoes, from which the whites appear to be departing.[3]

The life of the Negro in Syracuse is characterized by low incomes, unemployment, ill health, poor school performance and truancy, substandard housing, numerous brushes with the police, and heavy dependence on public welfare. Negro children tend to be victims of school segregation and have frustrating experiences in socialization.

What is true of the Negro in Syracuse applies generally to the Indians of the area. Mainly residents on the Onondaga Indian Reservation, they suffer all the social ills that befall minorities of low socioeconomic status.

Another dimension of the social profile of the Syracuse SMSA is education. By 1960, among persons twenty-five years old or over, 61 per cent had completed at least one or more years of high school. By

[3] Alan S. Campbell, et al., The Negro in Syracuse (Syracuse: University College, 1964).

the same census figures, approximately 1.7 per cent had no schooling, the number reaching almost 3 per cent in the city of Syracuse. In the area 10 per cent were reported to have attended college four years or more; Onondaga county, in which Syracuse University is located, is ahead of this percentage and Oswego county substantially behind. Within Syracuse the residential distribution of the uneducated and the highly educated is typical of the national urban pattern, revealing the usual de facto segregation by income, quality of housing, and color.

Distribution of personal income provides clues to the overall social profile of the area. By income categories Onondaga county conforms closely to the pattern prevailing in New York state. Madison and Oswego counties exceed the state level for the lowest-income persons and fall short in the high-income classes. In those counties marginal farming tends to depress the average income.

The thriving economy from which this income is derived or through which it is funneled to its recipients is dominated by manufacturing. The products that flow from industries in the metropolitan area run from pottery to silverware, paper cartons to chemicals, heavy military electronic systems to air conditioning machinery, and automobile parts to traffic control equipment. Automation is progressing, thus raising the specter of selective unemployment for the labor force, but the demand for skilled and trained labor is high. Trade unions are strong in the automobile and steel plants, but the electronics and related enterprises firmly resist their advance.

The economy has been bolstered by the growth of Syracuse University and Upstate Medical Center, which have steadily increased the outlays of funds received from such sources as federal and state governments and foundations, as well as tuition and gifts. The expenditures of Colgate University, State College at Morrisville, and Cazenovia College have had a marked impact in Madison county, as have those emanating from the State College in Oswego for that locality. Education is big business for the Syracuse area.

Much concern had been aroused in the city of Syracuse by the shift of industrial and retail operations outside the city. It is considered a serious threat to its tax base, though the advantages accruing to the revenue-starved counties are appreciated. Faced with competition for the local dollar from suburban shopping centers, the Syracuse leadership is attempting to project an appealing image of central Syracuse as a

vital regional metropolis, the hub of business and banking in upstate
New York.[4]

Behind the façade of these social and economic factors, one finds
deeper social sensibilities, an indicator of the quality of life in the
Syracuse area. In the twenties Syracuse was cited for the "interwoven
strands of idealism and of far-sighted planning which have gained for
Syracuse in at least one field—that of public health—a position of
preeminence." [5] However, the gulf that ordinarily separates the comparatively affluent and the misfortunate seems to be widening, especially
in its psychological dimensions. While sensitive to the troubles of others
the average citizen feels too baffled, embarrassed, or impotent to come
to the rescue. Human problems are being viewed as too complex for
the layman to grasp. They are thus turned over to committees of "experts" to study, in the tradition of the Fabians in Great Britain. In
recent years one report after another on community problems has
appeared. The flow of information, very little of which is new, tends
to outpace the efforts to implement the recommendations for action.
The resulting "response gap" supports the impression that this area is
slow in meeting the genuine social needs of its population and proceeds
to do so only in emergencies or after crises.

How competent the localities are in handling the problems raised
by mental disorders turns in a large measure on how adequate and
efficient they are in governing themselves and providing for the general
welfare. Equally germane is their adroitness in navigating the main
stream of relations among the local, state, and federal governments.

Approximately 228 general and special-purpose local authorities exist
within the Syracuse SMSA. The jurisdiction for these units of government closest to the people are the 4 cities accommodating daily far
more persons than those who obviously reside in them, 35 villages located inside the boundaries of 56 townships, the open space of which is
yielding inexorably to tract housing and suburbanization, and the 3
counties, among which Onondaga manifests noteworthy metropolitan
tendencies. The powers enjoyed by the governmental units, as well as
the forms in most instances, are largely determined by the state, as is

[4] *Central Syracuse Bulletin,* Sept. 15, 1964, prepared by the Metropolitan Development Association, Syracuse, N.Y.
[5] Winslow, *A City Set on a Hill,* p. 13.

amply demonstrated by the state laws on education, health, welfare, and mental hygiene.

The mayor-council form of government prevails in the cities and villages. The separation of executive and legislative powers has in recent years become more pronounced in both. It is more advanced where the mayor is elected by popular vote, is a dominant political figure, and heads up a substantial bureaucratic establishment, as is the case in Syracuse. The elected councils, capitalizing on their traditional prerogatives, exercise influence, especially through committees that scrutinize the activities of the executive branch and its subdivisions. Assisted by various commissions and boards, the municipal governments of the SMSA seem to satisfy a politically apathetic population that wants both more government and less government at the same time.

At city hall, the mayors of Syracuse, Oswego, Fulton, and Oneida preside over administrations entrusted with the maintenance of law and order, fire protection, garbage collection, provision of low-rent housing, urban renewal, upkeep of roads, parks, and certain other public facilities, and management of some additional amenities. Since the Syracuse school district lacks fiscal autonomy, the municipal government has the final say on the education budget. Public health has been a major responsibility of the cities but on January 1, 1967, Syracuse surrendered to the county government its powers in this field. Aside from certification for confinement in hospitals, the city health departments, as well as the town and village health officers, have provided no services for the victims of mental disorders. However, as a condition for the establishment of the county mental health boards in Onondaga, Oswego, and Madison counties, the city governments have had to agree, by formal action, to participate in countywide programs under the New York State Community Mental Health Services Act of 1954.

In the Syracuse SMSA, municipal government is a humdrum affair replete with city hall politics, arousing little interest in the population at large. It has earned little reputation for excellence. Imagination and foresight were consistently eclipsed by routine and feeble performance. However, in recent years personnel policy in response to state initiatives has increased emphasis on professionalism in the public service. Both staff and line departments have improved in quality of appointees, but the long-prevailing impediments to outstanding achievement continue to take their toll in frustration. The Syracuse government pursues fiscal policies that attest to the conservatism of the community leadership. It labors under the overriding fear that higher taxes will drive business away, though its willingness to borrow has also been constrained by state-fixed limits on municipal indebtedness. While it is the most developed of the primary level authorities in the area, even it lacks the requisite sophistication among its staff that is so vital for effective negotiations with the state and federal governments. Instead it relies heavily for this purpose on consultants, often persons of influence drawn from the economy, the bar, and occasionally Syracuse University.

With the urban governments baffled by the plethora of central-city problems and town governments enervated by the suburban explosion, the counties have begun to stir into action and display some verve. As Roscoe Martin, *et al.,* have observed,

Originating as an administrative district for convenience in executing a limited number of state functions, the county only slowly and over the course of decades established its right to consideration as a unit of general government. That trend indeed is still in process, although it is now clear that the county will maintain and broaden its position as a basic unit of local government.[6]

Until 1962 the three counties of the Syracuse metropolitan area conformed to the conventional pattern of county government in the state outside of the New York City metropolitan area. The central institution has been the elected Board of Supervisors, which in Onondaga, Madison, and Oswego counties has been structured around a definite rural bias. It has possessed the powers to tax and spend, which it has exercised with an uninhibited preference for frugality. To this body the departmental commissioners have been directly accountable, and committees of supervisors perform watchdog functions under a "strong" committee system. In the absence of a chief executive, the presiding officer of the supervisors has been the head of the county government. The county clerk and county attorney have handled the day-to-day tasks at the county hall or county court house. Frequently problems neglected by the county authorities have fallen on the shoulders of the county judges for disposition.

In 1962 Onondaga county parted company with its neighboring coun-

[6] Roscoe Martin, *et al., Decisions in Syracuse* (Garden City: Doubleday, 1965), p. 37.

ties when it adopted a strong executive form of government. Legislative and fiscal powers remain vested in the Board of Supervisors, which continues to operate through a "strong" committee system, but the new charter provides for a county executive, who is an elected official empowered to appoint the heads of the departments. The district attorney and sheriff continue to be elected. Departmental commissioners report to the county executive and through him to the Board of Supervisors (recently renamed the County Legislature).

A wide array of staff and line activities fall under the county executive. He is assisted by budget, personnel, planning, and research units. Departmental heads are for the most part professionals, and the regular employees possess civil service status as required by state law. In view of his responsibilities relating to the budget, policies, and programs, the county executive is in a position to play a leadership role rather than be a mere housekeeper. As a result of reapportionment, rural centers of political power have lost ground to the suburbs, a shift that is likely to open numerous opportunities for initiative to the county executive. Furthermore, the city of Syracuse is satisfied to have the county government serve as a metropolitan authority on a wider scale than ever before. Grants from the state and federal governments also strengthen the hand of the county executive and for that matter have turned county government into "big" government, a development that has not escaped the attention of local political circles.

Mandated by state law as the primary unit for local welfare administration, the county governments are no strangers in the field of social services. With roots in the poorhouse tradition, the county welfare departments have served the rural needy and poor. However, today, in Onondaga county in particular, urban poverty monopolizes the time, energy, and resources of the welfare authorities, confronting them with perplexing entanglements they are ill equipped to remedy or resolve. Though they have supported public health nursing, the county governments have been inclined to shun general public health responsibilities, leaving them to be discharged by city, town, and state officials. Nonetheless, the Onondaga county Board of Supervisors voted in 1966 to establish a county Health Department. In 1967, the newly inaugurated county Health Department succeeded the Syracuse Health Department and became metropolitan in jurisdiction and function.

New York mental health policy has gradually fostered creeping metropolitanism at the county level. Prior to 1945 Onondaga, Madison, and Oswego counties supplied no special services to the mentally ill and retarded but instead looked to the state institutions and clinics for assistance. Health officials, welfare administrators, probation officers, and judges channeled mentally ill persons into the state system. Mental health administration constituted no part of county government.

In 1947, the Onondaga county Board of Supervisors voted to create as an adjunct of the Children's Court a child guidance clinic staffed by a psychiatrist, psychologists, and social workers. State aid was available to finance it. The director was accountable to the county legislature, which also established a citizens' advisory committee for the clinic. Subsequently an adult psychiatric clinic was brought into existence; by that time the county had subscribed to the New York State Community Mental Health Services Act.

Responding to a rising crescendo of public enthusiasm and support, the Onondaga county Board of Supervisors approved in 1955 an ordinance to establish a mental health board that would be appointed, according to state law, by the chairman of the governing body of the county. Appointees were drawn from medical, psychiatric, business, legal, religious, and educational circles, and included the chairman of the Department of Psychiatry at the Upstate Medical Center. The mental health board had a part-time director, who was also the head of the Child Guidance Center. The board had the duties of developing programs, supervising service facilities, preparing a mental health budget, and rendering advice to the county government in regard to mental health.

Madison and Oswego counties waited until 1964 to establish similar mental health boards. In the meantime, Onondaga county had set up a department of mental health, headed by a commissioner, under the 1961 charter. The commissioner reports to the county executive. The Child Guidance Center and Adult Clinic, as well as all other community facilities receiving state mental health aid, fall within the jurisdiction of the department, as do all the earlier operating responsibilities of the Mental Health Board. The board itself has become an advisory body, though it is empowered by the county charter to recommend "rules and regulations concerning the rendition or operation of services and facilities in the community mental health program."

The powers of the commissioner of mental health are countywide. He advises, assists, and supports other departments of the county government and the courts in matters involving the mentally ill and retarded. His jurisdiction includes the city of Syracuse, townships, and villages, though he has no personnel on his staff to assign specifically to these localities except in an emergency or acute situation. He has sought to work out common procedures and standards throughout the county for the officials of all local authorities who encounter victims of mental disorders. In view of the presence of state and federal facilities serving such persons in Onondaga county, he has attempted to develop systematic and coordinated intergovernmental relations in the mental health field. His efforts to organize services along metropolitan lines have partially succeeded in surmounting county fragmentation only to be frustrated by the dispersion of authority at the state and federal levels.

Government fragmentation in Onondaga county is still a serious obstacle to the development of a general-purpose metropolitan government. It impairs the efficiency and effectiveness of the existing county government. To cope with this problem, the county executive has had several avenues open to him. He has been able to contact the town supervisors and village mayors directly, reviewing particular problems with them and their staffs. Or he has taken up matters with the town supervisors in their capacity as members of the county legislature. However, after November 1967 the nineteen towns in Onondaga county lost direct representation in the County Legislature, and, furthermore, the town supervisors are no longer eligible to sit in that body. A third course for him is to have the county party leaders or members of the county committee of the political parties serve as brokers between the county and local governments. The county executive, who was elected on the Republican ticket, turns occasionally to leaders of that party for assistance. Finally, over the past three years, the county government has sponsored general conferences and specialized meetings of local legislators and officials with the immediate objective of sharing information and developing a dialogue on problems of common interest. At these sessions countywide standards and practices are discussed; the conclusions that take the form of recommendations are by no means binding on the local authorities.

Mention should be made of the numerous special districts that render particular services in the three-county area. These include school districts, which also support interdistrict service organizations, for example, a special school for educable retarded children. District boards of education are empowered to levy taxes on property for educational purposes independently of the county governments.

Despite some progress, Onondaga county, to say nothing of Madison and Oswego counties, stands far from the goal of metropolitan government. Movement in this direction is negligible, although intercounty consultation on an ad hoc basis occurs with increasing frequency. Recently a formal planning committee was formed, consisting of representatives from the three counties and two neighboring counties with a full-time executive director. A regional committee on air pollution problems has also come into being. A heart–stroke–cancer region is currently being planned, with financial assistance from the federal government. Furthermore, the regional board of the state's Hospital Review Council has been transformed into a hospital review and planning corporation entrusted with regional responsibilities, although the boundaries of the Syracuse Standard Metropolitan Statistical Area and the Central New York Hospital Region do not coincide.

In actuality the only authorities with complete jurisdiction over the entire Syracuse metropolitan area are the New York state and United States governments. Located in Syracuse are several state operating units that report to the departments in Albany. The New York Department of Social Welfare works through a regional officer, whose powers are extensive. For example, he supervises the operation of child-care centers and foster homes licensed by the state. He is consulted not only on county welfare policy but also on the details of county expenditures in this field. Regional and district health officers do far more than simply serve as links between the state and local health departments. Their duties extend to environmental health, pure water supply, and the like.

By contrast, the state Department of Mental Hygiene, along with the Department of Education, maintains no regional officer in Syracuse. Each state mental hospital is situated in a "catchment area," which can be said to be regional inasmuch as it is delimited for a group of contiguous counties. However, that does not mean that the director of the hospital has the standing of or is accepted as a regional mental hygiene officer. Though Onondaga, Madison, and Oswego counties fall within the catchment area of Marcy State Hospital near Rome, New York, the hospital director is not perceived as the general supervisor or coordinator of mental hygiene activities for these counties. Nor has the government in Albany instructed him to serve in such a capacity. The New York State Committee on Mental Disorders in its report has proposed that the state be divided into regions and each region subdivided into areas. Under this proposal the Syracuse metropolitan area counties would be in a region that stretches from the Canadian frontier to the Pennsylvania line and would join Cayuga and Cortland counties to form an area. In the same report, no blueprint is offered for regional or area mental hygiene administration, but it does propose permanent planning committees for the regions and areas.

Conspicuously absent from the governmental scene is a specifically designated coordinator of state activities within the Syracuse metropolitan area. The governor himself has no personal representative stationed in the area. In daily affairs the state government communicates to the local authorities through several channels rather than a single one. In their turn, the local government officials employ the same channels, in addition to the state senators and representatives, who carry a heavy burden in this regard.

By political reputation the Syracuse SMSA is conservative. For a hundred years with few exceptions it has stood in the Republican column in elections for state and national offices. In 1964 President Johnson and Senator Robert Kennedy cut heavily into Republican strength, carrying on their coattails the Democratic candidate for the House of Representatives from Onondaga county. In 1966 this incumbent congressman won reelection with unusually strong support from rural and suburban districts ordinarily loyal to the Republican candidate. Yet, it is premature to conclude that political sentiment is changing drastically or permanently.

In local politics the Republican Party has consistently fared better than its opponents. For several generations it has been entrenched in the governments of the counties, most towns and villages, and the city of Syracuse. But Syracuse stands by itself in this respect, for it is the only city in upstate New York with a Republican administration. Even Oneida in the even more conservative Madison county and Oswego and Fulton in Oswego county elect Democrats as mayors. Today the Republicans feel more secure in the county than in Syracuse, and they have thus lent support to the evolution of the county government into a metropolitan government exercising powers over the city. However, the calculations of their political strength have been somewhat clouded by the reapportionment of the county legislature, which has increased the political weight of the suburbs now facing something of a services crisis. The political parties are currently adjusting to the new potentialities of local politics.

Closely related to the political culture and political organizations is the power structure in the metropolitan area. The power structure in Onondaga county has been studied and analyzed by various scholars.[7] Little is known of the power structures of Madison and Oswego counties through the findings of formal research.

If a power structure must be either monolithic or pluralistic, it is the latter characterization that most experts apply to the one in Onondaga county. Available evidence establishes beyond a doubt that many persons actually participate in community dialogues, and that several varied leadership groups exist or emerge when decisions on community problems are taken. No decision is in fact a monopoly of any single powerful figure or exclusive influential circle. Syracuse has no "boss," nor is its destiny shaped in secrecy in a law office, bank, or salon. However, if the basic social, economic, and political values or interests shared in common by the majority and minority leaders in this county are also taken into account, then a somewhat different picture of the power structure is a possibility. Where values are stressed, there appears to be a high degree of unity. In practice, the power structure tends to exclude from the direction of organizations under its aegis those persons in the community whose outlooks are considered deviant by local standards, for example, those favoring the direct provision of social services by the federal government. Current confrontations among the adversaries in the war on poverty in Syracuse have rendered more visible than ever the inner homogeneity of the power structure.

The power structure has changed in recent years and appears to be undergoing further transition. For their observation on this point, Martin, Munger, et al. chose as a base line an earlier period of Syracuse leadership when "there was a high concentration of community authority in the hands of a single man, simultaneously a political leader and public official." Likewise, Freeman, et al., accepted this portrayal, but with caution, indicating that it "may have made sense 20 years ago, but it is no longer adequate." Presumably the pluralism in decision making and

[7] Martin, *Decisions in Syracuse;* Linton Freeman, *et al., Local Community Leadership* (Syracuse: University College, 1960).

community leadership that these scholars detected took less than a quarter of a century to evolve.

Present representatives of the power structure quarrel with the accuracy of this particular base line for an analysis of the modifications that have occurred. They deny that a "boss" or a single clique ever ruled Syracuse, contending that the power structure has always consisted of several decision makers and leaders. In their view, while pluralism has tended to be centripetal in previous eras, today it is centrifugal. Expanding diversity of activities and responsibilities in Syracuse has presumably resulted in tiers and appendages being added to the power structure and the proliferation of its agents. Furthermore, in line with economic and social changes, new situations of power have over time succeeded those that have atrophied and expired. The process of displacement and replacement has produced a dilated rather than a compact power structure of both entrenched and virgin components.

Seen from another vantage point, the power structure is adjusting to the invasion by the giant corporations of national and international standing that have eclipsed and absorbed "old Syracuse." Where the vital interests of such mammoth enterprises are at stake, they are undoubtedly able to mobilize power that few communities by themselves can match and counter. Their management is alert and exercises very considerable influence over local decisions on matters central to their operations, such as certain public expenditures and taxation. On peripheral matters, such as the establishment of a new community hospital, they stand ready to make a contribution. However, if the item in the latter category is controversial, they tend to assume a posture of corporate aloofness and neutrality. Various executives personally may be inclined to apply pressure here and there in the community, but rarely is one willing or even able to commit the resources of the corporation in recurring community controversies.

The presence of these corporation managers has meant new blood, ideas, and strategies for the Syracuse power structure. However, the self-limitation on the use of corporation power leaves "old Syracuse" in a formidable position of strength to continue its influence over the decisions on health, education, and welfare. If some prominent families are participating less and less in decision-making sessions or rely regularly on surrogates, others still compete for official appointments in these areas. While their span of personal influence is generally diminishing, they are mastering the politics of community organizations and interest groups, to which they turn frequently to accomplish their ends. It should be mentioned that the power structures of Oswego and Madison counties are less touched by change than that in Onondaga county; traditional paternalism survives in both philanthropy and politics.

If the power structure is seen as comprised of various institutions or sectors rather than persons, as it is so described by Professor Charles Willie of Syracuse University, then the change that has taken place in recent years is both internal and external. In his opinion, the traditional institutions, specifically, business, government, and education, have grown in complexity and sophistication in their community roles. For example, no one company can any longer speak for business; spokesmanship is now organized through associations such as the Greater Syracuse Chamber of Commerce and Metropolitan Development Association. Moreover, professional consultants are retained by them to guide their participation in community affairs. At the same time, additional institutions are reaching the threshold of power. Professor Willie cites the example of the church. Similarly he attaches importance to the "poor" sector's expressing itself through community action and neighborhood organizations.

To a more dynamic community role for the church, the existing power structure in Syracuse can and is prepared to make appropriate adjustments. To the challenge from the "poor," its reaction is tinged with suspicion and resentment. The growing influence of the church, more negative than innovative in substance, raises essentially tactical issues that the parties are likely to resolve; none is unduly threatening. Where the "poor" insist upon "maximum feasible participation," strategic considerations are overriding. Faced with demands to surrender some measure of power, the community leadership of Syracuse, rather than capitulate, is prone to buy time with a modest expansion of social services. The present state of these services is a sound indication of how those who belong to the power elites discharge their responsibilities.

FACILITIES AND PROGRAMS

New York state prides itself on the assistance and protection it renders to the mentally ill and retarded. Its commitment is evident in the large expenditure of public funds for these purposes. Yet the existing local arrangements leave much room for improvement. The development of facilities and programs for the residents of the Syracuse SMSA who suffer from mental disorders has proceeded gradually and conservatively. After a century of largely episodic efforts, this is still a deficit area, with too many afflicted persons chasing too little effective care and treatment and with conspicuous gaps in the spectrum of services. Only a limited array of needs is met in the community. Those services that are available vary in sponsorship, accessibility, and convenience.

The facilities and services available for the treatment of mental disorders that occur in the Syracuse area operate close to full capacity given the prevailing condition of staff and bed shortages. What portion of the "needs" they actually meet at this high level of utilization cannot be specified because the real extent of mental illness and retardation in the area is unknown. How heavily the population is burdened by these infirmities or how widespread the various types are distributed remains a mystery. Nothing in the social organization or cultural pattern or stresses and strains of daily living suggests that the population suffers from an abnormally large quantity of mental disorders. Nor is there any indication that it is abnormally free of them.

To obtain some rough estimates, certain rules of thumb can be used. If one of every ten persons is in need of the services rendered by psychiatrists and psychotherapists, then approximately 62,000 persons in the Syracuse area (46,815 in Onondaga; 9,224 in Oswego; and 5,897 in Madison) would come under this rule. If one of every hundred persons is so emotionally or behaviorally disturbed as to require intensive or continuing treatment, the mentally ill would number approximately 6,200 (4,682 in Onondaga; 922 in Oswego; 590 in Madison). To quantify mental retardation, a 3 per cent multiplier is usually employed, resulting in an estimate of 18,500 persons who are retarded in some degree or other (14,045 in Onondaga; 2,767 in Oswego; 1,769 in Madison). If 0.5 per cent is so severely retarded as to constitute "problems" with which neither the individual nor his family can cope without professional assistance, presumably the Syracuse area population would contain approximately 3,100 cases (2,341 in Onondaga; 461 in Oswego; and 295 in Madison).

Mental disorders as indicated by the utilization of facilities and services fall short of these estimates. However, utilization statistics reflect little more than the traffic flow of patients according to the availability, capacity, and efficiency of existing programs. On March 31, 1967, there were 2,088 (337 per 100,000) Syracuse SMSA residents registered as inpatients and "leave" patients of the state mental hospitals other than the hospitals for the criminally insane. In this same year 1,296 residents of the metropolitan area were admitted to the state hospitals, in addition to approximately 1,000 admitted to nonstate institutions within Onondaga county. Over the past ten years the upward trend of admissions to state hospitals has been less steep for Onondaga county than the average for the state.

In March 1967 there were 1,157 inmates of the state schools for mental retardates from the Syracuse metropolitan area, at an estimated rate of 174 per 100,000 residents in Onondaga county, 230 per 100,000 for Oswego, and 220 per 100,000 for Madison. At this time, the school districts of the metropolitan area supplied special classes for approximately 1,600 mentally retarded children, classified as educable or trainable. To illustrate magnitudes again, in May 1967 there were 666 educable and 71 trainable retardates enrolled in the city of Syracuse school district.

These statistics rest on the acceptance of the conventional professional definitions or categories of "mental illness." Accordingly, if a person is diagnosed as a psychoneurotic or is "on the books" of a state hospital as a schizophrenic, he is a case of mental illness. In this sense the designation is applied to a wide spectrum of personal conduct or disturbance. However, the statistics are fatally compromised if one accepts the contention of Dr. Thomas Szasz, author of *The Myth of Mental Illness,* that "mental illness" as the term has come to be used in psychiatry and the community is fundamentally a matter of labeling behavior that society disapproves or proscribes rather than a matter of genuine pathological determination.

For inpatient services of extended duration the Syracuse SMSA has been served by institutions maintained by the state Department of Mental Hygiene and the United States Veterans Administration. A state school for retardates, soon to be rebuilt in entirety, a small state unit for the care of emotionally disturbed blind children, and a Veterans Hospital are located in the SMSA. The state mental hospitals that serve the area are massive in size and mainly custodial in performance, and they are situated beyond the boundaries of the SMSA. Normally these institutions receive patients certified by physicians, committed by the courts, or referred for observation. However, they have over the past decade experienced a sharp rise in their voluntary intake.

The state authorities have on several occasions been urged to construct a major mental hospital within the SMSA, specifically in Syracuse. Reluctant to add another monster edifice of the type under heavy attack in mental health circles and determined to improve its programs in existing facilities, the Department of Mental Hygiene countered with proposals to assign to Onondaga county whole units on the grounds of Marcy State Hospital. City and county officials, along with interested local parties, joined battle with state officials and carried their case to the legislature and governor, arguing for a suitable, modern, progressive facility within the county. Victory was achieved. Governor Nelson Rockefeller has included a state mental hospital for Syracuse in his capital improvement program, and the Department of Mental Hygiene has approved a site in the vicinity of the Upstate Medical Center. The size and exact purpose of the new hospital have yet to be determined, though presumably intensive treatment rather than custodial care will be the crux of the service.

The Syracuse SMSA lacks a long-term chronic care hospital for emotionally disturbed children. The Syracuse regional planning committee of the New York State Mental Health Planning Committee recommended the establishment of such a center. A unit of considerable size, probably two hundred beds, is now on the drawing board under the state's mental health facilities construction program.

When it comes to short-term inpatient services, the number of beds and services are gradually increasing in the Syracuse SMSA. The diversity of sponsors is worth noting. The state Department of Mental Hygiene operates a short-term care hospital for training and research at the Medical Center. The location of this hospital in Syracuse some forty years ago resulted from the initiative of a persistent band of health educators and social workers. The State University Hospital includes a psychiatric ward but has encountered delays in putting the beds into use, a matter to which the Onondaga county commissioner of mental health has drawn the attention of the public. The largest short-term care unit is to be found in the Veterans Hospital, a general hospital serving an area larger than the SMSA, however. Two voluntary community hospitals admit psychiatric patients, while a third is making a wing in its new building available for such patients, especially from low-income and welfare families. Finally, a private psychiatric hospital of twenty beds exists in the SMSA, staffed by psychiatrists who are also active in community psychiatry and who have played a significant role in the evolution of public mental health programs.

None of the county and city governments in the Syracuse SMSA possesses a short-term care psychiatric hospital of its own. However, the welfare departments and mental health agencies are sources of patients for the existing facilities. Since existing facilities are under different managements, it is difficult to find room for welfare clients. Multiplicity of units means multiplicity of styles and objectives, which proves troublesome to public agencies seeking to shape a consistent and economical set of community services. The Onondaga county commissioner of mental health, commenting in his 1966 annual report about lack of cooperation on the part of one hospital, said:

in the meantime we must express our grave misgivings about a program which does continued violence to the essential principle of comprehensive community mental health services, namely, full cooperation with existing community agencies. From the inception of the new program at Syracuse Psychiatric Hospital we have sought to establish a working relationship through a liaison committee. Our efforts have not been successful and our communications to the State Department of Mental Hygiene remain unununanswered.

Mention should be made of the roles played by some of the short-term care hospitals in the provision of emergency and partial hospitalization services, including day, night, and weekend care. It is generally recognized that expansion of these services is needed. From various local quarters has come strongly articulated support for them, but institutional separatism has not made the task of implementation easy. For example, no sooner had county officials designed a working arrangement for emergency services with the state's Syracuse Psychiatric Hospital than the administration and staff at that institution proceeded on their own initiative to experiment along quite different lines, narrowing its intake area drastically. It is clear that the benefits accruing to the inner city of Syracuse under various new programs fail to reach the population in the outlying sections of the SMSA. By themselves the local communities have virtually no way other than consultation, negotiation, and publicity to rectify this state of affairs.

Ambulatory clinical services are growing in importance. The use of

tranquilizers and other drugs, improved interpersonal and group therapeutic and educational techniques, and changing attitudes account for
the guarded optimism and enhanced confidence in the utility of clinical
services throughout the SMSA. It is the policy of the Onondaga, Madison, and Oswego county mental health boards to expand services for
ambulatory patients.

Some eighteen units supplying clinical services related to emotional disturbances and mental retardation are open to the residents of the SMSA
and are situated within its boundaries. In addition, the Syracuse school
district conducts classes for emotionally disturbed and mentally retarded children, while several voluntary agencies, by virtue of contractual arrangements with the Onondaga county Department of Mental
Health, are able to advise their clients on psychiatric services. Few of
the clinical facilities are multi-purpose; most are specialized. Some function on a daily schedule, others less frequently.

The provision of clinical and classroom services for ambulatory patients in the area manifests fragmentation that cuts across the entire
structure of American government and the voluntary system. No less
than fifteen governmental agencies or subdivisions and fifteen voluntary
organizations are involved in the direct delivery of these services. Conspicuously missing from the roster is Syracuse University, which adds
approximately ten thousand students to the population of the area but
operates no psychiatric facility to meet their needs.

No one level of government or agency enjoys a monopoly of clinical
services, nor is any one category of service totally and exclusively the
responsibility of a particular department or bureau. The clinical domain
of the local voluntary and private mental illness and retardation services
is basically pluralistic in structure and operation and does not present a
common front in dealing with the problems raised by mental disorders
in the SMSA. Communities seem unable to correct this situation. For
persons who can afford the fees private psychiatry is available.

Among the elements of comprehensive mental health services are
rehabilitative, precare, and aftercare services. There is a veritable pro-
fusion of organizations rendering these types of assistance. However,
only three or four minister exclusively to the specific needs of the
victims of mental disorders. The others, ranging from the Rehabilitation
Institute of the Upstate Medical Center to the Rescue Mission and including social service agencies, church charities, and community "char-

acter-building" groups accept formerly mentally ill persons as clientele. Most of these agencies are ill-equipped by professional standards and at best make rather marginal contributions. The insufficiency of aftercare in the area is, in the eyes of many careful observers, viewed as scandalous. The "revolving door" practices, with emphasis on tranquilization therapy at mental hospitals, result in the release to families of many anxiety-ridden persons whose further recovery and stabilization is contingent on easy access to appropriate local help of high quality. The load of aftercare is far heavier than the existing diffused structure of local social and health agencies can carry. Hence, strong misgivings have been expressed in Syracuse over the decision to locate a five hundred to one thousand bed state psychiatric facility in the city, a decision taken with little, if any, attention having been paid to the aftercare. Proponents of overall planning cite this matter as an example of how not to go about the development of community-based services. The relations between the several levels of government on such matters can stand much improvement.

In the realm of preventive mental health and precare some community entities including churches, boys clubs, probation agencies, and police function as points of contact between individuals in need of professional services and the systems that provide these services. Entry into the mental health traffic is often more difficult for the afflicted than the public realizes. Several local clergymen have worked steadfastly to bring about the formation of treatment centers. In Oswego and Madison counties it has been in the church buildings that the state adult clinic and child guidance staffs have met their patients.

Fragmentation of effort in the mental health field reaches its peak in the sectors of education, training, and research. It is futile to attempt to ascertain the exact number of organizations or persons engaged in relevant educational-propagandist activities, for in some respects all the participants in the field perform such functions purposely or unintentionally. It is a principal responsibility of the county mental health associations, which in turn have activated expatient groups to share the task with them. The staff of the Department of Mental Health in Onondaga county finds education of the community, its leaders, and professional population among its most time-consuming duties. As for training, the burden falls on the shoulders of the Upstate Medical Center, Syracuse University, Colgate University, Oswego State College, LeMoyne and

Cazenovia Colleges, and Onondaga Community College, in addition to
the state Department of Mental Hygiene. Programs are aimed at a wide
array of people, from psychiatrists through the residency programs to
mental health voluntary aides. Research is undertaken by the Mental
Health Research Unit of the Department of Mental Hygiene in Syracuse,
Upstate Medical Center, Syracuse University, and the Community Chest
Planning Department. No roster or inventory of projects is available.
Topics such as the content of dreams and "boundary consciousness" are
included, as are the biochemistry of alcoholism and delivery systems of
services. Many projects in progress are unknown to other researchers in
the vicinity. Consolidation of efforts is the exception rather than the
rule, though team research is often pursued. The involvement of the
Syracuse population in research undertakings of both behavioral and
nonbehavioral types occurs frequently.

Obviously the domain of mental health has elastic perimeters, encompassing innumerable backstopping, feeder, and supportive organizations. The success or effectiveness of certain mental health activities depends heavily on the performance of organizations in such other sectors
of society as education, housing, civil rights, and employment. In recent
years the Syracuse SMSA has witnessed a deepening concern for integrated education, nondiscrimination in housing, "one man, one vote"
in politics, and equal opportunity in employment. Although accomplishments in these problem areas have been substantial, there still remains to
be created a socially healthy environment as a proper setting in which to
combat mental illness and retardation and reduce their incidence.

Abbreviated as it is, this brief description of facilities and programs
suggests at least the breadth, width, and depth of the mental health field
serving the Syracuse SMSA. What accounts for its distinguishing dimensions, its strengths and weaknesses, and its potentialities for growth and
improvement? To which factors and influences can one trace its main
features?

Heading the list is the constitutional monopoly (and near monopoly
in practice) of New York state to provide care for the mentally ill and
retardates. With the failure of local communities in the nineteenth century to shelter and treat mental disorder victims humanely, the state
authorities assumed full responsibility. A state system was established
with a substantial investment in asylums and later mental hospitals and
schools, the evolution of the mental hygiene civil service, bureaucratic

regulations, budgeting practices, and attitudes toward local government, the public, and inmates that produced an autocratic style of operations. In the 1920s the new Department of Mental Hygiene inherited the system as well as its traditions, a legacy with which the department has had to live ever since.

In 1954 the era of community mental health officially began in New York state. In administering the Community Mental Health Act passed by the legislature in that year, the Department of Mental Hygiene scrutinizes local programs and activities closely. Inevitably in these matters the traditions of the system affect the professional perceptions and judgments of state officials, who themselves are products of the system or are entrusted with responsibilities for the welfare and development of the department's own facilities and programs. Even with a new team at the helm of the Department of Mental Hygiene in Albany, policy still favors a senior-junior partnership with the communities rather than total integration of state and community mental health services under a single local government unit.

Another determinant of mental health services for the SMSA population is the presence of the Upstate Medical Center. Oriented toward teaching and research, it is a system in its own right with internal interests, powers, and working rules. The constituent entities composing it hold their respective positions by virtue of their functions and by bargaining. Programs at the center reflect the pursuits and outlooks of the staff more faithfully than the needs of the metropolitan area. In reality the center has resisted becoming an adjunct of the Syracuse community. The pull of the center is gravitational, toward itself, resulting in a concentration of efforts in its immediate vicinity, often at the inconvenience of the SMSA population residing elsewhere. Counterpressures discourage rapport between the center and other bodies and impair community relationships. However, the center has teaching and research needs that the community can satisfy, and these mutual interests have led to service arrangements situated in facilities removed from "the hill," as occurs in the case of the Adult Clinic at the county Mental Health Department headquarters.

Growth without the benefit of overall planning is a third element in the area's mental health picture. Programs have been introduced piecemeal and tangentially, for example, to enhance the work of the Children's Court or to honor a political commitment or to strengthen an academic curriculum, without reference to the total requirements of the SMSA. Planned development of new services has been neglected or sacrificed to expediency or to emergency. At no time have the United Community Chest-Council, Community Mental Health Board, or the Department of Mental Health undertaken the comprehensive planning of services to combat mental illness and retardation in the area. In 1964–1965 the Syracuse Regional Committee of the New York State Mental Health Planning Committee missed a unique opportunity to attempt overall planning. Onondaga county's recently organized Community Health Information and Planning Service has given no indication that mental health planning enjoys a high priority on its agenda. In February 1967 the Community Problems Study Committee of the United Community Chest-Council proposed the creation of a super-agency for planning with respect to community services. If it is brought into existence, it may very well pursue overall planning for mental health services.

While the necessity for overall planning in the SMSA is more widely understood and accepted in influential quarters and in the public at large than ever, fragmentation, one of the major tendencies that it aims to counter, blocks its progress. With all levels of government and numerous social agencies operating in the mental health field, each from its own base and under its own policies, one can reasonably expect haggling over every aspect of the planning effort. Furthermore, the public is committed to the principle on which fragmentation feeds, namely, pluralism. In turn the relationship between pluralism on the one hand and federalism and voluntarism on the other is profound. In addition, competition between the public and private sectors is as welcome as cooperation between them, presumably to keep each "on its toes."

Out of adherence to the principle of voluntarism, the social services of the SMSA, including health and mental health services, have been compelled to endure fragmentation. Locally voluntarism, construed as synonymous with "nongovernment," is linked to charity rather than the democratic ethic. Some time ago the system of voluntary agencies was perceived as an arm of the Syracuse "power structure," but today this is not so evident. Traditionally the system has been donor-centered. With "maximum feasible participation" a major theme in the war on poverty, client representation is a legitimate subject for deliberation, and for that matter new client-centered agencies have taken shape, increasing the number of organizations in the SMSA.

An asset long heralded by the voluntary movement has been its capacity to show the type of sensitivity or sympathy that emotionally disturbed and retarded persons are most apt to lack in their lives, a "someone cares" attitude, a personal concern as evidenced by the presence of volunteers who are motivated to serve others. It is contended in some local circles that by contrast governmental agencies are overly bureaucratic and professional and, hence, impersonal in their assistance to patients. It is acknowledged more and more, however, that the voluntary movement is becoming bureaucratic and professional under pressure from funding bodies, professional associations, and the government. Furthermore, as they become more nonsectarian in reaching out for additional clientele, they manifest even less personal concern. Increasing case loads, perplexing problems, baffling clients, and conformity to the terms of government grants have dampened enthusiasm and dried up pools of sympathy. Moreover, it has been reported on the basis of information obtained from the welfare organizations operating in Onondaga county that

(a) agencies have a tendency to refer their most difficult cases to other agencies through various labelling devices and games; (b) agencies have a tendency to retain for themselves those simpler cases that promise a satisfactory outcome; (c) the more highly trained workers tend to be utilized in dealing with the easier or "less disturbed" rather than persistently intractible clients.[8]

Seen in a metropolitan perspective, voluntary agencies are reluctant to broaden their geographical jurisdiction for fear of acquiring more burdens but proportionately fewer resources. While Catholic Charities extends its services throughout the SMSA, which is part of the Syracuse Diocese, other Syracuse philanthropic groups assist individuals in Madison and Oswego counties only in rare instances.

The part public opinion in the Syracuse SMSA has played in the evolution of efforts to combat mental illness and retardation is hard to reduce to specifics. On mental health issues apathy has persisted. No bitter, extensive controversy has compelled the SMSA to take special notice of mental illness. What opinion has been mobilized is to be credited to the work of several highly motivated individuals, a few

[8] Claire Rudolph and John Cumming, *A Survey of Social Agencies' Perceptions of Community Mental Health Problems and Their Opinions About Solutions* (Syracuse: Department of Mental Hygiene, Mental Health Research Unit, n.d.), pp. 25–26.

public officials, journalists, and certain social workers, educators, and physicians, frequently acting in a personal instead of professional capacity.

To stimulate public attention and generate public support for mental health programs, institutional endeavors are increasing. The three county Mental Health Boards, the Department of Mental Health in Onondaga county, the chapters of the Mental Health Association, and expatient organizations are available for the pursuit of such activities. Although few citizens attend the budget sessions of the county legislatures, debate on mental health matters in the committees on health, personnel, and finance and on the floor reach the public through the press, radio, and television.

One may conclude that interest in mental health problems is still of a low order of involvement. No network of public and voluntary services exists in any meaningful sense in the Syracuse metropolitan area. The three counties are endeavoring to cope with the problems within their respective jurisdictions by developing their own community-based services with the help of grants from New York state and federal departments or under contract with nongovernmental facilities. So far there is no sign of the emergence of a metropolitan or regional authority to which the county, state, and federal governments can transfer their mental health responsibilities. In the meantime the various separate services continue to manifest overriding loyalties to the parent systems with which they are affiliated and which set the course of action for them.

Public agencies occupy so indomitable a position in the mental health field that independent initiatives of any great magnitude seem out of the question for the voluntary movement in the area. State and federal programs appear to have no voluntary counterparts. However, at the community level voluntary organizations are finding selected opportunities open for them to function in a variety of capacities to aid the mentally ill. Economy-minded county authorities are under pressure to forego services under their own direction in favor of those supplied by such voluntary bodies as the community hospitals.

In such a mixed governmental and nongovernmental structure of care and treatment for the mentally ill and retarded as the one that prevails in the SMSA, the service units tend to be narrowly problem-oriented or operate under highly confining terms of reference. Inasmuch as the field is broad, there is always plenty of room for additional specialized agencies that address their attention to unmet needs. The result is a plethora of organizations and participating systems that sponsor and nurture them. As experience in the SMSA indicates, the organizations have a propensity to compete with one another for resources, clientele, and reputation, while in their own inimitable fashion these systems have a tendency to extend their span of control and jostle each other to the point of hostile confrontation. Effective performance by them depends in the long run upon the "management of complexity," a formidable challenge to all the interested parties in the metropolitan area.

Where numerous agencies belonging to several systems are active, relationships of all kinds are formed among them by agreement and happenstance, by commission and omission. Such relationships inevitably result in forms of interdependence involving authority, policy, funding, facilities, personnel, and clientele. In turn interdependence opens the way for the decisions of one agency or system to affect the others. Thus, the mental illness and retardation services for the SMSA are exposed in entirety or in part to veto power and other influences exercised from hundreds of points, overt and covert, inside the mental health field and within the social and political structures which impinge on it. The mental health complex through which the population of the Syracuse metropolitan area obtains protection and assistance may be seen in the final analysis as the fruit of pursued aspirations and inflicted vetoes.

PLANNING, COORDINATION, AND DECISION MAKING

"Priority Problem Number One—The Lack of Comprehensive, Coordinated Community-Wide Planning" in Onondaga county is the unanimous verdict of the Community Problems Study Committee.[9] "Fragmentation, lack of coordination, duplication, wasted effort and lack of communication"—these words recurred again and again throughout the presentation as various observers and experts appearing before the committee reported not only on the essential social and environmental needs of people but also on specific functional areas. Regarding mental health, the committee said, "The fragmentation of mental health services and the lack of coordinated services for the mentally retarded were

[9] Planning Department, United Community Chest and Council of Onondaga County, Inc., *Report of the Community Problems Study Committee* (Syracuse: United Community Chest and Council, 1967), p. 11.

noted. Also mentioned was the lack of information on available local facilities and services in these areas."

Shortcomings and deficiencies along these lines are nothing new for the Syracuse metropolitan area. Typical rather than exceptional, they have arisen out of the piecemeal approach employed in arranging services for the sufferers of mental infirmities. So much effort has gone into the episodic creation of each facility or program that little has been devoted to the overall development of an integrated network of related services to meet current and future needs. No strategy has been designed for the acquisition and allocation of resources for a total war on mental disorders. Furthermore, the isolation of activities in this field from the other social services has added to the general chaos of the whole spectrum of services.

As an alternative to the piecemeal approach, systematic comprehensive programming for community mental health has never been tried in Syracuse. This type of programming, in its full dimensions, is a dynamic combination of planning, coordination, and decision making. Attempts at planning have occurred repeatedly with partial, short-lived success; barely has the surface been scratched by these experiences so far. Obviously decision making is also one of the critical processes in any system of community services. In Syracuse and its environs it has been practiced paternalistically, erratically, and divisively. Today the process is undergoing a transition that is rendering it more compatible with planning and coordination in a programmatic context.

Between 1926, when the Onondaga Health Association began to press for the creation of facilities for the mentally ill in Syracuse, and 1955, when the Onondaga county Mental Health Board was established, planning for mental health services was neglected. Only in the past decade has any progress been made.

In 1963 New York state accepted federal funds to undertake comprehensive, long-range mental health planning. In that year the commissioner of mental hygiene formed the New York State Mental Health Planning Committee to produce a master plan for the state incorporating a strong community mental health commitment. The state committee consisted of fifty-three members, twenty of whom constituted an executive committee. In addition, several task forces were assigned to assist the parent body, which included spokesmen for every major sector of the mental health field and every region of the state.

Ten regional planning committees were also established, mainly by designating the mental health regional advisory committees created in 1960 to serve in this capacity and adding members to their rosters. The Syracuse SMSA counties belonged to the Syracuse region, which included five other central New York counties in the catchment area of Marcy State and Utica State Hospitals. Of the sixty-five members composing the Syracuse regional planning committee, thirty were appointed from the three metropolitan area counties, nineteen from Onondaga county. The participants came from public agencies and voluntary organizations, as well as the private practice of psychiatry and psychology. To work with the regional committee, the Department of Mental Hygiene in Albany assigned one staff aide, who also served the St. Lawrence regional committee.

The meetings of the Syracuse regional committee afforded its members opportunities for expressions of concern and cooperation and exchanges of ideas and opinions. However, it may be legitimately asked whether it really engaged in planning of a professional character. The report of the committee itself is by no means a plan for the region as a whole or the counties in it. It is more of an inventory of deficiencies than a blueprint for the development and operation of services to combat mental disorders.

Several factors operated to deny the Syracuse regional committee a genuine planning role. First, its mandate was ambiguous since the emphasis was placed on vague goals rather than process or means in detail. Second, the regional committee was expected to contribute primarily to the formulation of the statewide plan, which the Department of Mental Hygiene had to develop in order to satisfy the requirements of the National Institute of Mental Health. Third, information for planning was woefully lacking, and the part-time staff member had no means at his disposal to remedy the situation. Fourth, participants were inclined to use the committee as a vehicle for broadcasting their personal judgments on mental health services and lobbying for more state assistance to their county programs. Fifth, consumer or patient representation was negligible. Sixth, it was known that the Department of Mental Hygiene was engaged in planning on its own initiative for the catchment areas with a strong bias in favor of the involvement of the state hospitals in community mental health programs. Finally, the Department of Mental Hygiene reserved to itself, rather than entrust the committee with, the full responsibility for the planning of facilities construction, thus by-passing the regional committees, as well as the communities and local authorities, on such vital matters as priorities, type of facilities, and allocation of funds and personnel. Certainly very few participants in the statewide planning effort from unofficial circles seem to have been aware at that time of the development of the construction plan or even the criteria for its development as specified by the Department of Health, Education, and Welfare in Washington. The construction plan that was submitted to the Secretary of Health, Education, and Welfare prior to the completion of the comprehensive plan was not distributed as a working document to the Syracuse regional committee. Though the state Department of Mental Hygiene encouraged community participation in the planning experience, its own report, "A Plan for a Comprehensive Mental Health and Mental Retardation Program for New York State," tended to overshadow those endeavors.

Consequently, the report of the Syracuse regional committee has been relegated to oblivion. Even mental health leaders of the communities know little about it. Though it brings together for the first time in a single document most of the ideas for the improvement of treatment and care for the mentally ill and retarded that have been in circulation in the metropolitan area for many years, it contains no new data, novel insight, or original findings. In any case it does not qualify as a "plan" and has virtually no standing as such in local public or voluntary agencies.

Upon the submission of its report, the Syracuse regional committee disbanded. It has not been reconstituted to plan for the local construction of new facilities under Public Law 88–164 or to review specific plans for community mental health centers. The New York State Mental Health Planning Committee in its report recommended the establishment of planning committees in each of the mental health regions, but the recommendation has remained a dead letter in the Syracuse region.

Without waiting for the state government to perfect its mental health planning arrangements, Onondaga county opened the way for local planning to improve the system of care for the mentally retarded. In 1962 the county Mental Health Board established the Committee on Mental Retardation with Dr. Sterling Garrard of the Upstate Medical Center, a widely recognized authority on mental retardation, as its chairman. Essentially a committee of experts, it viewed itself as a temporary body, charged with "preparing the way for specific planning in the county." To Dr. Garrard was given the specific task of preparing a document that could be used for obtaining funds for planning and might serve eventually as a guide for program development. In December 1963 he submitted his report, which has been described as "imaginative" and "pioneering." As a consequence of his labors, Onondaga county mental health circles presently possess a guide, based on expertness of the highest calibre, for action regarding mental retardation. Implementation is already under consideration in consultation with officials of the Department of Mental Hygiene.

For comprehensive planning on a continuing basis one must look to permanent agencies in the Syracuse community. With the creation of the Department of Mental Health in Onondaga county in 1962, planning became a function of the commissioner and his staff. He has demonstrated by his actions that he has an overall perspective, but he has had no penchant for the details of formal planning. His concern has been the whole spectrum of services, both public and private, not simply those under his jurisdiction. The department lacks a staff member with a full-time planning assignment. Moreover, the voluntary, state, and federal agencies in Syracuse have shown no desire to have the commissioner become the planning authority for all mental health services in the county.

After it surrendered operational responsibilities in 1962, the county Mental Health Board might have been converted into a planning agency, but this did not happen. Upon the establishment of the Department of Mental Health, the board lost its staff. It might have turned to the county planning department for assistance, but that department has been oriented toward physical planning. The board members, however competent, could not themselves have assumed the planning function since all have active careers and other obligations of their own. Moreover, the individuals now serving on the board are more committed to action than planning.

In Madison and Oswego counties the Mental Health Boards are staffed by executive directors, as was once true of Onondaga county. These officials have been so preoccupied with negotiations for services that they have had neither the time nor the staff for long-term planning.

Nor are the county legislatures in any better shape to assume the planning function. Each has a health committee, consisting of elected supervisors, but none has the inclination, experience, or expertise to play a major planning role for mental health services. The likelihood of planning for all three counties through this means or any other local mechanism seems very small indeed.

In the years to come, the communities may look to the recently organized local chapters of the Mental Health Association to mount a continuing planning effort. At the present time, however, these bodies do not view this as one of their prime activities. Their resources are too meager to pursue it in a professional manner. If they were to devote themselves to planning, their effectiveness as information and pressure groups might be severely impaired. Now their main task is to consolidate their position in each county, proving their utility through accomplishments of a practical nature, such as the training of home aides to assist the mentally ill.

One nongovernmental organization engaged in the planning of health services is the United Community Chest and Council of Onondaga county. This organization's planning department has within it a mental health committee, which has, during its tenure, tended to deal with specific problems rather than the field as a whole. In 1960 the Community Chest created a committee to establish priorities for services to serve as a guide to the community and its various appropriating bodies. While the report of the Community Priorities Committee was not a plan, it did include some aspects of planning. The committee, composed of "influentials" in the community, set its sights on a horizon well beyond the voluntary sector. Its findings extended to the responsibilities of the public sector, including those of state and federal agencies.

Various public officials in Syracuse are familiar with the priorities fixed by the committee but they do not feel bound by the report. In any case, it is one thing to set forth priorities in a comprehensive fashion, but it is quite another to obtain compliance from agencies that are not represented in the planning apparatus and belong to other "systems." Even agencies that belong to the Community Chest system have felt no obligation to concur in its recommendations when their own interests are threatened. For example, the nonprofit Crouse-Irving Hospital of Syracuse has demonstrated this attitude in its opposition to the report of the Community Chest Committee on Immediate Hospital Needs.

General dissatisfaction with its health planning and the recurring controversy that its hospital study committees engendered, led the Community Chest to launch a new agency in August 1965—Community Health Information and Planning Service of Onondaga County, CHIPS for short. It is an information-gathering and planning enterprise, the functions of which are both strategic (keeping the long-range health goals of the community under close scrutiny) and tactical (short-term developments). Those who brought CHIPS into being had a strong sense of urgency stemming from the following conditions: "chaos" in the modernization and expansion of Syracuse hospitals; addition of health services without much thought to the proper role of each type of service; construction of facilities under governmental auspices with little attention to the adverse consequences for existing programs or for the new burdens imposed on the voluntary structure; the need for a visible and viable community leadership in the health field to enable various institutions, loyal to their own objectives, to know the goals of the community; and to obtain for the community a voice in the local services complex in the face of an expanding state and federal involvement.

CHIPS has its own board of directors with an executive committee. Originally the directors were top community leaders invited by the Community Chest leadership to serve on the board. Those who advocated the formation of CHIPS sought persons of influence drawn from finance, business, labor, and the professions who could equip the organization with some "muscle." Operating health agencies received no representation on the board on the grounds that they might reasonably be expected to act as interest groups. Early in the history of CHIPS this position was abandoned and the board of directors was enlarged from eleven members to twenty-seven, adding the state regional health officer, health commissioner of Syracuse, Onondaga county commissioner of mental health, president of the Onondaga County Medical Society, and a hospital administrator to the roster. This change also brought to the CHIPS board several spokesmen for the governmental sector, who under the previous arrangement were to serve only on the task forces. It is interesting to note that on the seven-man executive committee are at least six of the original board members of CHIPS, giving a ratio of four top community leaders to three health professionals.

An important feature of CHIPS is its permanent professional staff. Recently it completed a base-line study of hospital utilization, including the utilization of psychiatric beds in all hospitals in Onondaga county. It has communicated to the Onondaga Department of Mental Health its willingness to assume the planning function for that agency. Presumably CHIPS responsibility ends with the recommendations that its board endorses. Since it is widely regarded as an arm of the "power structure," it may be able to dispose as well as propose. However, it is far too early to assess its strength. The test of its influence is still sometime in the future.

For mental health planning purposes, the Syracuse community can also turn to other local organizations. The Syracuse Governmental Research Bureau, closely identified with the Greater Syracuse Chamber of Commerce and the Manufacturers' Association of Syracuse, entered the mental health field in 1955 with a report that bolstered the case for the passage of the county mental health law. Another organization with growing capability in this field is the Syracuse University Research Corporation, which contributed heavily to the data processing required for the CHIPS base-line study. At this juncture mention should be made of the recommendation of the Community Problems Study Committee "that a new planning and coordinating organization be created with the purpose of uniting the entire scope of planning efforts at work in this community—social, physical and economic." Both mental health and mental retardation were listed as falling within the scope of concern of this novel agency.

Planning an arrangement of mental illness and retardation services for the Syracuse area is also a state government responsibility. During the tenure of the late commissioner, Dr. Paul Hoch, the Department of Mental Hygiene in Albany in 1962 produced the Master Plan for Mental Disability, under which it was proposed that the state and community services within each mental hospital catchment area be functionally integrated. The implication for the Syracuse area was that the public and voluntary community services be aligned with the services of Marcy State Hospital. "The New York State Program for Construction of Community Mental Health Centers," was prepared to satisfy Title II of the Federal Community Mental Health Centers Construction Act in 1965 under the acting commissioner of mental hygiene, Dr. C. F. Terrence, and Mr. Hyman Forstenzer, assistant commissioner for mental health resources and policy planning. In this plan the Syracuse metropolitan area was placed in the lowest category of "relative needs" for community mental health center projects. In this same period the New York State Planning Committee on Mental Disorders (originally known as the

New York State Mental Health Planning Committee) completed its labors with the assistance of the staff of the Department of Mental Hygiene. Its "Plan for a Comprehensive Mental Health and Mental Retardation Program for New York State" is intended as a guide for Syracuse no less than the rest of the state.

Because of its access to pertinent data, the Department of Mental Hygiene in Albany is the logical center for mental health planning throughout New York state. However, if it engages in detailed planning for the communities, it encounters the usual complaint that it lacks confidence in the competence of the localities to govern themselves, is depriving the local leadership of participation in the planning experience, and is attempting to dominate the mental health scene. Actually the commissioner has an equally difficult question to face in Albany, and that is the one of cooperation among the interested state departments—education, welfare, health, labor, vocational rehabilitation, and corrections—for planning purposes. The limits set on his own jurisdiction constrain him from resorting to total planning in depth throughout the state or in a particular area, such as Onondaga county. Not even the presence of an interdepartmental advisory council or the Advisory Council on Community Mental Health Centers appointed by the governor to advise the commissioner on "the orderly development and expansion of comprehensive mental health centers" has freed his hand for this kind of planning thrust at both state and local levels.

In summary, the status of mental health planning within the Syracuse metropolitan area is regarded with mixed feelings. On the affirmative side, it is accepted in principle as an appropriate approach to achieve a reduction of "chaos" in the provision of services. Interested parties are coming to realize that planning can result in improved communications whether or not a master plan is produced. The experiences involved in the process are in themselves valuable and can generate unintended rewards for mental health activities. On the negative side, planning is feared as a threat to the autonomy of various health organizations and a possible infringement on self-government. There is considerable anxiety over who is to be the planner. In some Syracuse circles planning is equated not simply with control but also with favoritism. Nonetheless, local sentiment for more and better planning of the social services is on the rise.

While the concept of planning leaves many people uneasy, coordination as another pivotal component of community mental health programing has the very opposite effect. Except in rare instances, it enjoys wide acceptance as the most adaptable thrust for countering fragmentation of the services in this field. It is commonly taken to be a process for piecing together the segments of an existing system and preventing competition that wastes resources and diverts effort from the pursuit of selected objectives. In contrast to planning, it connotes direct action in a practical, feasible, flexible, and cooperative fashion. As the mental health services for the Syracuse metropolitan area are provided through several separate organizations, some with autonomous subdivisions, coordination is a matter of increasing urgency.

The nearest thing to an areawide coordination unit for the Syracuse community is the regional advisory committee, members of which are the chairmen and directors of the county Mental Health Boards (the commissioner of mental health in the case of Onondaga county) and the directors of the state mental hospitals serving the region. Established in 1960, the committee was instructed to coordinate state and county programs. It has no authority over the facilities in the region, and it depends upon voluntary compliance with its recommendations. Moreover, it has failed to develop a regional outlook on mental health problems. The participants tend to be preoccupied with state-local relationships. It should be mentioned in passing that the county mental health officials also meet with some frequency to discuss common problems and work out a common posture for discussions and negotiations with the state Department of Mental Hygiene.

Under state law the county mental health boards in Onondaga, Madison, and Oswego counties have been entrusted with the task of coordination in their respective communities. By virtue of their diverse composition, for example, psychiatrists, Community Chest officials, educators, welfare commissioners, and health officers, they seem, at least on paper, to have more potential for this purpose than their accomplishments so far would suggest. In reality their legal powers are thin, their powers of appeal weak. They can do little more than open channels of communication.

In Onondaga county the commissioner and especially the deputy commissioner devote a substantial portion of their working hours to coordination. They are in constant contact with county, city, town, state, and federal officials, with the staffs of the Upstate Medical Center and state hospitals, and with spokesmen for community hospitals, clinics, voluntary agencies, educational systems, and professional associations, with the aim of linking up the various services for the mentally ill and retarded. Evidence of the extent and vigor of their approach is seen in the guidelines prepared for the Syracuse Policy Department, sheriff's office, and town health officers on the handling of emergency and acute cases of mental disorder.

In this time-consuming task of coordination, the commissioner is confronted at one point or another with every conceivable obstacle. If organizational ethno-centricism is not the hurdle, then personality conflict intrudes. On one occasion it is internal maladjustment of an agency, on another it is just bad timing or a staffing crisis. Or it may be a legal roadblock or legislative inconsistency. Within the county government it is acknowledged that coordination among the health, mental health, and welfare departments is imperative for effective programing, but the commissioner of mental health can attain it only through the cooperation of his fellow commissioners. At this level it is the county executive who emerges, or should emerge, as the chief coordinator.

Among the institutions that are vital to the county mental health program, the public schools, Upstate Medical Center, and Syracuse Psychiatric Hospital have been least responsive to the coordination efforts of the county government. There are several reasons for this. A separation of powers has traditionally made the school administrations independent of the county authorities. Moreover, the city and district school systems have tended to become self-contained operations subject to the mandates of the state education code and detailed directives and regulations of the state Department of Education. In the case of the Upstate Medical Center, its needs and objectives compel it to avoid becoming a community-centered facility. Another factor is the autonomy of the faculty projects, which militates against a concert of interests between the center and the community. The capacity of Syracuse Psychiatric Hospital to relate to local organizations has been seriously paralyzed by recurring identity crises. On its own initiative and with support from the state and federal governments it recently transformed itself into a "community mental health center" for Syracuse on an experimental basis. If it follows precedent, this present course will be abandoned with little, if any, advance notice to community agencies when the director or staff changes.

Outside the governmental sector, the United Community Chest and Council of Onondaga county have endeavored to fill the role of a coordinating body for health and welfare services. The capability of the Chest in this role rests on the prestige of its backers, experience of its staff, and the power of the purse. However, it is handicapped in dealing with other agencies by its own philosophy of autonomy. Moreover, so massive is governmental involvement in the provision of social services, especially mental health services, that the span of influence of the Chest is inadequate to effectuate a high degree of coordination among the many diverse public and voluntary organizations. Recognizing this insufficiency, the governing board of the Community Chest has approved the recommendation of the Community Problems Study Committee to develop a comprehensive planning and coordinating organization.

Another possible coordinating vehicle is the local chapter of the Mental Health Association in each of the counties. One of its prime tasks is to nurture sound relationships among the service agencies, but it is new at this pursuit. At present it lacks the requisite "reach" into the local-level, state-level, and national-level systems to effectuate coordination, largely because of its recent origins, understaffing, and inexperience.

What comes hard locally remains equally hard at the state level. Building integrated mental health systems in various regions of the state ranks among the most urgent responsibilities of the commissioner of mental hygiene in Albany. Within his department a division of community services is entrusted with the assignment to bridge state and local programs. However, so complex have these relationships become that a large number of specialized contact points are necessary for effective liaison. Thus, while on paper one division serves as liaison with local communities, in fact every division has its local contacts. Moreover, statutory construction and facilities agencies, with which the county authorities have to negotiate for assistance, have been created as adjuncts rather than divisions of the department. This simply adds to the confusion.

In 1960, by executive order, the governor created the Interdepartment Health and Hospital Council "in recognition of the need for the state departments to work closely in the areas of health, education, mental health, and social welfare." With a small staff, it has attempted to coordinate policy development in the health field, collaborating on occasion with professional and voluntary bodies. Inasmuch as the council has no powers of its own to compel departments that have been traditionally independent to work together, it has evolved more as a planning than as a coordinating agency.

By contrast, the Budget Division of the executive office and the Joint Fiscal Committee of the legislature wield wide influence over the departments. Their staffs are conscious of the tendencies toward fragmentation of government in the state. It is not unusual for them to reject budget items on the ground that coordination is missing from the proposed programs. To remedy cleavages and incongruities, the red pencil is as mighty as the sword. However, in the final analysis, the governor must settle interdepartmental disputes and attain harmony among his commissioners.

Like coordination and planning, decision making can be an event, an experience, and a process. Often the decision itself is less significant for community mental health programing than the interaction, the exchange of ideas, the personal contacts, and the negotiations that produce it. The process centers around communications, participation, and wielding of influence by a multitude of individuals with overlapping group affiliations. The mental health sector conforms to the same basic pattern of decision making that obtains generally for the social services. It utilizes familiar techniques and procedures for reaching decisions, but it manifests the emerging changes in the process of decision making that have occurred in the Syracuse metropolitan area. In fact it is in the avantgarde of change in this connection.

The actual arrangements for mental health decision making are diverse, though consensus has formed around a few fundamental values. No single authority or organization with supreme power is in this field. Interested parties are numerous. All operating agencies that provide services for the mentally ill and retarded are in a way decision-making units, although their decisions are largely of an internal administrative variety, concerned with such items as work schedules, office practices, and use of space. Ordinarily all these organizations belong to umbrella organizations: the Department of Mental Health and Onondaga county government in the case of the Adult Clinic and the Child Guidance Center; the state Department of Mental Hygiene and New York state government in the case of Syracuse Psychiatric Hospital; or St. Joseph Hospital in the case of the inpatient psychiatric services. Decision makers at this level have authority over personnel, salaries, treatment modalities, budget, new construction, clienteles to be assisted, and relationships with other organizations.

For the governmental agencies that organize and supply services, mental health is a "cause" behind which they have thrown their support. The New York state Department of Mental Hygiene and the Department of Mental Health in Onondaga county stand for changes in mental health policy, introduction of new services, and more ample funding of public and voluntary services. In the pursuit of their duties, their leaders have formed and cultivated contacts with leaders in every sector of society and are prone to utilize these contacts in decision-making situations affecting the mental health movement. When the county legislators are asked to approve the mental health budget, they know that local and state officials are watching them closely, prepared to emerge in the open as adversaries if a sponsored program is threatened with emasculation.

Numerous health and welfare organizations participate in decision making in various ways, exercising influence through their own programs, ideas and information that they circulate, public opinion that they alert and mobilize, and representatives who serve on boards and committees of public and other voluntary agencies. It is characteristic of this process that no single entity monopolizes and dominates it.

Political leaders in the metropolitan area indicate that mental health is a nonpartisan subject, which, unlike fluoridation, enjoys political respectability. They are willing to identify with it. For example, the Oswego Board of Supervisors voted unanimously to create a Mental Health Board in 1964. Expanded mental health facilities for Onondaga county was the number one item in the county Republican Party platform in 1964. A major figure in Syracuse and state politics, Senator John Hughes, has served as chairman of the mental health subcommittee of the Joint Fiscal Committee of the New York state legislature.

But if mental health is a nonpartisan matter there is still reason to believe that it will arouse political controversy in the future. In the first place, it requires heavy outlays of public funds for the construction of facilities and operation of services under state and federal programs. Second, mental health programing is a combined local-state-federal effort that may require party intervention to expedite intergovernmental decisions. Finally, as additional facilities are constructed in the Syracuse area, party interest and influence can be expected to figure in the allocation of contracts and jobs and purchases of real estate.

How mental health impinges on the realm of politics is illustrated in the recent establishment of a suicide prevention service. For three years the commissioner of mental health advocated the initiation of this type of service. In the spring of 1967 the Health Committee of the Board of Supervisors introduced the necessary legislation. At the request of the minority leader, the proposal was tabled for a month. As soon as the board postponed consideration of the bill, an active campaign was mounted in its support. Letters favoring the measure appeared in the local newspapers. Editorials raised the question of whether the minority leader, a candidate for the office of county executive, was not playing politics, furbishing his image as an economy-minded leader at the expense of "lives." The opposition was charged with insensitivity to suffering. At a subsequent meeting of the Board of Supervisors, passage of the legislation was achieved. The mobilization of public opinion for the suicide prevention service had all the marks of an organized effort. The Onondaga county Mental Health Association marshaled its forces for the measure and appears to have inspired expressions of support from other community circles.

Although traditional community leadership still predominates in the local power structure, county government officials and professionals are gaining in influence in the health and welfare fields, as well as in the community at large. The upgrading of county government partially accounts for this change, but there is a more significant factor. Today county government is a partner of the state and the United States governments. The county-state-federal relationship is now reshaping the pattern of community power to the advantage of the county executive in Onondaga county and the heads of several departments. To be a community influential one must be in a position to manipulate intergovernmental relationships. The Onondaga commissioner of mental health enjoys this standing, for he interprets the needs and inclinations of the county to state and federal officials and in turn interprets their policies to the community.

A crucial aspect of intergovernmental relations is the fiscal. In addition to increased local revenue, the Onondaga county executive has more state and federal funds to spend than ever before. There is no longer any comparability between the mental health, health, and welfare items in his budget and the outlays of voluntary organizations, the result being enhanced influence on the part of county officials in community decision making.

One consequence of local-state-federal relationships as a major determinant of influence in local affairs is that the formal processes of decision making and policy formation are being put to more genuine and less ritualistic use. Intergovernmental relations are also strengthening the standing of the state senators, assemblymen, and congressmen as community influentials. Traditional community leaders, if they are to be influential, must master the political and bureaucratic skills that are appreciated in governmental circles. If they cannot, they must then employ those who can. This practice is becoming commonplace in Syracuse, where various groups retain lawyers and other experts to wield their influence.

The deep involvement of modern government in the social services has also enhanced the status of the professional. His influence derives basically from his command of specialized knowledge, for which there is a growing demand in government and the economy. Public agencies and corporate bodies are staffed with professionals who share values and outlooks, as well as possess their own channels of communications. These channels tend to be beyond the reach of the ordinary run of community influentials. At the same time, they are significant parts of the decision-making machinery, to which the professionals have special access. Furthermore, they have professional confreres in all tiers of government. Hence, the commissioner of mental health locally has his counterparts in the Department of Mental Hygiene in Albany and the National Institute of Mental Health in Bethesda, Maryland. Through them he can bring pressure on local decision makers well in excess of that which his own power base generates.

In the face of these developments the traditional health and welfare influentials are displaying signs of uneasiness and anxiety about their own capability to discharge their usual responsibilities. They have detected the winds of change blowing across the metropolitan area. The nature of change is ambiguous, and this ambiguity, along with the concomitant tensions, disturbs them. A degree of strategic realignment is discernible, and in response the present community leaders have endorsed certain structural innovations as represented by the proposal for a comprehensive planning and coordination agency.

As the mental health decision-making system undergoes modification in the Syracuse area, it reveals its faults all the more starkly. There is ample evidence of obsolescence, duplication, petty competition for power, and personal antagonism. Mediators are sorely needed to cope with confrontations of interests and jurisdictional disputes. In most instances their task is to restore communications mainly by personal initiatives, thus relieving the stress and strain that eventually weaken services. Mental health in Syracuse has had its quota of crises, which it can ill afford in view of the precarious position of its programs for the mentally infirm.

Three brief case studies illustrate the interplay of community forces in the mental health area.

County Mental Health Board Crisis, 1959–1962. In 1959, "the wreckage of much of the county's mental health program" was evident. The Adult Clinic and Child Guidance Center had lost their directors; other professionals in the county program threatened to resign. It was even necessary to close the Child Guidance Center temporarily. Moreover, four years after birth, the county Mental Health Board was at loggerheads with its parent, the Board of Supervisors of Onondaga county. The supervisors had cut the budget of the Mental Health Board, presumably to discipline its staff. Charges and countercharges raised tempers to a boiling point.

The trouble seems to have had its origins in the creation of the county Mental Health Board, made up of professionals in health and education and "representatives" of the community. This board was entrusted under state law with quasi-legislative powers regarding budgets, personnel, and administrative regulations. Superficially these powers resembled those possessed by the Board of Supervisors. To be sure, appointments to the Mental Health Board were made by the presiding officer of the Board of Supervisors in 1955, but his hand was not altogether free in this matter.

It would appear that this arrangement brought professionals and politicians into a network of relationships for which neither was prepared psychologically. At this time there was a decline in public interest in mental health questions, which left the board in visible isolation.

Dialogue yielded to controversy as the politicians raised the banner of economy and professionals assumed positions behind the barricades of professional freedom, standards, and integrity. A debacle resulted with no one in a position to mediate the differences between the two boards.

With the loss of much-needed psychiatric services in 1960 and disillusionment and demoralization among professionals and citizens, a determined effort was finally made to remedy the situation. The Onondaga Health Association intervened. In 1958 the Metropolitan Health Council had been formed to support a metropolitan approach to the health problems of the city and county, but mental health was outside its focus of interest. However, its chairman, joined by various leaders in medical and medical education circles, undertook to get the public mental health clinics back into operation. Through contacts in professional and political circles, the fragile relationship between the Mental Health Board and Board of Supervisors was partially repaired. A formal way out of the crisis was provided by the reorganization of the county government in 1962. At that time the Department of Mental Health was established and it was given the powers of the Mental Health Board. Slowly, constructive relations developed between the commissioner of mental health and the supervisors.

Midtown Hospital Dispute. When the opportunity to obtain Midtown Hospital for use as a mental health center materialized in 1963, the county government acted with dispatch. The commissioner of mental health found the county executive receptive to the idea and encountered no serious objections from the Board of Supervisors. Quietly the county authorities executed a lease with the hospital's board for the rental of the entire building. It then spent a considerable sum to renovate, modernize, and brighten up the edifice, and by May 1964 the center housed the offices of the department, Adult Clinic, and Child Guidance Center. Space was also made available to the county public health nurses.

This adroit and successful operation by the commissioner of mental health aroused the opposition of a group of distinguished community influentials who protested the way the county government had taken action on Midtown Hospital. A few years earlier when the hospital was faced with closing, the Community Chest and local charitable foundations resuscitated it with a loan that was still outstanding at the time the county leased the building. These community influentials demanded that the loan be paid to the organizations they represented. Otherwise, they said the loan would become a hidden subsidy to the county. Thus the Midtown Hospital situation produced a confrontation between the voluntary and public sectors of the community.

Spokesmen for the voluntary groups complained that in this situation the county officials failed to consult citizen groups that shared responsibilities for mental health. It was argued that the decision to acquire and utilize Midtown Hospital as a mental health center was taken without regard to community health and welfare planning efforts and the report of the Community Priorities Committee of the Community Chest. County officials were also accused of showing no appreciation of earlier endeavors to rescue the hospital and of ignoring the intention to convert it into a much-needed care center for the aged. Finally, they were charged with failure to honor promises to keep certain community leaders informed of the future use of Midtown Hospital.

To justify its action the county government argued the protection of the public interest and implementation of public policy. It insisted further that as a public authority it could not submit its decisions for approval to community organizations or citizens' groups outside the normal channels of government.

In this dispute the county authorities found the press cooperative. A detailed story of their decision to lease Midtown Hospital was supplied to a newspaperman, and the resulting publicity strengthened the county officials in braving the displeasure of the elite of community leadership. Finally the storm subsided.

1,000-Bed Mental Hospital for Syracuse. At one of the first public meetings of the Onondaga County Mental Health Association in 1964, the county executive stated that the Syracuse metropolitan area was the largest in the state without a state mental hospital situated within its boundaries. Indicating that county officials were already discussing this deplorable situation with Albany, he spoke of a "1,000-bed" hospital as the remedy. During the next few months the county commissioner of mental hygiene mentioned the "1,000-bed" hospital on several occasions.

In September 1964 the Subcommittee on Mental Hygiene of the legislature's Joint Committee on Fiscal Affairs, chaired by Senator John Hughes of Onondaga county, held hearings in Syracuse. Aside from the usual formalities, the first order of business was a letter from

Mike Gorman, executive director of the National Association of Mental Health, opposing the construction. The assistant commissioner of the state Department of Mental Hygiene testified that agency opposed the construction of hospitals in metropolitan areas already served by an existing facility, as Syracuse was by Marcy State Hospital. He argued that it was far better to develop 1,000-bed intensive care units on the grounds of the established hospitals. Each unit would be assigned to a county and operate in close cooperation with its community mental health program.

The remaining witnesses fall into two groups. The mayor of Syracuse and commissioner of mental health of Onondaga county took up cudgels in behalf of the "1,000-bed" hospital in Syracuse. The other group, composed of representatives of the National Institute of Mental Health, Community Mental Health Board in New York City, the local chapters of the American Psychiatric Association and American Psychological Association, and the medical staff of a downstate hospital, wanted greatly enlarged community mental health programs. But some of them also supported the Syracuse proposal for a mammoth new hospital.

Subsequent to the subcommittee session the state commissioner of mental hygiene, Dr. Paul Hoch, argued that existing state hospitals should be revamped, and he opposed the idea of a new hospital in Syracuse. Nonetheless, in January 1965 the governor gave a firm commitment for the construction of the new hospital in Syracuse.

This *volte-face* took place within a month after the death of Commissioner Hoch in December 1964. About this time several of the regional mental health planning committees submitted their reports to Albany, with heavy endorsement of the community as the territorial base for mental health services rather than the isolated state hospital. In this period Senator John Hughes, who had presided over the subcommittee in Syracuse, intervened as a leader of the Republican minority between two wings of the Democratic majority over organization of the legislature. Hughes's support enabled one Democrat faction to win control.

Whether this event had anything to do with the selection of Syracuse as the site for the mental hospital is conjectural. Senator Hughes strongly supported the plan, which would bring jobs and contracts to his constituency. The senator is a shrewd and devoted participant in the political process. He commands virtually every skill of the political leader and mediator. To benefit his constituency he has put the art of politics to work on many occasions.

From these illustrations and other independent evidence, one is forced to conclude that community mental health programing in the Syracuse metropolitan area is haphazard. There is ample room for improvement in the clarity of purposes, identification of the need of clienteles, strategy in the management of resources, priority of services, attainment of consensus, excitement of leadership, sensitivity to changing needs, moods, and expectations, and cognizance of unintended consequences of the adopted policies. The quality of participation is too low for ample realization of the higher values of the mental health movement.

FINANCE

Funding is as integral a part of the mental health program of the Syracuse metropolitan area as treatment is, and the character of care is contingent on the fiscal patterns sustaining it. Funding involves more than the appropriation and expenditure of dollars for the construction of facilities and operation of services. It also reflects the forms of participation and attitudes of responsibility, as well as the intricacies of professional, organizational, and intergovernmental relationships. In an era of rapid change, financial arrangements can become as obsolete as therapy.

Services for the victims of mental disorders in the Syracuse metropolitan area have ordinarily been financed in several ways. While new ones have been added to the array, none of the traditional practices have disappeared. A common method that brings economic resources to the mental health field is the purchase of care through payments by patients to practitioners, hospitals, and clinics. In light of the high charges that arise out of private psychiatric treatment, presumably only persons in the higher income brackets make a substantial contribution in this category. Some minor relief from this type of financial burden can now be obtained through Blue Cross, Medicaid, and commercial insurance policies that provide for payments for psychiatric services in nongovernmental hospitals and the physician's office.

Public and voluntary programs expect reimbursement for services rendered if the patient or his immediate source of support are able to pay. New York state recovered 12 per cent of its expenditures on state hospital and school operations in this manner in the 1966 fiscal year. Usually this income is applied to internal improvements in the institutions. In 1966 Onondaga county clinics earned $14,000 in fees, roughly equal to 5 per cent of the total expenditures on the clinics.

Philanthropy constitutes another way of financing mental health services. In Syracuse contributions for this purpose have been meager, probably because charitable organizations have felt too inadequate to cope with the mentally ill. The now defunct Syracuse Dispensary depended heavily on gifts. The Association for Retarded Children engages in community fund raising. In its annual budget, the United Community Chest includes a line for mental health mainly to encourage innovation and also demonstrate to the county supervisors its commitment to the mental health programs of the county government. For new services certain local foundations have financially underwritten the initial stages.

In the public sector all tiers of government participate in mental health financing. The federal government bears all costs arising out of the construction, improvement, and operation of the Veterans Administration Hospital and clinic in Syracuse. Furthermore, it channels to the area federal funds for facilities, research, training, and demonstration projects relating to mental illness and retardation. Under the Hill-Burton-Harris Hospital Construction legislation Onondaga county, for example, received $146,445 in 1964 and $103,476 in 1965 for the construction of general hospitals that contain psychiatric beds.

Through June 30, 1967, the tri-county Syracuse area had obtained no federal assistance for the construction and staffing of community mental health centers contemplated under the 1963 Act. Though some steps have been taken to apply for a grant in support of a new mental retardation center, the application faces countless hurdles, including strict and possibly protracted scrutiny by various state authorities in Albany. Under Public Law 88–164 the federal government is to make a contribution of 37.6 per cent of the costs of construction of community mental health centers in New York state. To receive its share New York state and the Syracuse counties are obligated to put up 62.4 per cent of the costs. So far the much touted federal-state-local partnership on mental health center construction and operation has lain virtually dormant in Syracuse.

Whatever progress Onondaga, Madison, and Oswego counties have made with their own community programs, they still rely on New York state to finance institutional care. Marcy State Hospital, Syracuse Psychiatric Hospital, and the state schools serving the mentally disabled from these counties are carried fully on the state Department of Mental Hygiene "state purposes" budget, which totaled $253,044,661 or approximately 25 per cent of the entire state purposes budget for the 1966 fiscal year. In round figures, $10,000,000 is a reasonable estimate of the value of the annual state services to the three counties through its mental hospitals and schools. In addition, the Department of Mental Hygiene spends state funds for the Mental Health Research Unit situated in Syracuse. Various local organizations, Syracuse University and the Crouse Irving Hospital in particular, are direct beneficiaries of state support for training and demonstration projects.

Under the New York State Community Mental Health Services Act of 1954 the legislature annually appropriates funds for transfer to those counties eligible for this category of local assistance. Onondaga county has belonged to the program since 1955; Oswego and Madison counties are recent arrivals in this circle. In fiscal 1957 Onondaga county received $51,079 for its community mental health services. By fiscal 1966 the amount had grown to $293,958. But Oswego county received only $2,772 in fiscal 1966 and Madison county nothing.

Payments to the counties under the 1954 Act are authorized on a dollar-for-dollar matching basis. In 1964 the $1.40 per capita ceiling was removed on the condition that the local government agree to "extend or expand or otherwise improve its plan of the prior fiscal year in accordance with the commissioner's state-wide plan for state-local mental health services." Reimbursements are made for outpatient psychiatric clinics, inpatient psychiatric services in general hospitals, inpatient psychiatric services in nonprofit licensed institutions, psychiatric rehabilitation services, and consultant and education services. There are a number of exceptions, the most important of which are expenditures incurred for capital additions or improvements. To deal with this particular item, a Mental Hygiene Facilities Construction Fund has been created. Its relevance to the local scene remains to be clarified. Few county governments are in a strong enough position financially to commit capital funds to a large-scale mental health building program.

When the Department of Mental Hygiene renovates and modernizes the existing hospitals and schools or constructs new ones, it meets the costs out of the Mental Hygiene Facilities Improvement Fund created in 1963. In the late 1940s the people of New York by referendum approved the issuance of mental health construction bonds, which is one of the "earmarked revenue" accounts in the state treasury. This account shares with the War Bonus Account one ninth of the income tax and one cent per pack of the cigarette tax. Additional funds can be raised through the sale of other bonds that have been authorized but unissued so far. The construction of the new Syracuse mental hospital, state school, and unit for emotionally disturbed children will be financed with these resources.

New York state also subsidizes the local provision or purchase of care for the mentally handicapped through the diverse programs of such state departments as education, welfare, health, labor, and correction, and such divisions as youth and parole, and the State University of New York. A portion of the regular assistance paid by the state Department of Education to the school districts goes for the maintenance of classes for mentally retarded and emotionally disturbed children. These funds are incorporated in the usual state aid to schools and, therefore, are not considered special grants for these services.

Clearly massive financial involvement characterizes the concern of New York state for the mentally ill and retarded. It has a long history and will, in all likelihood, have a prolonged future. While the Department of Mental Hygiene is bound to alter its budgetary emphasis in favor of community mental health services, the state government has no prospect of escaping from the mental health business. Little enthusiasm greeted the New York State Mental Health Planning Committee task force recommendation that the counties assume the responsibility for reimbursing the state for institutional care rendered to its residents. In his annual report the Onondaga county commissioner of mental health noted, "There has arisen during the past year a vocal element in the county calling for the transferring of all community mental health services to the jurisdiction of the State of New York." So deeply rooted in tradition and the existing tax structure is the state's responsibility for the mentally disabled that the continuation of its fiscal roles can be taken for granted.

Overshadowed by the financial potency of the state government, local funding of mental health services is a recent development of growing importance. It has barely gotten underway in Oswego and Madison counties. Onondaga county is another story. Here "million dollar" budgets have been approved. In 1966 the expenditures within the jurisdiction of the Department of Mental Health reached the total of $829,213.60. Ten years earlier the comparable figure was $110,275.67, but ten years before that it was virtually nonexistent except for the expenses incurred in connection with court-ordered psychiatric examinations. A steady increase in outlays has occurred especially since 1962 when the Department of Mental Health came into being. Per capita expenditures on the county Mental Health Department activities rose from 35 cents in 1956 to over $1.75 in 1966, a fivefold increase in ten years.

A close look at the commissioner's "Expenditures and Sources of Funds" table in his 1966 annual report is revealing. It cites the expenditures by the county Department of Mental Health in addition to those by voluntary agencies in receipt of state community mental health funds under contract with the department. To illustrate, the roster contains the Adult Clinic, a local government facility, and the Elmcrest Children's Center, a nongovernmental facility. Furthermore, it records all expenditures of these organizations originating in the several different sources of financial support, from fees to state aid. Thus, toward the $829,213 total in 1966, county tax funds accounted for $251,636, voluntary funds $132,106, and state aid under the 1954 Community Mental Health Services Act $431,444, or slightly more than half.

In 1955 Onondaga county paid $35,000 out of its own revenues for mental health services. This figure excludes the payments to the state hospitals for the performance of court-ordered psychiatric examinations and hospitalization under the Code of Criminal Procedures. In the decade since 1955 the total county expenditures climbed to $195,000. In 1966 the county government spent $251,636 out of tax funds. While this rising trend, which is likely to continue, has caused some sharp questions to be posed in the Ways and Means Committee of the county legislature, the fact of the matter is that the actual expenditures amount to less than 1 per cent of the county budget. The growing sensitivity of the supervisors to expanding mental health commitments is in part indicative of the tradition of economy that is evident in local government circles. It also is aroused by staff shortages that interfere with the flow of services.

Though the mental health budget of Onondaga county is an instrument of policy and planning, it is not comprehensive. It fails to provide for the direct and indirect mental health expenditures of other county units, such as the departments of social services and health or the Syracuse school administration and district boards of education. By its shortcomings in this respect, it mirrors the prevalence of fragmentation. In this connection, a recent development of considerable significance is Medicaid, the administration of which has been lodged with the county Social Services and Health Departments jointly. In this program payment may be made to defray the costs of in-hospital psychiatric care. In effect Medicaid is subsidizing the very population ordinarily served by the county clinics to seek treatment in hospitals, which already shelter far too many patients with little need to be hospitalized. If Medicaid continues unmodified, its impact on community mental health centers threatens to be disruptive.

Constantly encountering emotionally disturbed and mentally retarded children, the school systems in the Syracuse metropolitan area find it necessary to budget school tax funds for "psychological services," "special education (handicapped)," and psychiatric consultation. Under a mandate from Albany to educate the "difficult cases" that are educable, these systems must pay for special teachers and other staff assigned to classes for these children without reimbursement from the state Department of Mental Hygiene. For this and related responsibilities some county school administrations have pooled their resources under boards of cooperative services. Despite the depth of their mutual interests, a conspicuous gap separates the Department of Mental Health and the school authorities fiscally, as well as operationally. The many attempts to achieve close collaboration have been frustrated by barriers of state law, administrative regulation, and local circumstances.

For the subject of funding, conclusions seem less appropriate than concluding observations. Financing the mental health services for the Syracuse metropolitan area is by no means an easy or simple undertaking in the prevailing condition of "multiple-funding." No one person or agency occupies a strategic enough position to unify or direct it. The power of the purse is so widely dispersed that the advantages of federalism and pluralism are sacrificed to the disadvantages. Funds are so scattered that those who control them can call the tune, though in actuality they may constitute minor participants in the whole system. Complexity is magnified without the parallel development in the management of complexity.

Personnel Puzzle

Mental health manpower in the Syracuse metropolitan area suffices to staff at least five community mental health centers according to the standards of the National Institute of Mental Health. This possibility implies that the area, unlike so many others in the nation, suffers no absolute or irremedial shortage of professional personnel, psychiatrists and psychologists included. Whether the staffing requirements of such centers can be satisfied at the same time that the heavy demand for private care is met and certain prime institutional commitments are pursued raises questions that shed a diffused light on the manpower issue. Quantity is not the only consideration. Equally important is the current state of the participating professions in their many dimensions, including diversity of practice, philosophies, attitudes, prestige, remuneration, and supportive conditions.

At the present time approximately fifty psychiatrists are actively engaged in practice or in administration, teaching, training, and research in Onondaga county. Madison county has three, Oswego county two. In addition, general practitioners, pediatricians, internists, and neurologists treat disorders with psychiatric components, probably retaining under their care far more emotionally disturbed and neurotic patients than they refer to specialists in psychiatry. The Syracuse regional committee of the New York State Mental Health Planning Committee reported that "it is becoming more and more apparent that the nonpsychiatric physician is extremely important in the total planning for Community Mental Health."

As more than half the patients at Marcy State Hospital are from the Syracuse area, the staff of that institution may be counted among the mental health personnel of the area. Including the director and assistant director (medical), the hospital has twenty-five psychiatrists on its roster, with authorization to appoint up to thirty-four. Five psychologists are employed there, as are sixteen psychiatric social workers.

Virtually 90 per cent of the psychiatrists of the three-county area hold full-time or part-time salaried appointments at the Upstate Medical Center, including the Veterans Administration Hospital, county Mental Health Departments or Boards, public clinics and voluntary programs supported out of public funds, state hospitals and schools, nonprofit and proprietary hospitals, and boards of education. In most instances they wear more than one hat; some administer programs, serve as consultants to other programs, teach, and engage in research, in addition to their participation in clinical psychiatry. Most also maintain a private psychiatric practice.

Only five or six psychiatrists devote their full time to private patients. The other practitioners with institutional appointments vary drastically in the patient load that they carry. It has not been possible at the present time to ascertain the number of private patients in the Syracuse area.

While there are the usual differences of approach to psychiatric knowledge, doctrine, and technique, Syracuse has seen the psychiatric profession divide dramatically over the public role of psychiatry. Professor Thomas Szasz, in the Department of Psychiatry of the Upstate Medical Center, has been an implacable foe of community psychiatry.[10] He contends that community psychiatry is in essence an instrument of social control rather than a channel of genuine assistance to a person. He perceives mental health under public and community agencies as reaching the "misfits" and "deviants" whose individual conduct inconveniences and offends the family, school, police, employer, or neighbor, and contravenes the prevailing norms of society. Its purpose, in his view, is to deter, discipline, or punish such persons in violation of their individuality, interests, and even rights to the satisfaction of the aggrieved unit of the community. Postulating that the "mental illness" involved in these cases is a myth, that psychiatry is legitimate only when utilized by the individual who voluntarily seeks and chooses what it has to offer, and that a psychiatrist is legitimate only when he acts as the agent of the patient, not the society or a third party, Dr. Szasz condemns community mental health as a menace to the values of freedom. He cites, for example, the suicide prevention idea as a threat to the personal liberty of any person who telephones for assistance.[11]

Dr. Szasz is not alone among the local psychiatrists in the posture he has assumed. Others who exhibit less extreme reactions to community psychiatry have nonetheless indicated their discomfort in treating patients under the auspices of community agencies. The constant threat to the confidentiality of the physician-patient relationship is often pointed out as a ground for concern. Their preference for an entirely private relationship is evident.

[10] Thomas Szasz, "Mental Health Ethics," *National Review*, June 14, 1966, pp. 570–72.

[11] Personal conversation, May 5, 1967.

Community psychiatry has equally staunch proponents, especially in the former Onondaga commissioner of mental health. A civil libertarian, he finds Dr. Szasz's observations an exaggeration of what actually occurs in the clinics and agencies for which he has full or partial responsibility. In his view, safeguards have been built into community mental health programs for the protection of the individual. Moreover, it is his opinion that community psychiatry is in reality and potentiality a vast improvement over futile and degrading hospitalization in a state institution. Apparently community psychiatry is, to judge by the number of psychiatrists affiliated with local agencies, professionally respectable.

Dr. Szasz's style of polemics, as well as the content of his argument, has influenced the organization and operation of services locally. One matter on which he is an outspoken critic is the involuntary admission of persons into psychiatric facilities. This he proscribes as unjustifiable deprivation of liberty. Some psychiatric residents at the Upstate Medical Center have been reluctant to sign commitment documents for the involuntary admission of persons into Marcy State Hospital. They justify their attitude on the ground that any person who is not willing to commit himself on a voluntary basis is unready for genuine therapy.

However, public authorities are compelled by court orders or administrative decisions to proceed with "emergency" and involuntary commitments. Many local psychiatrists hold that it is more desirable for a person in need of therapy to be placed in the custody of a hospital or clinic than a local jail or county penitentiary. In recent years, the "libertarian" psychiatrists have been relieved of commitment responsibilities in the agencies in which they serve or they avoid appointments in agencies that require them to act in contravention of their own professional and ethical position.

For his testimony in a "fit to stand trial" proceeding that was highly critical of the policies and practices of the state Department of Mental Hygiene, Dr. Szasz lost his status as a consultant at state hospitals. This cancellation of his privileges triggered some hostility at the Upstate Medical Center. In the course of the episode the chairman of the Department of Psychiatry resigned his post and also surrendered his appointment as director of Syracuse Psychiatric Hospital, thus ending an administrative experiment in collaboration between the two institutions. Moreover, the commissioner of mental health in Syracuse came in for severe criticism by several faculty members, which also damaged the relationship between the Upstate Medical Center and county facilities.

Some indication of the antipathy that has enervated Syracuse psychiatric circles is revealed in the regional planning committee report:

It was Dr. Hollander's feeling that the present status of psychiatry in Syracuse has gone through a crisis itself and that it would take years for the debris and the bitter feelings to be cleared away so that a better level of psychiatric practice could be reinstated. Some discussion of personalities, domain jealousies and areas of legitimate disagreement were discussed and some of these areas seem to be critically involved in changes taking place in the Medical School itself.

It is one of the purposes of a university to encourage intellectual ferment. Although the turmoil was difficult, the Upstate Medical Center has on balance helped rather than harmed community mental health efforts in Syracuse. It has proved useful in at least three respects. The three-year psychiatric residency program that it sponsors has increased the professional manpower pool out of which local clinics and other mental health facilities have been able to draw staff. The *quid pro quo* is training experience and additional income for the residents. For example, in 1966 the Adult Clinic of Onondaga county employed eight residents. Also, four attained the status of ward directors in the community mental health center at Syracuse Psychiatric Hospital. The future of these relationships is, however, ambiguous. Now that the University Hospital has opened its own psychiatric clinic, fewer residents are available for staffing the existing agencies.

Another way in which the center assists Syracuse mental health programs is in attracting staff to the metropolitan area. Clinical appointments, research opportunities, seminar participation, and intellectual stimulation that the center provides appeal to psychiatrists and psychologists seeking professional recognition and advancement. For example, psychiatrists at the Veterans Administration Hospital and Syracuse Psychiatric Hospital also hold appointments at the College of Medicine.

Mental health programs require staff other than psychiatrists. Approximately forty-five licensed psychologists reside in Onondaga county, six in Oswego, and the same number in Madison. Most are in the employ of the universities, colleges, state hospitals, Syracuse State Schools, clinics, city and county boards of education, industry, and youth and probation agencies. Seventy-five per cent have had more than five years' full-time clinic and hospital experience. Given the present professional trends, it comes as no surprise that most are also engaged in private practice, though only a quarter devote more than ten hours a week to it. Local agencies often turn for psychologists to the Department of Psychology of Syracuse University. Moreover, the School of Special Education at Syracuse University has trained psychologists for rehabilitation assignments, reading and speech therapy, and special care for retarded children, all of which utilize special skills in very short supply. The other universities and colleges are also sources of psychologists for the metropolitan area.

Other personnel in mental health programs include psychiatric social workers, psychiatric nurses, occupational therapists, work counselors, nutritionists, ward attendants, and aides of various types, in addition to administrators. Ordinarily where training is required, the Syracuse metropolitan area is adequately equipped to provide it. A critical vocation is nursing. An overall shortage of qualified psychiatric nurses prevails and threatens to grow as beds in hospitals are opened for short-term, and day and overnight care. Public health nurses are gradually being drawn into mental health activities, but opposition has been expressed to any move that entrusts to them official jurisdiction over aftercare.

An innovation in the health care field, a small group of home aides recently received instruction for duty with families in which some member suffers from mental disorder. The Onondaga county Mental Health Association has started to train volunteers who wish to work with mentally ill or retarded persons. Local cognizance has been taken of the frequent contact between teachers, clergymen, and policemen and victims of mental illness. While the talents and energies of the metropolitan community remain to be fully mobilized, more roles for the nonprofessional are in the process of development.

Every major mental health program and facility in the area has a psychiatrist as its administrator. The Onondaga commissioner of mental health and the directors of the Mental Health Boards in Madison and Oswego counties must be psychiatrists. As state law mandates their employment in this capacity, it imposes a requirement that diverts a scarce psychiatric resource into administration. The soundness of this practice is doubted. Onondaga county is temporarily departing from it in an interim appointment of a nonpsychiatrist as the acting commissioner of mental health, pending the selection of a replacement for the original commissioner, whose grasp of the professional, fiscal, legal, and political aspects of the local mental health problems has been exceptional.

On several occasions, psychiatrists who are filling administrative posts have mentioned the need for training in management and executive leadership. While the universities in Syracuse conduct no degree program in hospital or clinic administration, administration is the speciality of the Maxwell Graduate School of Public Affairs and Citizenship at Syracuse University. Consultation between the school's faculty and administrators of psychiatric facilities is increasing in scale and depth.

Another component of the personnel sector is the professional organization. During the recent staffing crisis in the Onondaga County Department of Mental Health, the Central New York branch of the American Psychiatric Association was requested to assume responsibility at least for temporary coverage of the clinical vacancies. Agencies look to this and similar bodies, such as the local chapters of the American Psychological Association and National Association of Social Workers, for assistance in staff recruitment. In addition, these organizations exercise a general responsibility over the professional standards and conduct of their members. Here as elsewhere, their concern also extends to the conditions of employment in the various mental health institutions.

A condition that is considered unsatisfactory is the level of salaries in the county clinic and related voluntary facilities. It is charged in professional circles that the staff shortage exists in the program only because the salary level is minimal or in any case too low to be competitive. Discontent is evident over the manner in which the Boards of Supervisors in the upstate counties have begrudgingly and belatedly increased the remuneration of their professional employees in this field. The attitude of the supervisors has seemed unduly parsimonious in view of the fact that the state government reimburses the county fifty cents on a dollar spent on salaries in the Department of Mental Health. On their part the county legislators are dismayed at the twenty thousand dollar, and higher, salaries that are paid to senior psychiatric personnel, salaries in excess of the county executive's. They are also dismayed at the turnover in the county services, resulting from the more attractive salaries offered by other mental health institutions in Syracuse. Confronted with a tight professional market, some officials are wondering whether the county government should even endeavor to operate clinics. The question remains unanswered.

So jumbled is the personnel situation that the community mental health centers emerging in the Syracuse area will face difficulties in staffing. The more personal attention modern care dictates for mental disorders, the more crucial are the needs for quality and versatility of mental health manpower. Each program implementing the "bold new approach" has its concomitant personnel problems. Moreover, continuity of care demands that one practitioner cooperate expeditiously with the next, thus linking up all efforts expended on behalf of the recipient of care. Only if the staffing arrangements satisfy these and related conditions can Syracuse reasonably expect to attain its mental health goals.

IX: BOSTON

ROBERT H. MARDEN

METROPOLITAN Boston, situated in eastern Massachusetts, covers a semicircular area extending roughly fifteen to twenty miles from the northeast to the southeast of the city of Boston, around Boston Harbor and Massachusetts Bay. The early settlements in the Massachusetts Bay area were along the coast, at such places as Boston, Dorchester, and Salem. By the late seventeenth century, the "frontier" had been extended throughout most of what is now the Boston Standard Metropolitan Statistical Area (SMSA).

The important units of local government in Massachusetts are the incorporated municipalities, namely the cities and the towns. Counties exist primarily as judicial districts. The Boston SMSA includes seventy-seven municipalities, seventeen cities, and sixty towns. The "central city" is, of course, the city of Boston itself. Next is the "urban core," consisting of those cities and a few towns that are adjacent or close to Boston. Surrounding the "core" is the "inner band," a ring two or three municipalities deep which is quite densely settled. Outside the "inner band" is the "outer band," an area of many municipalities that are generally oriented to Boston as a center.

The topography of the Boston area has influenced the pattern of settlement. Low but clearly defined hills and bluffs ring the "Boston basin." Early urbanization occurred almost entirely in this area, while the small villages beyond continued in their placid way. A basic shift in the relation of residence and work location during the nineteenth century changed all this. The development of cheap means of mass transportation made it possible for anyone to live at increasing distances from the office, store, shop, or factory. Later, the automobile made the choice of residential location even more free. The burst of population

The field work underlying this chapter was greatly aided by the energetic work of Joan B. Goldstein and John E. Hambright, who acted as research assistants. Dr. Jack Ewalt, Director of the Massachusetts Department of Mental Health, was helpful in ensuring that matters of fact set forth in the initial draft were correct.

growth after the Second World War led residential developments to "spill over" the surrounding hills, much to the surprise of the residents of many rural towns, who were ill prepared for the physical, economic, and political results.[1] In addition, there also has been considerable movement from the older areas of Boston, Cambridge, and Somerville into the next ring of cities and towns. The consequences of such changes have been particularly marked in the period since 1940, as Table 1 shows.

Table 1: Population Growth in the Boston City
and Metropolitan Area, 1940–1960

Location	Population			Per Cent Change	
	1940	*1950*	*1960*	*1940–1950*	*1950–1960*
Boston city	770,816	801,444	697,197	+4.0	−14.0
Area outside city	1,438,792	1,609,128	1,892,104	+11.8	+17.6
Total	2,209,608	2,410,572	2,589,301	+9.1	+7.4

While in 1940 Boston city had about one-third of the metropolitan area population, by 1960 this proportion had declined to one-fourth. Moreover, the city experienced an absolute decrease in population.

In 1960 the population of Massachusetts was 5,149,317, of which about 50 per cent lived in Boston. Foreign-born residents and those with one or both parents of foreign birth composed less than 20 per cent of the state's population, but over 40 per cent of metropolitan Boston's. The nonwhite population of Massachusetts was almost 125,000. Of these, 70 per cent lived in the Boston SMSA, and 50 per cent in the city of Boston. It is therefore not surprising that the most vigorous fight in Massachusetts over de facto school segregation occurred in Boston.

The Boston area is one of the oldest settled parts of the United States and one of the first to be recognized as a metropolitan area. The need to organize basic public services within the growing metropolitan area was accepted in the late nineteenth century, and several unifunctional agencies were established. These were merged into the Metropolitan District Commission (MDC), which acted as a wholesaler for water supply and sewage disposal and provided a system of parks and

[1] Robert C. Wood, *Suburbia—Its People and Their Politics* (Boston: Houghton Mifflin, 1959).

beaches for many of the municipalities within the Boston region. Thus, it might be said that Boston has had a metropolitan government of a sort for over half a century.

Nevertheless, the seventeenth-century pattern of local government has continued with only minor modifications. The original concept of local government was that of unified religious, political, and economic communities termed towns, which were established by permission of the provincial or state legislature as sufficient settlers moved in. Eventually the entire area of Massachusetts was divided into towns, and while some of them grew in population sufficiently to lead to transformation into cities, their boundaries remained largely the same. The only exception was the absorption of a few adjacent towns by the city of Boston prior to the First World War when it provided better public services at low tax rates. Thus, Massachusetts is blessed (or cursed) with an array of 351 municipal governments: 39 cities and 312 towns.

The Boston SMSA adjoins four other SMSA's: Lowell-Lawrence on the north, Worcester on the west, Providence (Rhode Island) on the southwest, and Brockton on the south. Its geographic growth is consequently limited unless economic warfare pulls some bordering municipalities from one metropolitan area into another. The Boston area's seventy-seven municipalities have long civic traditions, and their differentiation embodied or shaped many psychological, political, economic, ethnic, and religious cleavages. However, these differences became less acute as massive migration from one part of Greater Boston to another took place, as confidence grew among suburbanites in the quality of Boston's government, and tensions between various religious groups steadily declined.

County government came to be of little importance in Massachusetts except as the areal basis for the organization of the judicial system. The limited government functions performed on a county basis could well be transferred to appropriate state agencies, and the sentiment is growing that Massachusetts should follow the example of Connecticut and abolish county governments altogether.

Only a few special districts are to be found in the Boston SMSA, other than the Metropolitan District Commission. The most important is the newly created Massachusetts Bay Transportation Authority (MBTA), an expansion of the Massachusetts Transportation Authority (MTA) which served Boston and thirteen other cities and towns close to Boston. This new agency is wrestling with the major problem of mass transportation over an area of eastern Massachusetts somewhat larger than the Boston SMSA. A few other special districts are to be found in eastern Massachusetts, composed of two or more municipalities for such purposes as health services, mosquito control, and the like. The public schools are formally dependent parts of city and town governments, although as local agencies of the state government they have a considerable measure of autonomy. There are, however, some autonomous regional high school districts within the Boston SMSA. Thus, the government within the Boston SMSA can be considered as having three levels: the state and its agencies; the two metropolitan service agencies (MDC and MBTA); and the seventy-seven cities and towns. Retail public services, as contrasted with the wholesale services (of the MDC and the MBTA) are provided by the highly fragmented cities and towns. The organization of any public service that is to be provided on a more limited area basis than that of the entire state must take into account the "building blocks" of the cities and towns, or possibly, as in the case of Boston proper, parts of the city. This is true not only for public agencies, but also for private service agencies. Municipal fragmentation is, then, a basic fact of political life in Massachusetts and is of particular importance for any public service that is oriented to the concept of community organization as in the case of mental health. But all this fragmentation is on a single level of organization. Massachusetts has been spared the plague of the numerous and often overlapping special districts which developed in so many American metropolitan areas. The traditional Massachusetts penchant for a multiplicity of autonomous elected boards and commissions and latent hostility to being planned or managed, however, makes this advantage more apparent than real in many cities and towns.

The limited government functions performed on a county basis could well be transferred to appropriate state agencies and the sentiment is growing that Massachusetts should follow the example of Connecticut

MENTAL HEALTH ORGANIZATION

A study of mental health programs in the Boston metropolitan area logically should begin with an assessment of the extent of the problem of mental illness. Yet two practical difficulties stand in the way of any complete statement. The first is the elastic definition of who is mentally ill or who requires some type of professional attention. The

William Ryan in his study of the problem within the city of Boston used a very broad definition to include all those who have "emotional problems that interfere in their lives, handicapping them in their work, in their social relationships, and in dealing with members of their own families. These problems range from being nervous and making mistakes when the boss looks over their shoulder all the way to believing that the Communists are putting bad thoughts in one's mind with atomic machines.[2] Ryan estimated that between 20 and 25 per cent of those living in the city of Boston might fall within this category. It is hardly surprising that many local authorities in the field of mental health have questioned Ryan's definition. Furthermore, even should his estimates be approximately accurate, there is considerable doubt that everyone needing help should be defined as mentally ill. Such a figure certainly is not a sound basis for estimating the total demand to be met because, as Ryan noted critically, many of those concerned with expanding mental health services base their arguments upon a "hidden assumption . . . that all persons who are handicapped by emotional disturbance are entitled to services to lessen their handicap. In practice, society has made no such commitment and there is no mechanism for providing such services to all who need them, or even to all who request them." Finally, even were Ryan's very broad definition accepted as valid, the range of intensity and length of help or treatment would be very great, with the result that little could be concluded about total requirements.

The only firm data available on the extent of mental illness in Massachusetts was a study of first admissions of adults to state, private, and Veterans' Administration hospitals over the three-year period 1959–1961. For an area which is substantially the same as the Boston SMSA, the figure was 10,418. But the relation of an admission figure to total need is subject to widely differing interpretations. The critical shortage of available children's facilities and the long waiting lists discourage many parents and school authorities from seeking such services. Despite the lack of evidence, the accepted "rule of thumb" that 10 per cent of all children require some assistance was utilized in planning for Massachusetts. As of 1960, metropolitan Boston had approximately

William Ryan, Distress in the City (Boston: Community Services, 1965), pp. 389–396.

272,000 children under age five, and approximately 456,000 age five through fourteen; 10 per cent of the total would be about 73,000. In contrast to this figure, the thirty-six clinics of the statewide Department of Mental Health served over 8,000 children under eighteen in 1964; possibly as many as two-thirds of these were from the Boston SMSA because of the number of clinics in eastern Massachusetts.

A statewide survey conducted in 1965 identified more than 135,000 mentally retarded children and adults[3] who were being served in the state. It was estimated that if those with milder forms of retardation were included the total would be 165,000 persons requiring assistance. Since the Boston SMSA has approximately half the state's population, it is conceivable that over 80,000 persons in the area might be designated as mentally retarded. Many of them receive some degree of help because of the substantial facilities in the area. Additionally, there was a detailed survey of the number of mentally retarded children on the waiting list for admission to state schools. The waiting list for the cities and towns in the Boston SMSA totaled 532. A more significant indication of unmet need in 1965 was that there were plans for at least four more state schools for the mentally retarded.

Taking all these figures and estimates into account, it would seem that the only sound conclusion is that there is far more need than is currently being met. The state as a whole is considerably better provided with health and mental health resources than is the United States, and within the state the Boston SMSA is far better provided than other parts; 88 per cent of the psychiatrists having a private practice who responded to a 1965 questionnaire practiced in this area.

The Mental Health Planning Project recommended thirty-seven community mental health centers for the state of Massachusetts, of which fifteen would be located in or would serve the Boston metropolitan area. The greatest need was reported within Boston and the adjacent urban areas of Lynn and Cambridge, plus that part of the Boston SMSA to be served by the Plymouth center. The suburban areas are relatively well provided for, although they are still lacking in mental health resources in comparison with the potential demand.

The formal organization for providing or affecting mental health

[3] Herbert C. Schulberg and Henry Wechsler, "The Uses and Misuses of Data in Assessing Mental Health Needs," *Community Mental Health Journal*, Winter 1967, pp. 389–396.

services in Massachusetts and the Boston SMSA is vertically dispersed along federal, state, and local levels. At the federal level, there is, first of all the NIMH, administratively a part of the Department of Health, Education, and Welfare. Most of the activities of the NIMH in the Boston SMSA are coordinated through the Region I office of HEW, located in Boston. One member of the regional staff is an NIMH representative. The regional staff has been particularly helpful in mediating the views of state and local officials, which are sometimes sharply divergent from opinions in Washington.

Other federal agencies involved in mental health matters within the Boston SMSA include the Veterans Administration, which maintains three hospitals in the area (Bedford, Boston, and Brockton) with a large outpatient clinic in Boston. It has virtually no operational or technical relationships with other mental health agencies in the area, although the state hospitals occasionally refer veterans to VA hospitals. The federal Office of Vocational Rehabilitation and the Children's Bureau are interested in various types of mental health problems or activities, but such functions within the Boston area are supervisory or advisory. Thus, in the context of meeting mental health requirements within the Boston SMSA, direct federal activities are of limited importance.

In the past, there seems to have been only very limited communication between the several federal operating agencies involved in mental health activities, nor is there much formal contact between them and the regional office of HEW. Even within the regional office of HEW, more vertical communication (state-region-national) was evident within the several specialties than across specialties in respect to common problems.

Because of the increasing scope and complexity of federally aided projects, such as the antipoverty programs, urban renewal, urban transportation, and civil rights and their relationship to many existing programs, such as public assistance, education, public health, and mental health, it has been recognized that it is highly desirable to have more internal communication at the regional level. Consequently, vigorous efforts have been launched to overcome the isolation of many functions and programs that was evident in the recent past.

Massachusetts was perhaps the first state to take official action in respect to the mentally ill. The colonial General Court (as the state legislature is still termed) passed a law in 1676 empowering the "select-

men" of each town, who were the elected governing officials, to care
for the "insane," and this original assignment of responsibility persisted until the twentieth century. In the meantime, Massachusetts also
was developing hospitals for the mentally ill; the first devoted exclusively to this purpose was the private McLean Hospital in suburban
Belmont, opened in 1818. The city of Boston opened what is now Boston
State Hospital soon afterward, and eventually this municipal institution
became a part of the state system of mental hospitals. The first of the
mental hospitals established by the state government was that in
Worcester, in 1833; others were added and they now total thirteen.
In the early 1900s the state established four state schools for mentally
retarded children.

Until 1904 the state hospitals took care of patients referred to
them by the cities and towns, and charged the community from which
each patient came. Traditional Yankee thrift led local authorities to
seek the earliest possible release of such patients. However, many municipalities and some counties preferred to care for their "lunatics" close
at home, which was cheaper. Evidently in many places it also resulted in
appallingly bad treatment, which obviously had limited therapeutic value.
A reform movement led to the passage in 1904 of a law that is often
described as establishing a "state monopoly" in the public care of the
mentally ill. Chapter 123, Section 2 of the Massachusetts General Laws
states:

The commonwealth shall have the care, control and treatment of all mentally
ill, epileptic and mentally deficient persons and of alcoholics and drug addicts,
the care of whom is vested in it by law. No county, city or town shall
establish or maintain any institution for the care, control and treatment of
mentally ill, epileptic or mentally deficient persons or be liable for the board,
care, treatment or act of any inmate thereof.

To carry out this responsibility, the state government had available
a large but somewhat unwieldy organization composed of the state
hospitals and state schools. These had been established as independent
entities, each with a governing board, and to some extent were regional
agencies with a high degree of autonomy.

The state had showed its early concern with the kind of care the
mentally ill received when it established the Commission on Lunacy
in 1854. This was the first of a long series of state commissions and
study committees. In 1879 the Board of Health, Lunacy, and Charity
was established to give some small measure of unity to state activities.

The legislation of 1904 cited above authorized a separate department to carry out the state's exclusive responsibility for the treatment of the mentally ill in Massachusetts under a state Board of Insanity. The present Department of Mental Health was authorized in 1938. This department is administered by a commissioner who is appointed by the governor for a term of four years, coterminous with the governor's four-year term. Until 1965 such appointments had to be confirmed by the elected Governor's Council (an institutional relic from the colonial period) but public dismay at the apparent "wheeling and dealing" of the council led to massive approval in 1964 of a referendum proposal stripping the council of most such powers. The governor now has sole responsibility for this key appointment. The Department of Mental Health employs about one-third of all state employees and the total number of patients reported for June 30, 1966, was 23,147. The budget for fiscal 1967 was $91,200,000, the second largest item in the state budget that year.

Within the Boston SMSA, the effect of the state's assumption of primary responsibility for the mentally ill in 1904 has been that the major mental health units (that is, the area are state hospitals and state schools, and a considerable number of outpatient and service facilities largely or wholly supported by the state. In addition to those institutions located within the Boston SMSA, a number outside it serve certain cities and towns in the metropolitan area or serve certain categories of patients, drawn in part from the Boston SMSA.

The development of mental health programs in Massachusetts has been substantially affected by the so-called Anti-Aid Amendment in the state constitution, which is similar to those enacted in a number of other states during the latter part of the nineteenth century to block the use of public funds, either state or municipal, for direct fiscal assistance to religious, educational, or other nonprofit groups, associations, or institutions. Amendment XVIII of the Massachusetts constitution reads as follows:

No grant, appropriation or use of public money or property or loan of public credit shall be made or authorized by the commonwealth or any political subdivision thereof for the purpose of founding, maintaining or aiding any school or institution of learning, whether under public control or otherwise, wherein any denominational doctrine is inculcated, or by any other school, or any college, infirmary, hospital, institution, or educational, charitable, or religious undertaking which is not publically owned and under the exclusive control, order and superintendence of public officers or public agents authorized by the commonwealth or federal authority or both.

The sentiment was reaffirmed in the 1919 constitutional convention, and indeed a constitutional amendment adopted at that time excludes any matters affecting religion or religious institutions and state appropriations from the provisions of the popular initiative and referendum amendments. The only way in which these constitutional provisions could be changed, therefore, would be in a state constitutional convention. This is one of the reasons for continuing opposition in some quarters of Massachusetts to such a convention.

The constitutional provision is significant for two reasons, so far as mental health in Massachusetts is concerned. First, some have held that there is doubt about the constitutionality of the law enabling state and local payments in support of local mental health clinics that are operated by local mental health associations. This practice has never been tested in the courts, but it is possible that if proposals were made for large-scale payments for community mental health centers under control of private agencies such as local mental health associations, their constitutionality would be challenged. For similar reasons, the proposal that community mental health centers should be constructed and operated as integral parts of existing private general hospitals and subject to the control of such hospitals—which the federal act permits—would seem barred by the state constitution. The only exception would be in the case of municipal hospitals, of which there are seventeen in Massachusetts.

Another provision of the same amendment of the constitution, however, provides a possibility for reaching some type of compromise:

Nothing herein contained shall be construed to prevent the commonwealth or any political subdivision thereof, from paying to privately controlled hospitals, infirmaries, or institutions for the deaf, dumb or blind not more than the ordinary and reasonable compensation for the care and support actually rendered or furnished to such persons as may be in whole or in part unable to support or care for themselves.

The purpose of this provision was to enable the state to continue to pay for the care of the blind at the famed Perkins Institute for the Blind. It has been suggested that the words "mentally retarded or mentally ill" could be added to this provision, but constitutional amendments take several years to be enacted. However, it is contended by other legal authorities that this change is not necessary since state and local agencies have been making such payments for the care of the mentally ill for many years, on the theory that the phrase "privately controlled hospitals [and] infirmaries" can be separated from the phrase "institutions for the deaf, dumb or blind" in the amendment. Indeed, the practice of making such payments has been validated by several advisory opinions of state attorneys general, and any change of this interpretation would wreak havoc with welfare and medical programs throughout the state. A secondary question then remains of how much can be paid; obviously for "privately controlled instiutions," whether nonprofit or proprietary, part of the "ordinary and reasonable" operating costs reflected in charges for patients is to pay off the costs of capital investment. Hence, it would seem that the financing of care for mental patients in segments of private general hospitals through payments of fees for services is as constitutionally valid as payments for the care of the aged in nursing homes, emotionally disturbed children in special schools, and indigent patients in hospitals.

Mental illness is closely related to a number of other health, welfare, and law enforcement activities. Thus, the Department of Mental Health has a role singly or in collaboration with other state agencies in such fields. It has been increasingly aware of the problem of the older persons who need some degree of care, but who are not really mentally ill. The development of Cushing Hospital in Framingham for older people is the result of this concern. More facilities of this type may well be added in other parts of the state.

In recent years, Massachusetts has gone far to provide classes for the mentally retarded, by requiring that each city or town in which there are a certain number (now five) of children with special problems must offer a special class for them or must send them to a nearby community in which there is such a class. Special state financial assistance is available for these classes. The program is administered by the Department of Education with some collaboration with the Department of Mental Health and serves over 12,000 pupils, providing a major relief for the overcrowded state schools for the retarded.

The Department of Mental Health has initiated a program of nursery schools for retarded children, usually associated with mental health clinics. This statewide system of 32 nursery schools in 1964 cared for about 330 children; there are waiting lists for most of them.

A recent study indicated that twelve state agencies are in one way or another involved in coping with alcoholism. The central responsibility for treating alcoholism lies with the Division of Alcoholism, located in the Department of Public Health, which operates the major centers for the treatment of alcoholism. The Department of Mental Health is involved to an increasing degree with alcoholism. For instance, the number of patients admitted to mental hospitals for temporary treatment of alcoholism increased from 282 in 1958 to 667 in 1963, and there are also many longer-term patients. Furthermore, it is estimated that one-third of the patients have some degree of a problem with alcoholism, and that about 8 per cent of the total department budget of $72 million in 1964 was assignable to alcoholic patients.

The primary state agency in respect to juvenile delinquency is the Division of Youth Service, nominally located within the Department of Education, but "not under its control," to conform to a constitutional limitation on the number of state agencies. The division operates four correctional state schools with a capacity of about a thousand, two reception and diagnostic centers, and two detention centers for juveniles awaiting disposition of their cases by courts. The division also has about two thousand children on a parole or aftercare basis. Many of the children in the division's institutions come from the Boston metropolitan region since the various units differ in type of service, not in geographic coverage.

The division's concerns for mental health mainly relate to the children under its control. Its staff positions for mental health services are described as grossly insufficient in number, and inadequate in pay levels to attract or hold the staff required. The Department of Mental Health provides psychiatric consultation to institutional staffs, psychological services in the reception centers, and psychiatric social work in the aftercare program. Specifically, in which there is such a class, a nearby community in which there is such a class. To some extent, the division utilizes local child guidance clinics in its aftercare program. Due to the heavy load of such centers and divergencies in approach, such services seem limited, but possibly the proposed community mental health centers would be more effective in this regard if they are staffed with this function in mind.

It is evident from this description of state mental health activities that they are scattered among a number of agencies, depending upon how one defines mental health. Many of the problems which the state government faces involve from two to ten existing agencies. Each agency has staked out its own "domain" and tends to be jealous of what it may interpret as efforts of others to move into that field. Agencies that once had clearly distinguishable but narrow areas of operation have broadened their activities and consequently overlap along their functional perimeters with other agencies. The field of mental health well exemplifies these problems, as well as efforts to deal with them. For instance, the care of the mentally ill who need institutionalization may not seem an insurmountable problem, for that was the basic function upon which the Department of Health was founded. But part of this responsibility involves care of the criminally insane (shared with the Department of Corrections); care of tubercular patients (requiring special units in cooperation with the Department of Public Health); and providing increased care of the aging even though they may not be mental cases (a concern shared with the state's Commission on Aging as well as with local welfare services).

Alcoholics constitute the most rapidly growing segment of the short-term population of some mental hospitals, as well as requiring long-term care in some cases. Twelve state agencies are involved in one way or another in dealing with alcoholism, which affects perhaps 200,000 persons. However, the more than $12 million which is spent annually is used chiefly to cope with the *effects* of alcoholism. Many argue for increased expenditure to deal with the problems of the alcoholics.

The treatment of mentally retarded children is another widely dispersed concern. The Department of Mental Health has for many decades operated four state schools for the mentally retarded and a fifth unit has been opened at Danvers State Hospital. However, the Department of Education directs and supports the public school special classes for the high grades of mentally retarded, as well as the emotionally disturbed. The Department of Public Health is responsible for the screening of all newborn babies for PKU, a physical cause of retardation that can be remedied; it also may contribute to diminishing the incidence of mental retardation by providing or aiding services to expectant mothers through various public health and public welfare activities.

It should be evident that considerable fragmentation exists within the state government in matters affecting "mental health" and the "mentally ill," broadly defined. Several alternative methods have been used to deal with the problems caused by this fragmentation. One alternative was to set up a special unit with a controlling group drawn from those agencies most concerned, assigning the unit to one or another agency for "housekeeping" purposes. This is the pattern used to cope with drug addiction. A board consisting of the commissioners of public health, mental health, and corrections was established, and the unit was located in the Department of Public Health for administrative and budgetary purposes. This option seems to work well enough for an operation that does not need large appropriations and hence need not be concerned with its base of political support.

A second possibility was to assign the function primarily to one agency but provide for consultation with one or more other interested agencies. Thus, the Department of Mental Health was supposed to work with the Department of Education on the special classes in the public schools, but this seems to have been very much a *pro forma* relationship involving infrequent contacts between agencies. On the other hand, good cooperation existed in the review of cases of emotionally disturbed children who were proposed to be sent at the state's expense to appropriate private schools.

A third option was to establish an interdepartmental advisory committee for a particular project or function. When controversy developed in Massachusetts in 1964 over whether the Department of Public Health or the Department of Mental Health should be responsible for the federally financed planning project for mental retardation, Governor Endicott Peabody resolved the conflict by designating the Department of Mental Health as the responsible state agency. However, he also established an Inter-departmental Advisory Committee on Mental Retardation, headed by the commissioner of public health and comprising the commissioners of all state agencies directly or tangentially concerned with mental retardation, plus representatives of various concerned institutions and citizen groups. Such an arrangement could be mere "window dressing" but both planning projects actively utilized this group.

A fourth alternative was to assign members of different state departments and agencies to work on a specific problem. This device was used in a study of alcoholism requested by Governor Peabody. Representatives of twelve state agencies worked under the assistant to the commissioner of administration to prepare a comprehensive report on what was being done and to recommend the steps that various agencies should take in the future. A modification of this device was used by the Mental Health Planning Project and the Mental Retardation Planning Project through the formation of specialized "Task Forces," which normally included one or more members of relevant state agencies, to develop detailed proposals in major areas of concern.

A fifth means for attacking the problems of fragmentation was to have a central agency in the state government, often the budget bureau or a similar agency, suggest the need for coordination whenever it appeared necessary. This process evidently was effective in respect to naming the Department of Public Health as the "responsible authority" for the Mental Retardation Planning Project. However, generally the state budget bureau is so involved with fiscal estimates and so understaffed that it cannot be relied upon to fulfill this function nearly as effectively as the federal Bureau of the Budget.

A development of interest was the designation by Governor John Volpe of Elliott Richardson, his lieutenant governor, in 1964–1966, as coordinator for health, education, and welfare matters in Massachusetts; some staff assistance was provided for this activity. This was particularly appropriate in view of Mr. Richardson's experience as Assistant Secretary of Health, Education, and Welfare in Washington. Whether this assignment will be made for other lieutenant governors in the future is questionable.

The creation of a state monopoly on mental health services in Massachusetts by the 1904 Act might have eliminated local activity in mental health entirely, but it did not. There have continued to be local mental health activities. These have been conducted in some cases by public agencies, and in others by a curious amalgam of public and private groups.

Some of these local operations were outpatient services, as an alternative to institutionalization. An outpatient clinic was established at the Massachusetts School for the Feebleminded (now the Fernald School) in 1891, and Dr. Walter Channing directed an outpatient clinic at the Boston Dispensary as early as 1897. Northampton State Hospital provided outpatient service in 1910, and the outpatient department of the Boston Psychopathic Hospital (now the Southard Clinic of the Massachusetts Mental Health Center) opened in 1912. The experience with these outpatient centers led the State Board of Insanity to suggest in 1914 that each state hospital should serve as a mental health center for its district and establish outpatient departments and clinics in nearby cities. However, this proposal evidently was not pushed very vigorously since relatively few of the state mental hospitals in Massachusetts today serve as mental health centers for their areas, although there are some outstanding exceptions.

Beginning in 1919, however, the state hospitals and state schools did organize traveling teams to visit neighboring school systems and examine those children who were three or more years behind in their school work in order to determine whether they were mentally retarded or merely lazy. In 1917 Dr. William Healey established a private clinic for children in Boston, which developed into the noted Judge Baker Guidance Clinic. Beginning in 1922 the state provided mental health clinics for children in various cities under Dr. Douglas Thom of the Division of Mental Hygiene; these were called "Habit clinics" because of the belief at the time that what was needed was the development of the proper "habits" in children. The exigencies of the Second World War forced the elimination of the traveling teams and the closing of most of the children's clinics.

Prior to the war, however, a new and much broader concept developed of a desirable range of mental health services within the local areas or what was loosely termed the "community." In that period there had been limited experimentation in Massachusetts with community mental health clinics for outpatient care. These pioneering ventures conducted valuable research on the relationships between social structure and emotional well-being. This experience was of considerable importance in leading to the federal proposals embodied in the 1963 legislation.

During and immediately after the Second World War, there was a notable increase of interest within Massachusetts in providing more mental health services within the community. Under the leadership of Dr. Clifton Perkins, then commissioner of mental health, the department began developing such services along a new pattern. The former practice of sending traveling teams out from the central office to locations within the state for part of the week was abandoned in favor of establishing permanent clinics with their own professional staffs.

From an organizational and legal point of view, the most interesting thing about the new community mental health concept was the ingenious way in which it attained two goals. First, persons in the area to be served had a substantial part in starting the new clinics and in controlling their policy. Consequently the clinics were not state institutions merely located in the community, but were, to a large degree, local organizations. Second, they required an initial and continuing local financial contribution. By providing that the local group sponsoring the clinic be a private association, it was possible to receive both individual contributions and fees for services from local governmental agencies, despite the ban in the 1904 Act on local activities concerning mental health. The significant Mental Health Act of 1946 amended the general laws to allow the expenditure of city or town funds for this purpose. The belief that mental health centers which were merely physically located in the community, but had no real ties to the community, could not become true community agencies was the reason for the new system. It had been observed, for instance, that local clinics established before the war wholly with money from the Commonwealth Fund had not developed any local roots and there had been no local willingness to take over operations when the grants were terminated. The new approach was to be a "partnership" between local communities and the state, with both playing a role but allowing a large degree of local flexibility.

This is how the plan worked. Local mental health associations could be established by interested citizens. The Department of Mental Health relied heavily upon such groups, active, self-directing, and effective citizen units. The ideal population base for such units was 150,000 people but on occasion areas with smaller population were approved if there was intense local interest. The Brookline clinic was a case in point. Services of local clinics were available only to residents of the municipalities within the organization. The department wished to avoid dictating what the areas should be, but also sought to have these areas developed so that no communities were left out. Nevertheless, some of the local units left a considerable amount to be desired so far as area coverage was concerned. A more basic criticism of the reliance by the department upon "citizen" leadership was that such individuals were much more common in some areas than in others. They were more influential in the affluent suburbs or smaller cities. Consequently, the early mental health clinics were frequently established in the areas that needed them least, while the large cities, which needed these services most, were less likely to be organized. Some places were never provided for adequately, and probably never would have been if this pattern of developing local services had been the only one used. Furthermore, it has been charged that this type of development led to an anarchistic situation in which any determined local group, whether qualified or not, could set themselves up as the exclusive partner of the state.

The continued efforts of the Department of Mental Health, however, supplemented until recent years by the sporadic missionary work of the Massachusetts Mental Health Association, led to coverage of substantial areas of the state by local mental health associations and limited service clinics.

Once a local association was established and showed the department that it could provide logistic support for a local clinic and could persuade its local legislators to support state help for the clinic, the department would request money in its budget for a "block" of professionals. The early concept of a block was three persons: a psychiatrist who was also head of the clinic, a psychologist, and a social worker. This was soon expanded to include a junior mental health coordinator. Such departmental requests usually were approved by the governor and legislature, although not always at the time of the first appeal. This professional block would then be assigned to the local clinic and paid by the state.

Virtually all of the local centers in the Boston SMSA started as "child guidance clinics," because this type of service had general public acceptance growing out of the guidance work in the public schools. Furthermore, very few private psychiatrists devote much time to children, and consequently state-supported clinics for that purpose were viewed as only a minimal threat of "socialized medicine." It was hoped that as the services of the clinics became appreciated in the community, demand for adult services would develop as well. Indeed, this was what occurred in a number of areas, notably the South Shore Mental Health Center. As a need for a larger staff developed, it was the responsibility of the local citizens to generate sufficient political pressure upon the legislature to augment their basic block. Some needs were met by loaning the blocks authorized for new centers to existing centers. The South Shore Mental Health Center seems to have been most notably successful in utilizing this method.

The financing of the local share of the cost of mental health clinics has been somewhat aided by the payment of fees for services to children by local school departments and boards of health. In 1964 such payments amounted to 9 per cent of the total reported expenses of $3 million for all the local clinics in Massachusetts.

In planning for the development of community mental health centers in Massachusetts under the 1963 federal act, both Commissioner Solomon and his departmental staff and the members of the Mental Health Planning Project sought to provide as many alternative ways of establishing community centers as possible. This varied approach left unresolved the status of the local mental health associations and their present clinics after a new community mental health center is established in their area. Avoiding rigid definitions in the planning process has considerable merit, particularly because it is likely that the actual development of a statewide system of centers will take years. Consequently, most of the existing local clinics will be needed for some time.

Some local mental health associations, however, developed proposals to establish full-blown community mental health centers operating on somewhat the same "partnership" basis as the present clinics, but with a much larger contribution of state funds. The Department of Mental Health contended that it could not legally provide direct state support to either local nonprofit hospitals or to private nonprofit groups, no matter how praiseworthy or capable they might be, because of the constitutional prohibition cited above. At the same time, there was strong feeling that the proposed community mental health centers should not be merely regional outposts of the department, or of the state hospitals. The solution was to propose a system of regional centers controlled in many respects by a board of local citizens appointed by the governor, but basically responsible to the Department of Mental Health. Thus, it has not been possible in Massachusetts to translate into action the concept contained in the 1963 federal legislation of local mental health clinics supported jointly by the state and the local community but operating substantially under local control.

It has long been observed in Massachusetts that some of the cities and most of the towns are too small to serve as efficient units of local government, even though they may have other virtues. They tend to require an inordinate number of public officials, and yet often cannot afford to pay salaries that will attract or hold really capable people. Most of the objective studies of public schools, for instance, suggest that for maximum efficiency a system should serve about 10,000 students. Very few school systems of this size are found in Massachusetts; indeed, only about 60 of the almost 400 existing school units have as many as 1,000 elementary or 100 high school pupils. Similar recommendations for larger service areas have been made for health functions. On the other hand, many per-

-sons are sufficiently attached to the presumed virtues and benefits of small municipalities to deliberately select them for residence according to their reputation for public services, tax levels, and the like. Consequently, while there may be optional or forced adjustments or coordination in certain functional areas, it is very unlikely that the basic municipal structure in Massachusetts will be radically changed.

In respect to mental health, it is obvious that so far as localized services are concerned, most of the state's 351 municipalities are far too small to serve as the population base for either the existing mental health or child guidance clinics or for the proposed community mental health centers. The Department of Mental Health suggested a population base of about 100,000 persons and the federal regulations for community mental health centers suggested a range of 75,000 to 200,000. In the case of most of the existing mental health clinics, two or more cities and towns are included in the area of the local mental health associations fostering them. The clinics' governing boards are normally drawn from all the participating communities, except when there are many small towns involved. Thus, the danger of excessive fragmentation of local government in Massachusetts has been dealt with by using aggregations of municipalities, or, as in the case of the city of Boston, parts of a municipality.

The second type of fragmentation at the local level is *within* a municipal government. This can be a serious problem in Massachusetts, in the towns, because a considerable number of functions are controlled by independently elected boards or committees. So far as mental health is concerned, these bodies normally include the School Committee, which runs the schools, the Board of Health, which operates such local health activities as exist, often a separate governing board for municipal hospitals, and a Board of Public Welfare to administer what is largely a state and federal program within the municipality. Some degree of fiscal coordination is provided in the towns by the locally selected finance committees, which review all budget requests and make recommendations to the town meeting. In the cities, the mayor and council (with their larger professional staff and often a city manager) carry out the task of integrating the many requests and programs of the various agencies, with widely varying degrees of competence and judgment.

So far as mental health activities within the city of Boston are concerned, fragmentation between municipal agencies is not a severe problem because the city government has done very little in this field, with the exception of services at the Boston City Hospital. Services are provided directly by the state in such centers as Boston State Hospital, and the Massachusetts Mental Health Center, through largely state-supported centers such as the Dorchester Guidance Center and the North Suffolk Mental Health Center, and through substantial activities by private or university hospitals such as the Boston University Medical Center, Massachusetts General Hospital, Boston Dispensary, Boston Floating Hospital, and New England Center Hospital. In addition, there is a considerable number of small private clinics and services.

In summary, the fragmentation of responsibility for mental health within federal and state and local governments is overcome to varying degrees and by varying methods. At the federal level, only recently has there been much activity by operating agencies that have diverse responsibilities, yet make relatively little impact on the total mental health problems of the Boston SMSA. Within the state government a number of different devices for overcoming fragmentation have proved effective to the extent that the participants wish them to be. Until very recently, however, only sporadic coordination resulted from the direct collision of competing agencies, or from the incidental observations of the state budget authorities. At the local level, coordination is largely informal and limited in the towns, although the occasional town manager may exercise more persuasive power. In the cities, the formal machinery for coordination is used with more or less insight and effectiveness by mayors and city managers; in the central city of Boston, municipal participation in such activities has been very limited and there have been few problems.

A second major resource is the very large number of medical facilities. The analysis of federal, state, and local activities in mental health in Massachusetts has been structured upon the traditional "layer cake" concept of federalism, but the account has indicated the complex relationships between officials at the various levels, and between private groups and individuals. Many influences and pressures are transmitted from local to state to federal officials or from state to federal officials, as well as operating in the reverse order. This is in accord with conventional concepts of the developing web of the modern federal system. Of particular interest in Massachusetts is the extensive contact between certain individuals in the Boston mental health community and the officials of the NIMH and related agencies in Washington. This contact might be viewed as separate from the state government and the Department of Mental Health as such, although individuals in that department, notably former Commissioners Ewalt and Solomon, have exercised considerable influence in Washington. This is attributable primarily to their personal effectiveness rather than their official positions in the state. Most of the individuals in the Boston mental health community who have had a major role in defining federal policies on mental health are also persons who actively participate in shaping the policies of the state Department of Mental Health. This does not mean that departmental action is always entirely in tune with that of Washington, and certainly it is not the reverse. On the whole, however, there is a considerable degree of harmony, which some informed observers believe more evident than in most of the states.

The extent of private mental health services in this area is somewhat difficult to assess, because it depends upon what is defined as a "mental health service" and what is viewed as "private." The mental health clinics and centers largely supported by state funds may be viewed as "public." The major private hospitals and centers within the city of Boston have been noted above; others in the Boston SMSA that provide mental health services of varying types are Mount Auburn Hospital in Cambridge, college health centers providing extensive services to the large number of students at Harvard and the Massachusetts Institute of Technology in Cambridge, and McLean Hospital in Belmont. In addition, other private hospitals provide some measure of mental health service to patients of their doctors. No detailed information is available on the extent of these services.

A second major resource is the very large number of private psychiatrists in Greater Boston and especially in Boston itself. Based upon Schulberg's study already cited, more than 80 per cent of the three or four hundred psychiatrists in private practice in Massachusetts work in the Boston SMSA. Many of them devote much of their time to teaching, clinics, or other related work.

In addition to what may be viewed as specific mental health services in the private sector, there are many other private resources which Ryan reported as providing a substantial amount of mental health service in varying degrees. He believed that the primary private resource was composed of medical doctors who provided some measure of mental health service to their patients as a component of their concern for their health generally. Another source of assistance is comprised of the larger social agencies such as the settlement houses, YMCA, and so on. Finally, Ryan identified seventy-three smaller social work agencies that performed some sort of mental health service, even if it was only referral to other agencies; undoubtedly there are more such agencies now.

INFORMAL STRUCTURE OF MENTAL HEALTH

The state Department of Mental Health is the dominant force in Massachusetts; consequently the major part of this consideration of individual and group behavior and interaction will deal with the state level of activity. However, the local mental health associations also have significant aspects that will merit consideration.

It is common to think of a governmental agency or department as having a single point of view toward its major function in which its staff all concur. In numerous instances, however, groups or subunits of a public agency have diverse or even clashing objectives or attitudes. Such diversity is not necessarily harmful, but it should be noted that it exists in the Massachusetts Department of Mental Health.

Former Commissioner Dr. Jack Ewalt has described the Massachusetts Mental Health commissionership as "the most powerful in the country"; Dr. Harry Solomon, his successor, was clearly conscious of this and at the same time was aware of the limitations in his position. Both in technical matters and in the external relationships of the department, the commissioner has extensive powers. Furthermore, Dr. Solomon and the department were respected throughout the state government and carried weight with the legislature and with governors. While members of his department may have differed from time to time on matters of policy or organization, they were enthusiastic in supporting the commissioner. Such attitudes were in part a result of Dr. Solomon's administrative style, which has been described as being in "the Franklin D. Roosevelt tradition." In order to encourage diversity of opinion and the fermentation of new ideas, patterns of organization and of responsibility were purposely kept unclear and frequently similar tasks were assigned to more than one unit or individual. Policy was developed through "seeing how things will work out" rather than by a formalistic process of definition of goals, development of projects, and detailed follow-up. This approach led to bustle and conflict, and it offered considerable scope for individual enterprise.

The commissioner was ready to impose his will only when it was absolutely necessary. This free-wheeling approach was much like that of his predecessor, Dr. Ewalt. The sense of energy and excitement in the department might pain the orthodox administrative analyst, but it gave the mental health agency undoubtedly unusual vigor.

While the commissioner has extensive formal power, he is by no means omnipotent. There is a considerable amount of tension in the relationship between the central office staff and the superintendents of the state hospitals and state schools. The department does have stringent budgetary and fiscal controls, but this does not automatically provide control over policy and practice. The state hospitals and schools each have boards of trustees appointed by the governor, and this provides each hospital or school a source of support and an avenue of appeal against the decisions of the commissioner. Furthermore, the staffs of many of these institutions maintain effective contact with the legislators from their service areas. Relatives of patients offer another source of support, particularly in the case of the mentally retarded children. Finally, most of these institutions are physically removed from the Boston headquarters and sprawl like baronial estates upon many a hilltop throughout Massachusetts. Consequently, the superintendents have a considerable degree of autonomy within their own institutions, and they tend to stick together when they feel their collective interests are threatened by the central office.

A second division is the divergency of views between the staff of the Division of Mental Hygiene, who manage the present community clinics, and everybody else in the department, including the superintendents of the state hospitals. The commissioner has described the Division of Mental Hygiene as "a separate kingdom" although in view of the commissioner's extensive powers, "barony" might be a more appropriate term. The staff of the division is committed to developing localized services within the "community" for the mentally ill, the mentally retarded, and the emotionally disturbed. The agency which is thought best for such activity is the local mental health clinic or center, and Dr. B. R. Hutcheson, present director of the Division of Mental Hygiene, would like to rename his unit the "Division of Community Mental Health Services." The basic concept of the division has been described as "community oriented," "social-work oriented," "taking a 'functional' view of psychiatry,' getting away from the one-to-one doctor-patient relationship," seeing the broad range of social ills as both caused by and causing a broad range of emotional disturbances, and so on.

The vigorously expressed views of the staff of the Division of Mental Hygiene have at times placed them in opposition to others in the Department of Mental Health on such matters as the nature of the proposed community mental health centers, the relationship of such centers to nearby state hospitals, and the relationship between medical and nonmedical staff in treating mental illness.

Perhaps of most significance has been the basic conflict over whether the new centers should be small-scale and dispersed versions of the existing state hospitals, wholly subject to the control of the central staff of the Department of Mental Health, or whether there should be a substantial measure of local influence on the policies and practices of such centers, and an extensive pattern of working relationships with the whole range of community agencies in the area served by the centers. This issue was basically resolved in the *Report* of the Mental Health Planning Project, which supported a considerable measure of local participation in the proposed centers.

This recommendation also disposed of an earlier conflict with the superintendents of some of the state mental hospitals, who wished to have control over centers in their areas. The *Report* recommended that hospitals might operate centers "on their own" grounds, and that the centers and the state hospitals should cooperate in offering the full range of mental health services in their service area. This is quite different, however, from viewing all community mental health centers as satellites of the nearest state hospital.

A related debate seems more semantic than real, but it aroused considerable emotion. The more enthusiastic advocates of the new community mental health centers envisaged these units as able to deal with all the mental health problems of the state. Therefore, they took the view that once these centers are in operation the large state hospitals would "wither away." The hospital staffs retorted that there was no firm evidence to support that conclusion. The new centers, they said, would treat a new group of patients, and thus would have little or no effect upon the demand for services at the state hospitals and state schools.

A final area of dispute between the Division of Mental Hygiene and

Massachusetts Mental Health Planning Project, *Mental Health for Massachusetts* (Boston: Massachusetts Department of Mental Health, 1965).

the rest of the department, as well as with private psychiatrists, concerned the relation of "medical" and "nonmedical" personnel in the
treatment of mental illness. The view which dominates the department
is that treatment of mental illness must be closely directed by a medical
doctor who is a psychiatrist. Furthermore, institutions dealing with
mental health must be directed by psychiatrists. The contrary view is
that properly trained and capable "nonmedical" personnel, primarily
psychologists and social workers, must assume an increasing role in dealing with mental illness, especially as the trend toward "community mental
health centers" is accelerated. This attitude derives from experience and
necessity, for if the division's concept of comprehensive community
mental health centers, which is substantially the same as that proposed by
the 1963 federal legislation, is to be realized, the problems of staffing
such centers must be solved. In the view of many in the Division of
Mental Hygiene this can only be accomplished by revising staffing
patterns to utilize more nonmedical personnel. Another source of
grievance in some quarters is the superior authority of any medical
doctor—no matter how junior—over any nonmedical person—no
matter how eminent. To the extent that community mental health centers
may in the future increasingly be staffed by nonmedical professionals, this
feeling might well grow.

Most discussion of "interest groups" arouses images of lobbyists,
marches on the State House, and other expressions of organized political
or social fervor. While these have figured in the history of mental
health in Massachusetts, perhaps the largest interest group concerned
does not operate at all in this way. It is composed of a large number of
professional men and women engaged in teaching, research, and practice relating to the prevention and cure of mental illness.

Boston is well known as one of the medical centers of the world, and
closely associated with most of its great hospitals are noted medical
schools with clinics devoted to mental health. Probably the best known
is the Massachusetts Mental Health Center (formerly the Boston Psychopathic Hospital), at which hundreds of the leaders in American mental
health activities have been trained. The present commissioner, Dr. Harry
Solomon, was formerly superintendent of this institution; his predecessor, Dr. Jack Ewalt, became superintendent when he ended his term as
commissioner. Other institutions in the Boston area concerned with
mental health include the medical schools of Harvard, Tufts, and Boston

University; the Boston Psychoanalytic Society and Institute; and extensive training programs for clinical psychologists and psychiatric social workers at Boston University, Boston College, Harvard, and Simmons. As a consequence, the "mental health community" is a very considerable interest group.

This nominal "group" is by no means a monolithic entity, and only a limited number of its members usually influence public policy about mental health in Massachusetts. The majority of psychiatrists and related groups in the Boston area evidently are sufficiently engaged in their own pursuits so that they have not been active, even in respect to the controversy over the location and control of community mental health centers. Members of the Associated General Hospital Psychiatrists are not engaged in public mental health activities, and the leaders of this group commented upon the political apathy of most psychiatrists. Similarly, many staff members of the teaching hospitals in the Boston area have not concerned themselves with public mental health policy, although the developing linkage between these hospitals and the proposed community mental health centers in Boston may change this. Consequently, the active leaders in the shaping and developing of mental health policy for Massachusetts are a relatively small group of able men who have dominated the field for a considerable time.

Ideological divisions exist in medical theory and practice as well as in the relation between public and private activities in the field of mental health. Views diverge over the nature of mental illness, the types of effective therapy, and which professional group should have authority in this area.

Many doctors oppose the extension of "state medicine" or "state psychiatry," and they see the proposed system of community mental health centers as a major step in that direction. Included among the opponents of such a system are a number of private psychiatrists who are organized as the Associated General Hospital Psychiatrists. They welcome an expansion of community mental health services but insist that any such services should be a part of the program of private general hospitals and under the control of the hospital boards. Their attitudes and activities are described in some detail below, but this group seems to be a distinct minority within the mental health community. Many psychiatrists work at least part of the time in state hospitals or state-supported clinics; others are engaged in research that is supported by

governmental grants in whole or in part. But there is a considerable body
of psychiatrists who do not seem to care much whether more extensive
government-supported programs are adopted or not. Apparently they
have more patients than they can take now and expect little change in
the future. Thus, while the mental health community exercises a considerable degree of influence generally in support of mental health activities, it is divided over key questions of the organization and control of
the projected community mental health services.

The psychiatrists within the mental health community are of course
also members of the medical profession and consequently the Massachusetts Medical Society is a relevant interest group. Its Committee on
Mental Health is responsible for linking the two activities and for keeping an eye on what has been predominantly a socialized activity in
Massachusetts. Generally this committee has supported the policies and
practices of the Department of Mental Health, although at times the committee and the society have questioned the proposals for community
mental health centers. Yet while the state medical society is respected,
it does not have much political power. The society has not been able
to present any serious obstacles to the current developments of community mental health centers along the lines favored by the department.

A second major category of interest groups are those who benefit,
directly or indirectly, from the services of such agencies, or who support such services for a variety of reasons. At the state level the
Massachusetts Association for Mental Health (MAMH) is such a group.
However, while some local mental health associations are its affiliates,
others are not, either because they feel they do not derive any particular
benefit from the state association or regard it as ineffective, or disagree
with its policies. A particular source of local unhappiness with the
state association is the latter's doctrine that what is needed most for
mental health is 'education' and 'new services.' Consequently it seeks
to have its local associations drop their responsibilities for the local
mental health clinics, which the Association believes should be publicly
supported, that any such services should be a part of the program of priv-

One source of power for the state association is the practice of the
Greater Boston United Fund organization of using the Massachusetts
association to distribute money ($45,000 in 1963) for local mental
health clinics. This money goes only to the affiliated local associations,
and United Community Services officials have not encouraged the affilia-

-tion of new mental health associations. The only exception to this practice is a small amount of direct United Fund support of the pioneering Wellesley Human Relations Service, which was established before the Massachusetts Association for Mental Health was formed.

So far as political effectiveness is concerned, the Massachusetts Association for Mental Health is rated by many observers as having little influence. It tends to support the requests of the Department of Mental Health but tries to retain freedom of action. Consequently it is not a fully reliable auxiliary of the department, and past friction on its self-defined role as the organizer of local mental health associations left scars which are still evident. While one of its major concerns is supposed to be with legislation, its efforts on specific bills are described as "too little and too late." It does not seem to be able to mobilize its local members effectively to apply political pressure. While its leadership is earnest, the Massachusetts Association for Mental Health does not seem to have much influence at the State House.

The Massachusetts Association for Retarded Children (MARC) stands in marked contrast to its mental health counterpart. It has a steadily growing number of local affiliates, which work well together as a politically potent group. It was started in the 1950s to bring together parents whose children were mentally retarded. One of its first successes was the law requiring local school systems to provide special classes for children who were retarded, emotionally disturbed, or who had other problems that prevented their participation in regular school activities. The law originally required these classes when there were ten such children in a city or town; later the minimum number was reduced to five. It is said that this law was introduced and passed without the knowledge of the Department of Education, which was to administer the act. In 1964 the association generated sufficient pressure upon the state legislature to effect a massive upgrading in the state schools for the retarded, over the objections of the governor and the plans of the Department of Mental Health.

The United Community Services, which is the central staff agency for several hundred private social-service agencies receiving funds from the Greater Boston United Fund, was extended in 1964 to cover a large part of the Boston SMSA through merger with the South Shore and Greater Lynn area Funds. In 1964 the UCS sought a grant from the National Institute of Mental Health to plan for the coordination of public and private agencies for mental health. This request was rejected because it conflicted with the activities of the Mental Health Planning Project. However, members of the UCS staff and representatives of some of its constituent agencies have worked on a number of the task forces of the project, and greater confidence now exists that future relationships of public and private agencies in the mental health field will be good.

Recently, United Community Services organized the Mental Health Planning Committee of Metropolitan Boston, composed of about fifty prominent figures from public and private agencies and institutions. This was intended to be a significant step in developing a metropolitan "interest group" in the mental health field. The committee's basic staff will be provided by United Community Services with the assistance of the Mental Health Planning Project and various other organizations. The purpose of this committee is to take the basic proposals of the Planning Project as they apply to the Boston SMSA and work out the roles of the public and private agencies involved in mental health activities.

The committee membership is dominated by representatives of social service agencies, but it does tap the power structure of the multiplicity of associations and organizations in Boston, as well as of the medical community. It could provide the basis for a metropolitanwide concern for mental health, which up to now has been conspicuously lacking. Hopefully, it will become the vehicle for top-level policy formation and program planning for dealing with the range of emotional disturbances that Ryan set forth so persuasively in his study, *Distress in the City*. This committee makes possible the linkage of more than a nominal sort between "community agencies" and the new community mental health centers. Finally, it provides a means of focusing the attention of representatives of many types of agencies upon problems of emotional disturbance.

The major influences upon mental health activities in the Boston SMSA are those bearing upon the Department of Mental Health or other state agencies and officials. Lively activity at the local level revolves around the organization and operation of local mental health associations, local child guidance or mental health clinics, special classes in the schools for mentally retarded or otherwise "exceptional" children, nursery or preschool organizations for mentally retarded children, and related programs.

The interest groups most prominent in respect to mental health are f course the local mental health associations, of which there are currently seventeen within the Boston SMSA. These tend to consist of hree types of persons: the enthusiastic and vigorous leaders who often ave relatives who have experienced mental illness; members of various rganizations in the community with an interest in mental health; and . larger number of persons who are somewhat interested and provide ome measure of continuing support. The formal leadership of the local ssociations naturally is drawn from the first two groups, with the addiion of local notables and usually one or more local physicians.

Governmental fragmentation in the Boston SMSA is reflected in he organization of public and private service agencies. Municipal oundaries are usually followed by these agencies. The city of Boston s the largest public unit serving about 700,000 persons, but some mental ealth organizations in Boston serve only parts of the city. In the other arger cities in the Boston SMSA, such as Cambridge, Lynn, Quincy, nd Newton, most mental health organizations serve areas coterminous ith municipal boundaries. In all the cities and towns, local governmental ervices are usually limited to a single municipality. A general law ermits cooperative arrangements between two or more communities, ut this rarely has been used except for a few regional high schools and ocational schools. The multiplicity of small municipalities means that uch services as require a large population base for efficient operation —most notably in the health and social service fields—must be organized y the voluntary or mandatory aggregation of a number of municipalities. The United Community Services (UCS) has been instrumental in helping constituent agencies organize in more rational and economical patterns. A number of cities and towns have community councils that eek to coordinate the various public and private social services.

In establishing child guidance clinics or broader mental health clinics, he state Department of Mental Health set an arbitrary minimum population to be served at around 100,000. Under this standard, only about half-dozen municipalities in the Boston SMSA could have their own linics. The remaining cities and towns would have to join with their eighbors in order to comprise an adequate population base for clinics. n view of the antagonism that exists between certain communities, one an understand why the process by which these service areas were ormed has been characterized by some observers as "anarchic." True, almost all the municipalities are now embraced within existing or proposed geographic consortiums, but some of these did not make for viable organizations. The criterion for the population base for the new community mental health center is larger than that for a clinic, and therefore the Mental Health Planning Project has devoted considerable attention to the development of new service areas for the centers, which in most cases are composed of aggregations of municipalities.

The extent to which the service areas of the social service agencies conform to the service areas of the local mental health clinics varies a great deal. Only in the larger towns and cities are they substantially coterminous. Consequently, the staff of local clinics may deal with as many as four family service groups, and conversely a family service group may have to deal with two or three clinics.

Fragmentation of municipal government and the necessity of combining two and frequently more municipalities in the service area of the present local mental health clinics poses problems to the governing boards of such clinics. Each municipality must be represented on the board. Furthermore, in seeking initial support or continuing appropriations for the services rendered, it must maintain working relationships with a multiplicity of municipal agencies and officials. Undoubtedly, these complex relations require a considerable amount of time and diplomacy, and may limit the attention that leaders of the local mental health associations can give to general policy issues and legislation. This necessary preoccupation with the sometimes mundane details of the local clinic is the reason the Massachusetts Association for Mental Health maintains that local associations should drop their responsibility for the clinics once constituent agencies organize in more rational and economical...

How does the marked degree of political fragmentation in the Boston SMSA affect the efforts of the local mental health organizations to secure support of community leaders? Obviously, the few community leaders work within the several municipalities. Relatively few leaders represent the metropolitan area as a whole and little occasion arises for metropolitan leadership. When issues or problems develop on this scale, they tend to escalate to the state level for resolution. Thus, whether the mental health unit in question serves only a single municipality or several, mental health advocates must deal with the leaders of public and private agencies in each municipality involved. Because of the long...

tradition of local particularism, this "federative" activity takes a good deal of time.

The support that is needed is of two types. The first might be termed moral support, an endorsement of the necessity or value of the local mental health services. The second is tangible support in the form of public funds, provision of public facilities, or other types of cooperation in the operation of the local mental health clinics.

Since in Massachusetts the state has for so long exercised a monopoly in mental health, most local governmental leaders consider it outside their responsibilities. The heavy load of local real estate taxes required to support the functions that have been traditionally local means that any proposal to pay for new and expensive functions arouses violent opposition. The fact that the bulk of the cost of the existing type of mental health clinics is paid for by the state, however, and that some support comes from private sources with the remainder generally split among several municipalities means that the cost of limited municipal participation is small. For instance, the recently opened clinic in the city of Newton involves city funds of about $30,000 annually compared to a total city budget of almost $29.5 million.

It is easier for the advocates of local mental health programs to secure the support of local officials and other notables for the present type of mental health activity, since they are not very costly. Massachusetts so far has not experienced any of the vitriolic right-wing attacks on the concept of "mental health" that are reported from other states, and only a very few persons seem to be "against mental health." Finally, the initial request for local mental health activities is usually for child guidance clinics. This need usually is supported by both the schools and the police departments and is not opposed by doctors or psychiatrists. Thus it is not difficult in most Massachusetts communities to secure the open support of community leaders for the current type of mental health clinic.

Were the costs to be significantly higher or the local program significantly broader—as would be true under the 1963 federal legislation and if the community mental health centers were to rely heavily upon local funds—then it is likely that the fiscal and local antagonisms would lead to much sharper opposition and more controversy. The marked degree of political fragmentation in the Boston SMSA would create even more difficulties for the advocates of mental health because there would be many individuals and agencies in the territory of the proposed centers who would have to be consulted and persuaded.

COMMUNITY PATTERNS OF INFLUENCE

In the Boston metropolitan area, "community" has a more precise meaning than is true in many other parts of the United States because of the role of the municipalities—cities and towns—as the provider of most public services. Furthermore, Boston, the largest city, is a single community for the provision of municipal services, but also it embraces many sociologically and psychologically identifiable subcommunities such as the North End, South Boston, Roxbury, Brighton, and the like. Over the years these areas have had a distinctive ethnic significance, some of which is changing now.

There is a second level of "community" comprising the areas covered by the voluntary mental health associations. Thus, a set of special "communities of interest" for mental health has arisen, composing segments of the city of Boston, the larger single municipalities (Newton, Brookline, and Cambridge), and aggregations of two or more smaller municipalities. Presumably, these will be superseded by, or incorporated into, "communities" of the projected mental health centers.

Finally, there is the larger "community" of "Greater Boston," with varying boundaries, perhaps more a mystique than an actual entity so far as specific action is concerned. Its major organizational expression is the Greater Boston United Fund. It is perhaps only a coincidence that this United Fund expansion occurred at about the same time that a metropolitanwide advisory planning agency was authorized. The other organizational expression is the Greater Boston Chamber of Commerce, which has a good deal of influence and stimulative effect but not much power.

Policy decisions about the city of Boston are made by three groups. The formal governmental structure of officials includes the mayor, City Council, School Committee, and the Boston Redevelopment Authority under the dynamic Edward J. Logue. The second group is comprised of the leaders of private interests in Boston and include banking, business, and industrial leaders whose joint efforts find formal expression in the Chamber of Commerce, taxpayers' and civic associations, and so on. The third influence group is the state government, including the governor, legislature, and state agencies, which have exercised strong controls over cities and towns generally and Boston in particular, although a recently approved "home-rule" amendment to the state constitution has modified this somewhat. The local newspapers are not particularly effective or influential, although they have improved somewhat in recent years and seek to support progress. Labor is important on bread-and-butter issues; although labor leaders are becoming more aware of the benefits to their members of improving governmental services such as education, most opposed the state sales tax required to pay for such improvements. Neighborhood political leaders in Boston are considerably less influential since the City Council and School Committees were shifted from ward representation to election at-large.

Surprisingly few studies have been made, and none in depth, of the nature and effects of patterns of influence in Boston. However, informed observers are of the opinion that there is no single power structure of the continuing and pervasive sort described by Hunter and his followers. The business-financial-industrial community can be mobilized from time to time on specific issues and will provide strong and continued support for such policies as urban renewal. Particular segments of this community will support projects which particularly benefit them. However, their support must be sought; rarely do they initiate, and they do not veto. Furthermore, on occasion they will be split because of conflicting interests, and their effectiveness is virtually nullified. Much of what initiative and communication exists within this broad group comes from the technical and staff people who regularly talk with each other, formulate proposals, and seek the support of their superiors for particular projects. A great many of the business leaders of Boston live outside the city, which diminishes their political importance and provides them with another set of local concerns in their residential location. Consequently, they speak as leaders of economic organizations operating in Boston, rather than as citizens of the city.

These Boston economic leaders evidently have not been brought into the mental health picture as such. Many individuals are active in public or private social service agencies (of which Boston has a great many), but theirs is a personal, rather than an institutional, interest. Mental health services have been to such a large extent state-operated that neither the city government nor general-purpose groups within the city have seen them as a local concern. Mental health is, then a peripheral concern for the multi-centered power structure of the city of Boston. Of the sixty-five persons on the Advisory Council of the Mental Health Planning Project, only six came from business firms and three others were lawyers.

The second level of community, the mental health communities, have developed extensive ties with the people and organizations of their areas. Yet virtually all of the clinics are basically "service-area" units that touch the lives and sentiments of only a small minority of the people living within their territory. Apparently, they usually are quite unrelated to any local power structure, although they are in most cases claimants for limited amounts of financial support from local governing bodies. Consequently their professional and lay adherents constitute small pressure groups, which usually do not need to press very hard because their requests are quite modest.

The third level of community, Greater Boston, is a vague geographic expression. Except for the exponents of regional planning, and the advisory committees for such metro organizations as the Massachusetts Bay Transportation Authority, it would appear that no power structures are organized or operate in Greater Boston as a whole. Either such interests and groups are organized within separate municipalities, or they operate at the state level where most matters of concern affecting Greater Boston are decided. No general governmental agency other than the state operates throughout Greater Boston. The MBTA is an innovation, but any pressures on it will be transmitted through the ambassadors from the constituent cities and towns. The Metropolitan District Commission is essentially a state agency with a limited service area and one which is not entirely limited to Greater Boston. The new metropolitan planning council is advisory, and it is unlikely to be the scene of fierce conflict.

Decision making concerning mental health in Greater Boston is based on a series of decisions stretching into the past. In respect to mental health, probably the primary decision of public policy was made in 1904, when mental health became an exclusive concern of the state government. In consequence, all the major decisions concerning public mental health services in metropolitan Boston have been, and still are, made at the state level. Since public activities in the mental health field account for the great preponderance of mental health care, it is fair to say that these state policy decisions are the only ones of major significance.

In addition to the 1904 legislation, other basic decisions include: (1) the development of the concept of community mental health units; (2) the decision to involve local citizens and agencies in the founding and operation of such local clinics through the means of the mental health association; (3) the requirement that local schools provide education for various types of mentally retarded and emotionally disturbed children; and (4) the planning for substantial community mental health centers as an alternative to the expansion or multiplication of the large state mental hospitals.

The second type of decision implements these basic policy decisions, determining how these policies will be carried out, what the priorities are, and where specific projects will be located. Subsidiary to these implementing decisions are specific questions such as location, area served, staffing pattern, location of authority, and means of financing for community mental health centers.

Mental health is similar to any other function of government in that it is only a single segment of the total political environment inhabited by legislators, governors, and reporters, even though it bulks very large in costs and personnel. While the Department of Mental Health and its commissioners have been well supported, and currently the department spends more than any other state agency, this does not imply that it has a blank check. Its budget requests often have been cut substantially, so that proposed improvements in services or expansion into new fields have had to be deferred in many cases.

Once the department's budget request is worked out internally, which must involve many balancings of relative needs and choices of priorities, it must run three gauntlets. The first is review by the budget officials in the Commission on Administration, which is the central administrative arm of the state government and compiles the governor's draft budget; the second is review and decision by the governor, who necessarily must be concerned with the overall budget proposals; the third is action by the General Court when the legislators have a crack at the department's budget. It appears that formerly there was considerably less supervision or intervention by the Budget Bureau into the budget requests of the Department of Mental Health than in the case of other state agencies. This testifies both to the high regard for the department within the state government generally, and for the hesitancy of state officials to delve very deeply into what they regard as a "medical" area. However, in view of the major long-term expenditures in the mental health field, an increasing concern of the state budget officials with the major policy and program issues underlying the specific budget requests of the department is quite natural.

The final decisions about the total level of the state budget and the allocation of resources must be made by the governor in formulating his executive budget. The expansion of demand for existing programs and a chronic shortage of tax revenues has been a continuing problem in Massachusetts, and consequently governors have been forced to restrain departmental spending, especially for new enterprises. In consequence, the budget of the Department of Mental Health as presented in the executive budget has often been substantially less than was originally requested, and many desirable projects have had to be deferred.

The last hurdle for the department's budget comes from the General Court. On the whole, the requests for mental health services submitted by the governors have been approved by the legislators, and indeed the legislature has from time to time increased the departmental budget over what was requested, most notably in 1964. However, many problems of the Department of Mental Health are the result of more general conditions in the state government. For instance, the perennial shortage of sufficiently trained personnel in large measure has stemmed from civil service salary schedules that are not competitive, especially for professional personnel, and the department has recurrent difficulty in explaining to legislators why it wants funds for added positions in new programs or institutions when it is unable to fill the positions it already has been granted.

Thus, for the most part, the Department of Mental Health may propose, and the elective officials (governor and legislature) dispose. The most significant developments of public mental health practice—such as the development of child guidance clinics, the expansion of some of them into broader-spectrum clinics, the concept of community mental health centers serving a smaller area on a more intensive basis than the state hospitals or local clinics could—have come from the Department of Mental Health. Such departmental ideas have not always gained immediate or complete acceptance, but eventually some small measure of approval was secured; the process from then on was one of gradual expansion.

The marked success of the department in securing such large appropriations is remarkable compared with the difficulties encountered in financing mental health in many other parts of the country. Reasons for this success include the following: (1) Massachusetts was one of the first states to take seriously its social welfare responsibilities. In the late nineteenth and the first part of the twentieth century it was a leader in the nation. This is now an established tradition and would be virtually impossible to change. (2) The early assumption of complete state responsibility for the mentally ill led to relatively large expenditures for this function on a statewide basis. On the average this probably was substantially more than it would have been had this continued to be dealt with by local governments, many of which had severe fiscal problems. (3) The state government was somewhat more free of conflicting demands and somewhat better able to levy taxes for this function than many local governments would have been. (4) The widespread location of state hospitals, state schools, and of local clinics provided both an extensive, direct legislative interest and increasingly broad public support. (5) The high professional reputation of the department led to both governmental and public support, especially for proposals to improve and expand service.

All these factors contributed to developing a very large "going concern" that now employs about 15,000 persons, about one-third of all state employees. Merely the maintenance and minimal increases to keep up with rising costs lead to a very large standing fiscal commitment. When, despite such investment, there are recurrent charges of poor conditions in the state hospitals or state schools, and when there is professional and citizen pressure for improved and expanded services, the basis for the size of the state mental health budget is obvious. In fact, had it not been for the introduction of tranquilizing drugs and more intensive treatment so that the number of patients in state schools and hospitals has declined from 33,000 to an average of 23,000 since 1957, departmental costs probably would be higher by more than $50 million.

Governors have been influential in shaping or accelerating public policy regarding aspects of mental health, though few have made it a major issue of their programs. Governor Paul A. Dever in the late 1940s became aroused by conditions in the state's mental institutions and particularly the state schools, and secured major improvements through increased appropriations. One of the four schools for mentally retarded children is named in his honor. Subsequent governors have recognized the increasing importance of the mental health function—who could fail in view of its massive significance in the state budget? They have all included recommendations for improvements. While Governor Endicott Peabody was a member of the board of the Massachusetts Association for Mental Health and expressed much interest in both mental health and mental retardation matters, this was not reflected in any major effort on his part in the mental health field. Indeed, one of his more notable battles was in opposition to an unrealistically rapid expansion of the budget for education of mentally retarded children. On the other hand, in another bitter controversy, the "Battle of Mission Hill," he supported the expansion of the Massachusetts Mental Health Center. Governor John A. Volpe did not demonstrate any particular interest in mental health through 1965, but in 1966 he called the legislature into special session to reorganize the Department of Mental Health, including provision for a system of community centers as recommended by the Planning Project. In summary, it is fair to say that the governors of Massachusetts only rarely have taken a prominent part in the expansion and improvement of mental health services or facilities. On the other hand, they have been generally sympathetic to the requests of the Department of Mental Health and have allocated very considerable portions of the growing state budget to it.

Legislative groups of primary concern in the field of mental health are of two major types, standing committees and special committees or commissions. The Massachusetts legislature has a rather unique and time-saving practice of conducting much of its committee work by joint committees of the House and Senate. Matters affecting mental health usually are referred to the Joint Committee on Public Welfare. It is surprising that so important a function has not had its own committee, as do rather less significant concerns—agriculture, for instance—since welfare is a sufficiently massive problem in itself. Issues related to mental health also might be considered by the Joint Committees on Public Health or Education. Particular problems may be made the subject of study by special commissions or special committees drawn from both branches; such units are usually provided with funds for a staff and consultants and may be continued from one year to the next. The Special Commission on Mental Retardation was extended for many years; another commission on revision of laws relating to mental health and mental retardation was also productive in recent years. Over the decades, there have been many such special commissions, which often have been of substantial significance in laying the groundwork for later legislative action.

Three special commissions of significance to mental health have functioned in Massachusetts. The first was the Special Commission on the Reorganization of State Government (the "Little Hoover Commission"); its staff prepared an extensive report on the Department of Mental Health but the commission decided not to issue it. The second special group, the Special Commission Relative to Training Facilities Available for Retarded Children (hereafter referred to as the Special Commission on Mental Retardation), was established in 1952 and was revived semi-annually ever since. While this commission presented a number of reports and secured some action, none of them made the deep impression of its comprehensive *Report* issued in May 1964, which reported appalling conditions and desperate inadequacies in the state schools for the retarded. The third legislative group of significance is the Special Commission on Mental Health, first authorized in 1962. The charge from the legislature to this commission was for a far-ranging survey of the Department of Mental Health, but when it was learned that the Mental Health Planning Project soon was to be launched, the special commission shifted most of its attention to improvements of the laws governing the committal and release of mental patients. Finally, the Legislative Research Council, a staff agency of the legislature that makes factual reports but no recommendations on such matters as may be directed, submitted a report in the spring of 1964 concerning the possible merger of the Departments of Mental Health, Public Health, and Public Welfare.[5] While the report came to no conclusions on the matter, it quoted the views of authorities that complete merger tended to lead to serious administrative bottlenecks.

The report of the Special Commission on Mental Retardation, referred to above, offers an interesting case study of what might be called ward

[5] Commonwealth of Massachusetts, Senate, No. 850, *Report Submitted by the Legislative Research Council Relative to Combining State Departments of Public Welfare, Public Health, and Mental Health* (Boston: Legislative Research Council, 1964).

politics in the decision-making process. The commission was directed in 1963 to make a study of the state schools for the retarded. In 1964 it presented a vigorous and angry *Report,* whose main conclusions are as follows:

With profound regret we report that Massachusetts . . . has yet to emerge from the dark ages with regard to the quality of care offered to those unfortunate retarded individuals who require placement in a residential school.

*   *   *

Commission members were appalled at the very critical state of conditions within the state schools of the Commonwealth. Human beings are existing in an intolerable living situation, provided with totally inadequate shelter, within antiquated buildings.

*   *   *

In every school, there is only a handful of dedicated nurses, attendants, social workers, teachers and therapists attempting a job which actually requires hundreds of additional skilled personnel.

*   *   *

Currently, there is no coordination of educational and vocations programs in three of the state schools and though the fourth school is making an admirable effort to achieve this, the lack of staff prevents a fully integrated program.[6]

The *Report* included a comprehensive set of nineteen bills to carry out its recommendations. The principal items were for extensive construction and renovation of buildings at the four state schools, and a massive expansion of professional and supporting staff. The proposals were referred to collectively as the "Ward Bill" because of the chairman and principal legislative exponent, Senator Joseph Ward of Fitchburg, once a Democratic candidate for governor. The main bill was introduced as an "emergency law necessary for the immediate preservation of life and safety," which ensured its consideration despite late filing; legislation on staffing was introduced as an amendment to an existing bill.

The hearing on the several bills was held in the large Gardner Auditorium. The bills had not yet been printed, so hardly anyone except the members and staff of the special commission knew their contents in detail. Another notable aspect of the proceedings was that the Massachusetts Association for Retarded Children (MARC) and its chapters secured the attendance of large numbers of citizens, more than any other public hearing in many years had enjoyed, according to one experienced

[6] *Report* of the Special Commission Established to Make an Investigation and Study Relative to Training Facilities Available for Retarded Children (Boston: Wright & Potter, 1964), pp. 9–17.

observer. A further advantage for proponents of the legislation was the election-year sensitivity of politicians. About 150 of the 280 state senators and representatives appeared to express their support for a set of bills they had not yet seen, and which some observers felt contained a number of questionable items.

A majority of the Committee on Welfare was at first inclined to approve all the bills as they were written, but this action was forestalled and four of the bills were referred to the Committee on Education, three were rejected, two were returned for further study, and others were somewhat amended. However, the major proposals were approved. The total costs of all the proposals were estimated at over $19 million above the already precariously balanced state budget. While Governor Peabody was sympathetic to substantial increases if the legislature would approve the necessary revenues, he opposed appropriation of the full $19 million on the logical ground that new buildings required a considerable time for planning and construction, and there was no point in authorizing the staff for new facilities that would not exist during the budget year. However, the representatives of the Massachusetts Association for Retarded Children were adamant in their demand that the full amount should be granted, as recognition of past inequities. Feeling their new sense of political power, they threatened a "march on the State House" by 7,000 parents and their retarded children to emphasize their feelings. The governor stood firm, and although the "march" occurred, its numbers were nearer 700 than 7,000. The logic of the governor's position was evident to Senator Ward, however, and he accepted a scaled-down appropriation of about $9 million for renovation and the start of construction, and about $1 million for immediate staff increases; the remainder of the recommended funds was to be covered in subsequent budgets.

Two new positions in the state government were authorized by the legislature; the first was assistant commissioner for mental retardation in the Department of Mental Health, and the second assistant commissioner for special education in the Department of Education. The position in the Department of Mental Health was proposed partly because of the increase in the department's work in this area and partly to assert the importance of this aspect of the department's responsibility, which mental retardation groups were convinced had been neglected as compared with mental illness.

The proposed position of assistant commissioner in the Department of Education was also a move to enhance the importance of this function. It was greeted with a notable lack of enthusiasm within the department. While some additional staff positions are desperately needed, it was considered a poor administrative move to place a particular service dealing with a minute fraction of the state's school population in a position higher than any other function. The bill was amended to insert relevant professional qualifications for this position, but in an evening meeting of the legislature late in the session these qualifications were struck out, and the eventual appointee to the position was the director of the Division of Special Education, who had been a member of the special commission since its founding in 1952.[7]

The political steam pressure was high as the heat of both the voters and the summer weather beat upon the legislators to respond to a very real and emotionally appealing demand in an election year. The strategy of the special commission, the effective public response organized by MARC, and the astute political leadership of Senator Ward combined to secure a marked increase by the legislature of the executive budget recommendations. At the same time, the recommendations in many respects accorded with prior proposals of the Department of Mental Health. The Boston *Herald* commented:

The most phenomenal individual performance of the 1964 legislative session was turned in . . . by . . . Sen. Joseph D. Ward (D-Fitchburg). . . . Ward, armed only with his forensic ability and the knowledge gained from years of experience on Beacon Hill, singlehandedly steered to enactment an $8,200,000 program to improve the lot of the mentally retarded in the commonwealth. . . .

In the opinion of observers, it was the most startling exploit by an individual legislator in at least the recent history of the legislature.

It appears, then, that in the field of mental health the technical decisions usually are worked out by specialists and experts in this field—sometimes with the participation of influential laymen and legislators—and then are legitimized by the formal decision-making processes of the state government. The legislative commissions that have made some notable contributions to services for the mentally ill and mentally retarded, as in the Ward bills, have in most cases utilized the service of one or more of the informed professionals within the Boston mental health community. It

[7] This position was abolished after a heated fight and close vote in the complete reorganization of the Department of Education in 1965.

appears that there have been no successful legislative proposals of any significance in this field which have been initiated by individual citizens, although the right of free petition is one of the pillars (some would term it a major harassment) of the state's legislative processes.

The traditional sources of informal pressures are, of course, the representatives of the various organized interest groups. Such pressures in Massachusetts can be divided into those relative to the local mental health centers as they find expression at the state level, and those concerning the activities of the Department of Mental Health or other state agencies. The primary sources of informal pressures concerning existing or proposed local mental health centers are the local mental health associations. Those associations that already have a center seek to enlarge their state-supported staffs; those just getting underway want an initial allocation of a block of professionals. The Division of Mental Hygiene insists that any local request for staff, whether for an initial block or for expansion, must be supported by the state legislators representing the service area. Obtaining such support is a responsibility of the local associations. It is possible for a legislator to put in a request for added local staff during the legislative action on the department's budget or supplemental budget without securing departmental approval. In practice, however, this is rare; for one thing, the lack of such approval is a good out for legislators in dealing with their constituents on a technical matter.

Pressure from outside interest groups may deal with the policies of the Department of Mental Health as well as with budgetary requests. Perhaps the central policy issue of recent years has revolved around the department's proposals for an extensive system of community mental health centers, antedating but similar to the concept embodied in the federal Act. The debate has concerned the basic concept of such a state system, the relationships of these proposed centers to the existing means of dealing with mental illness, and with other agencies, and in one case at least with the location of a proposed center.

Opposition to aspects of the proposed program that developed within the medical profession, however, has hinged upon two related, but separable, viewpoints. The first was the hostility of many doctors, and of the organized medical profession generally, to direct governmental provision of medical services; the second was the contention that if community mental health services were to be provided (and there seemed to be general agreement that they were needed), they should be integral parts of general hospitals. President Kennedy's message to Congress specified that there could be a variety of local organizational arrangements; among the possible arrangements were such service psychiatric units. Medical spokesmen in Massachusetts combined ideological opposition to expansion of the state's mental health system through community mental health centers with the assertion that such services would be more accepted in the community and hence more effective if they were part of a general hospital than if they were separate. Furthermore, there was apprehension that local physicians would not have access to the centers.

The early views of the medical profession on these points were shaped in the Massachusetts Medical Society's Committee on Mental Health in the spring of 1963. In May 1963 the council of the Massachusetts Medical Association adopted a resolution at the suggestion of the committee, which urged that the proposed new centers be attached to general hospitals and under the control of the boards of such hospitals. Also the resolution recommended that no action be taken by the Department of Mental Health until a study of the whole proposal could be made by a committee that would include a representative of the medical association.

The continuing agitation within the medical profession over the nature of the proposed system of community mental health centers was expressed by Dr. Robert E. Arnot, president of the Associated General Hospital Psychiatrists, in a letter published in the *New England Journal of Medicine*. While he accepted the need for such centers, he commented, "Unfortunately, psychiatry by necessity has been under government ownership and control, largely through default. Recently, however, psychiatry has been developing under private auspices in the general hospital, so that now a welcome alternative to state psychiatry is offered." [8] An editorial in the same journal's issue of January 2, 1964, restated the criticism of the medical profession, raising four questions:

Is a state-directed, supported and controlled network of psychiatric centers the best way to treat the mentally ill?

Should mental health clinics be distinct and separate from general hospitals or part of a general hospital's facilities?

How can the state, which cannot staff satisfactorily its existing mental hospitals, construct and staff an extensive network of community mental health centers?

[8] *New England Journal of Medicine*, Vol. 270 (April 16, 1964), p. 853.

Is the Commonwealth of Massachusetts concept of community mental health centers consistent with President Kennedy's recommendations?

The several task forces of the Planning Project attempted to overcome these objections of the medical society but without much success. During the winter of 1964–1965 the state society transmitted the substance of its earlier resolutions to the American Medical Association for possible national action.

The position of the Department of Mental Health on the issue was that regardless of what might otherwise be desirable, the state constitution barred the direct distribution of state funds to nonprofit organizations of any sort to build facilities or conduct activities under their own control. Consequently, the integration of community mental health centers and private general hospitals was not possible. However, the legal opinions cited above relative to state contracts with private agencies for mental health services did allow the coordinated use of public and private resources under public direction.

The role of lay leaders generally in respect to state mental health matters in Massachusetts has been quite limited. The Massachusetts Association for Mental Health came into being long after the establishment of a strong state mental health program and professional service. This eliminated the possibility of its spearheading a great crusade to "wipe out the snakepits" as such associations had done in other states. The Massachusetts association therefore has had an uphill fight to establish itself. During most of the last two decades, its leaders evidently have felt that they were competing with the Division of Mental Hygiene in stimulating the organization of local mental health associations. The result has been the development of two distinct groups of local mental health associations, only one of which is affiliated with the state Association for Mental Health. For the most part the association has supported departmental program and budgetary requests, but it has been in the position of a late and not very potent quasi-auxiliary to the department.

Thus, at the state level leaders in mental health find it difficult to harness their full political potential. The basic problem, however, traces back to the high degree of political fragmentation, which has centered so much citizen attention on the local clinics and has demanded so much from the leadership in related local issues. This same phenomenon has already been noted in respect to the absorption of the political interests and energies of many able persons in the affairs of the individual cities and towns, rather than in metropolitan Boston or the state as a whole.

Because of the preponderant authority of the state in mental health activity in Massachusetts for the last sixty years, state planning has been of paramount importance. In fact, were it not for the decision of the state Department of Mental Health to encourage organization of local mental health associations and clinics, there would be no planning to discuss within the Boston metropolitan area other than that done by the state.

Any consideration of the influence of state planning on mental health in the Boston area must distinguish between the planning of earlier decades and the efforts under the Massachusetts Mental Health Planning Project (MHPP) and the Department of Mental Health in the mid-sixties. Planning is, of course, one of those all-purpose words that can mean whatever one wishes it to mean. Here it is used to refer to the conscious definition of alternative courses of long-range action or development, estimates of costs, and follow-up to improve the provision of mental health services. Early planning efforts involved three types of mental health activity: first, the development of the state hospitals and state schools which serve this area; second, the provision of local mental health services; and third, the provision of various other services.

The first type of planning is done initially in most cases by the superintendent of the particular institution and his staff. This may range from modest steps toward improvement to major program developments or requests for larger facilities. So far as the impact upon services in the Boston SMSA is concerned, state planning of this type has only the peripheral effect of enlarging or improving services available to residents of the "feeder area" of the particular institutions.

There was no predetermined statewide plan for the development of local mental health clinics in the past, but often there was considerable discussion between departmental personnel and local leaders in working out rational and viable units that would fit into those already existing. The only firm requirement was that the proposed unit should serve at least 100,000 persons. On the whole, the Department of Mental Health sought to avoid dictating to local groups, and sought flexibility and spontaneity in the new local organizations: "The function of the Department is to remove obstacles to the natural, free, easy and spontaneous entering into active participation by many groups." No doubt one reason for this policy was the unsuccessful experience of the Massachusetts Department of Public Health during the 1950s in attempting to force every city and town either to establish its own public health department or to join in some regional grouping. The Department of Mental Health did not wish to be caught in the same trap; consequently it insisted on a considerable degree of community study and participation before approving a new unit.

It obviously takes a good deal of time to develop a high degree of community understanding and to shape a proposal. Indeed, five years was regarded as normal for this process, and some places have taken twice that long. Consequently, not only were the service areas of local mental health clinics flexibly negotiated by the Department of Mental Health, but the timing of establishing local clinics was more dependent upon local processes than upon departmental action. This might be viewed more as the gradual carrying out of a policy, than a rigorous planning activity.

Finally, the department has controlled the development of outpatient services by the state hospitals, to the extent that it required specific enlargement of the hospital staffs, through budgetary processes. Planning of this character varies from none at all for some institutions in the Boston SMSA to a very considerable operation in others.

An innovation of major significance in state planning for mental health in Massachusetts was the organization of the Massachusetts Mental Health Planning Project in 1963, supported by federal funds. The goals of this activity in Massachusetts were defined as: developing a comprehensive plan of mental health service for Massachusetts; involving community and professional leaders in its formulation and implementation; and developing a planning mechanism that could later be integrated into the organizational structure of the Department of Mental Health. The project was headed by Harold Demone, Jr., a sociologist and head of the Medical Foundation, and had a staff of full- and part-time workers from psychiatry, law, biostatistics, clinical and social psychology, social work, sociology, and health education. The planning project was aided by problem-area task forces, whose members were drawn from voluntary groups, professional organizations, health insurance companies, communication organizations, federal agencies, and representatives of cities and towns, religious groups, and the schools. The task forces met at frequent intervals to determine the issues in their respective fields, and used personal interviews and detailed questionnaires to secure information.

The task forces were organized on topical rather than geographic lines. In addition, an overall Advisory Council was created, composed of both medical professionals and laymen, with the responsibility of approving or revising the plan developed by the task forces and the project staff. While the Planning Project staff realized that they would have to grapple with the thorny issue of a more rational definition of areas each center would serve, they avoided a direct approach to this problem. Instead, they organized the study on a statewide basis.

The result was to achieve a very considerable degree of consensus within most of the advisory study groups, and this was of critical importance for the future of the Department of Mental Health. The time was deemed ripe to present proposals for the proper operating areas of centers to be developed in the future, and for more rational clientele areas for the state hospitals. So long as it was a matter of local option whether or not local mental health clinics were to be established, how they would be supported, and what the service areas and functions of such clinics should be, the Department of Mental Health could leave it to "citizens" to define areas. Now that the concept of eventually providing local mental health services throughout the state was accepted, more logical service areas became possible.

The product of this massive effort by the Massachusetts Mental Health Planning Project was a plan that covered all aspects of the provision of mental health services in Massachusetts. It proposed a statewide system of thirty-seven mental health centers of quite diverse types: some to be parts of existing state hospitals, such as Boston State; others to be an expansion of existing facilities, such as the Massachusetts Mental Health Center; new units in conjunction with major private or university hospitals, such as Boston University and Tufts; existing area mental health centers, such as the new Lowell unit; and entirely new units in other areas. Planning for mental retardation was to be coordinated with the subsequent report of the Massachusetts Mental Retardation Planning Project.

The *Report* also contained a number of recommendations for reorganization within the central office of the Department of Mental Health, with the addition of a deputy commissioner and several assistant commissioners. Finally, to provide for closer coordination of the department's activities in the field, it was proposed that there should be six regional offices for administration of all departmental resources within their respective territories.

Decisions on site location of the new community mental health centers, it is expected, will be quite different from the methods used to determine the locale of clinics in the past. The initial decision as to the location of the local mental health clinics in the past was made primarily by local leaders who organized local demands upon the Department of Mental Health and through it to the legislature. Usually, they sought inexpensive or free space in a reasonably central location. There was some review of relative claims and priorities by the department, but on the whole the demand developed slowly enough that requests could be handled as they came to fruition. Consequently, it may be concluded that decisions about the service area and site of the clinics established by local mental health associations were initiated locally and validated by the department, the legislature, and, at times, the governor.

Decisions on the location of the full-fledged community mental health centers as they were conceived early in the 1960s (before federal action in this field) were made by the Massachusetts Department of Mental Health, largely on the basis of objective need and partly in response to the developing plans of several hospital complexes in Boston. The first state-planned centers were in areas that had concentrations of population and high need for mental health services, and had insufficient facilities presently at hand. Often such locations lacked vigorous citizen organizations that could pressure the legislators. Two and possibly three of the centers planned in Boston will be related to hospitals and universities. Other community mental health centers were planned by the Department in other cities and were to serve surrounding areas as well; the first to begin operations was the unit at Lowell. So far, it would appear that there have been only two arguments over the location of mental health facilities, both within the city of Boston; another issue concerned proposed service areas in the city.

Part of the widely heralded rebirth of the city of Boston has involved the razing of a grubby area of amusement parlors, bars, and cheap rooming houses in the Scollay Square area near the State House. A massive rebuilding effort is underway, involving a new City Hall, a very large federal office building, a twenty-two-story state office building, and another state government unit termed the health-education-welfare unit, which will include several state agencies plus several privately financed office buildings. Present plans call for the construction of a community mental health center as part of this health-education-welfare building, with a staff linkage to the Massachusetts General Hospital situated a quarter-mile to the west.

One of the first political efforts of the Associated General Hospital Psychiatrists was to reverse this decision. They urged that it would be much better to have the proposed center physically a part of the Massachusetts General Hospital complex to enable closer contact between the staff people concerned. This feeling was shared by some of the staff at Massachusetts General. Furthermore, it was urged that patients would prefer to go to a clinic that was part of a general hospital complex and that it is not wise to segregate mental patients. Finally, it was argued that most of the care at the proposed government center unit would be by state-salaried doctors and that this would intrude on the role of the private psychiatrists in the West End renewal project, whose services could be secured for a center next to the Massachusetts General Hospital.

These views were urged upon Governor Volpe during his first term. While he was sympathetic, he concluded that planning was too far advanced to change. A similar appeal to Governor Peabody led to a new review of the site decision. Agencies controlling the adjacent land were loath to sell, although it is possible that a strenuous campaign could have overcome these objections. One advantage to having this community mental health center as an integral part of the government center rather than being a separate item in the capital outlay budget is that the construction cost is thus provided in the total bond issue for the larger building.

The other conflict over a mental health site is not solely about a community mental health center, but it is of great political interest nevertheless. This concerns plans for building a $7-million addition to the Massachusetts Mental Health Center on Fenwood Road in Boston as one of the five community mental health centers in the city. The center is located within one block of the famed Peter Bent Brigham Hospital, which, in turn, abuts the Harvard Medical School and a large complex of other medical and teaching facilities. Dr. Jack Ewalt, superintendent of the center, has urged that it be linked physically with the general hospital area.

The difficulty is that the intervening block is occupied by a number of three-story houses in reasonably good repair, and the adjoining block already is being leveled to provide for an expansion of Harvard facilities. All told, about 200 families are involved in this institutional expansion, and many of them are members of a Catholic parish, Mission Church, which had been considerably affected in the past by other renewal projects. A strenuous fight against the Fenwood Road project has been led by Representative William D. Carey (Boston); in 1964 Carey tried to persuade the legislature to repeal the 1961 act that appropriated $650,-000 for this land acquisition. The next obstacle has been the state's elected Executive Council, which would not allow expenditure of the funds appropriated for this project by the legislature in 1961. When the powers of the Executive Council were reduced by a popular referendum on the November ballot, Governor Peabody directed the attorney general's office to proceed with the acquisition. This led to a massive "march on the State House" by 3,000 persons from Mission Hill, led by the parochial school's drill team and band, but Governor Peabody would not be moved.

The wide-ranging battle has involved peripheral attacks upon mental health in general and Dr. Ewalt's proposals in particular, and upon Harvard as well because it has taken over a former Catholic institution on the other side of the center. It was suggested that the center should expand in that direction instead of toward the hospital area. The Boston Redevelopment Authority was also involved because of the charge that it favors the Fenwood Road land-taking because this would produce large federal credits for the city even if it meant wiping out a nonblighted area. The Boston Redevelopment Authority administrator denied this and stated that the Fenwood Road plan was only one of dozens of possible institutional expansion projects within Boston, all of which produce federal credits.

A third controversy related to state planning resulted from the proposal of the Mental Health Planning Project to divide Boston into five mental health service areas. These would be centered on the existing units at Boston State Hospital, the Massachusetts Mental Health Center, the Boston University Medical Center adjacent to Boston City Hospital, and the Tufts Medical Center in the South End, with the addition of a new unit in the North End at the government center, affiliated with the nearby Massachusetts General Hospital.

It was argued that the proposals of the Planning Project gave some centers a considerably heavier population load than others. Furthermore, a disproportionate number of persons probably requiring the most service were assigned to the proposed Boston University Center. Among other groups in this area were a very large number of Boston's Negro population. In contrast, the Massachusetts Mental Health Center drew less than 10,000 of its proposed 210,000 persons to be served from areas of high levels of need for social services (as defined in a study by United Community Services), while it had over 54,000 from the town of Brookline, an area of relatively minimal need. The Boston University Center, in contrast, drew 121,000 of its proposed 169,000 potential clientele from areas of high need, and the other 48,000 from areas of strong need. Furthermore, the Boston State Hospital Center would draw its entire 230,000 persons to be served from an area of strong need.

It was argued that if the UCS estimates of needs for services were at all accurate, the facilities and staff required by the Boston State Hospital and Boston University Centers would have to be very disproportionate to those at the other three centers. The Tufts Center was smaller because the population in its service area is much smaller, and it was intended to use existing facilities insofar as possible.

The Boston University staff suggested several alternatives that would present a more balanced clientele for both its center and the Massachusetts Mental Health Center. These suggestions had only a limited effect upon the planning of service areas within Boston during the early stages. In following years, however, the rigorous application of the federal maximums for populations to be served by a single mental health center led to some adjustment of service areas and some equalization of the service load. These changes moved in the direction suggested by the Boston University Hospital staff.

FINANCING MENTAL HEALTH ACTIVITIES

At least three major aspects of the financing of public functions can be identified. First, there is the amount being spent. Second, there can be significant differences in the allocation of that total amount between particular parts of the organization, service areas, or types of activity. Third, there is the important question of the source of the funds being spent for the purpose.

It has long been accepted in Massachusetts that there should be state-operated facilities for the care of those persons who must be institutionalized, where they can receive the type and degree of treatment required. While this service was originally for adults, it was expanded about the turn of the century to include mentally retarded children; more recently it has been recognized that other children and adolescents may need treatment. Finally, it gradually has been accepted that treatment should be provided for individuals with mental problems that are not yet so severe as to require hospitalization or full-time institutionalization. Such less severe problems traditionally were viewed as an individual matter, but there is now a willingness to look upon this type of mental illness as a proper public concern. In part, this seems due to a changing public view of the nature of mental illness; indeed, in some circles or communities it would seem that to be in the care of a psychiatrist is a status symbol.

The primary determinant of expenditure for mental health at a given time is the need, both quantitative and qualitative, of the population served. The capacity of current institutions and service centers is a limiting factor on the basic *quantity* of mental health service available. The *nature and quality* of service is the result of professional opinion and recommendations modified by the willingness and fiscal ability of the supporting unit of government. The "adequacy" of this service is usually measured by reference to national standards developed by the particular professional group in question. What is provided is almost always below such standards. Public mental health is a particularly notable example of "gaposis" between the proposed standards and what exists because of the high costs of service.

Pressures for increasing expenditures come from a variety of sources and, while these demands may not be immediately met, they have a glacier-like quality once they are enunciated and some support is organized. A major source of such proposals is from the professionals in the particular service who perceive a need and try to secure approval from political authorities for the necessary funds. A second source of pressure is from clientele groups. A third source of pressure is the adoption by legislators or political executives of "mental health" as an issue or a program item. The fourth pressure for expansion of mental health programs at any particular time is the availability of money from some higher level of government. The distribution of current funds among mental health functions reflects many decisions about theories of therapy in mental illness, the type of services to be provided, concepts of the type and extent of services required, and so on. If funds are limited, then only the highest priority needs (as priorities were perceived at some time in the past) will be met.

Who is to pay for what, and how any existing or potential expenditure can be shifted elsewhere, in whole or in part, is a continuing concern of almost all governments. At any given time there is a pattern of sources of funds for mental health services based upon earlier decisions as to what the need was, how it should be met, and who was responsible. The most significant decision of this type in Massachusetts was embodied in the 1904 legislation that stated that the counties, cities, and towns should withdraw from the field entirely and the state should become the exclusive agency in the mental health field.

The Massachusetts Mental Health Planning Project's *Report* noted that "there is a large sum of money now being expended from many sources to finance mental health care . . ." yet "there is a substantial unmet need for additional financing." The *Report* continued:

The additional operating and capital funds needed probably will exceed the amount of tax funds, whether federal, state, or local, which will be available for these purposes. It is equally unrealistic to expect traditional voluntary and charitable resources alone to provide these needed funds. . . . A method of expenditure of state-federal tax funds should be used to work most effectively in encouraging voluntary additive financing of the mental health program, both operating and capital. . . . Insofar as he is able to pay, the basic responsibility for meeting the cost of treatment rests with the individual, his family and private resources, including insurance . . . (although) present insurance coverage often is not sufficient to meet potential mental health needs of the great bulk of the citizenry.

While the thrust of this argument was directed at expanding both the role and the fiscal contributions of nonpublic agencies to meet mental health needs insofar as possible, the *Report* concluded that "increased needs and rising costs suggest that, for the foreseeable future, voluntary financing will supply . . . [a] smaller share [though the absolute amount in dollars may continue to expand] of the funds for support of services and facilities in the mental health field. In turn, government at all levels will have to bear an increasing portion of the financial load."

The study recognized the major and continuing role of the network of voluntary agencies, which it urged should be coordinated with, rather than being supplanted by, the proposed community mental health centers. It also noted that a change was occurring in respect to hospitalization for mental illness. "Prior to the last few years, hospitalization for mental illness was predominantly in hospitals maintained by the public . . . [but] nationwide statistics suggest that as many psychiatric patients are now cared for in general hospital psychiatric services as in tax-supported hospitals." Not only does this diminish the load upon public facilities, but also

in general hospitals, the duration of stay has been reduced to an average of fourteen days which compares favorably for hospitalization for somatic illness and represents a great saving of time away from the family, work and the community. . . . Psychiatry in general hospitals, while still new, seemed to establish one principal fact: the majority of acute mental illnesses can be short-term.

While it undoubtedly was gratifying to the private psychiatrists in Massachusetts to have their developing role recognized in the *Report*, the significant aspect of this approach was the full acceptance of a "mixed economy" of public and private effort for mental health—hopefully to be better coordinated than in the past and much more comprehensive—and with a continued mixture of individual, philanthropic, and public financing as well. This approach to the financing of mental health costs seems to have been impelled more by recognition of the very large costs of the proposed expanded program, however, than by specific acceptance of the views of the Department of Mental Health of the desirability of mixed financing of a community facility as a means of involving the entire community in the enterprise.

Substantially all public funds spent for mental health services in Massachusetts (aside from the considerable expenditures by the Veterans Administration hospitals and clinics) are state funds, because of the assumption of state responsibility for the function in 1904. To the extent that local governments have been involved in supporting mental health activities, this has been through limited contributions to the operating costs of local mental health clinics, which in fiscal 1964 totaled approximately $600,000.

The operating budgets of the Massachusetts Department of Mental

Health have risen from $72.4 million in 1965 to $91.2 million in fiscal 1967. The governor recommended $105.5 million for fiscal 1968. Thus mental health would be the first departmental *operating* budget in Massachusetts history to rise above $100 million.

During this period, which saw a decline of about 10,000 in the number of patients in the state's mental hospitals as a result of the increasing use of tranquilizing drugs and expanded rehabilitation programs, there has been some shift of the allocations of the department's operating budget. The first major change was a greater expenditure for state schools for the mentally retarded, and for special hospitals for the aging, epileptics, and others. More recently, there has been an increasing variety of functions directed at service in communities and to various outpatient groups, such as those in courts, and to alcoholics.

In fiscal 1959 almost 65.5 per cent of the department's $57.2 million budget went to the state mental hospitals; by fiscal 1965 this had diminished to about 61.5 per cent. The budget of the Division of Mental Hygiene, concerned with community clinics, which was about 1.3 per cent in 1959, comprised more than 4 per cent of the proposed fiscal 1968 budget.

Large allocations of state funds have been made for capital outlays by the department to provide new facilities for state hospitals and state schools and to modernize some of the structures built in the latter nineteenth and early twentieth centuries. Since the reawakening of governmental and citizen concern about mental illness following World War II, Massachusetts spent over $90 million for capital expenditures. About $4 million of the capital outlay authorizations through fiscal 1965 was for community mental health centers, prior to federal action on this matter.

In fiscal 1964 the Division of Mental Hygiene spent close to $2.5 million for community clinics. Of this, about $175,000, or 7 per cent, came from federal grants. The contributions of municipal governments and private sources amounted to $800,000, or about 32 per cent. Consequently, state support of the local mental health clinics was about 59 per cent of their total cost. In addition, the clinics benefited from a program of training grants administered by the division, which cost about $114,000; almost three-quarters of this was provided by the federal government. Thus the Division of Mental Hygiene was successful in drawing about two-fifths of its cost in fiscal 1964 from sources other than the state government.

No public function or service can be adequately considered alone. All exist within a total political context and a total political economy, and the fortunes of each are in some degree affected by what happens to others. This may occur within a particular governmental unit, as for instance when a city needs both new schools and new sewers at the same time but cannot afford both. It is notably true in respect to single-purpose state-aid or federal-aid programs that offer subordinate units of government matching funds on varying bases and in varying amounts for particular types of activity, rather than others.

Massachusetts has spent very substantial sums of money for mental health activities over the years. While these amounts steadily increase, the availability of vast federal sums for the defense highway system on a 90 per cent matching basis has tended to raise state highway expenditures. Yet it is difficult to prove that the state's spending for mental health would have been substantially increased if this highway program had not existed. The requests by the Department of Mental Health have consistently run well ahead of the governor's recommendations, but both the requests and the budget recommendations have steadily climbed.

Education appears to be the major new claimant for state funds, largely as a result of the two-year study by the Massachusetts commissioner of education.[9] It may well be that the projected tapering off of the federal highway program in the next few years will be matched by increasing state expenditures for public education, leaving mental health in substantially the same position it is today—one of the top three or four claimants for state funds in a steadily expanding state budget. The sharp rise in the education budget was primarily due to the expanded state aid program made possible through the enactment of the sales tax in 1966, which led to increases from $60.5 million in fiscal 1966 to a proposed $98 million in fiscal 1968.

Consequently, it would appear that in Massachusetts the state budget will respond to a particular stimulus on a particular category of expenditures somewhat independently of other programs, although there are

[9] Special Commission Relative to Improving and Extending Educational Facilities in the Commonwealth, *Quality Education for Massachusetts—An Investment in the People of the Commonwealth* (Boston: General Court of the Commonwealth, 1964).

obvious limits both as to number and size of departmental increases that are possible in a given year. It is likely that municipal spending for mental health will not increase significantly, and indeed, if the dominant organization for community mental health centers follows the pattern being established in Lowell, local spending for this function, limited as it is, might even decline, as state-supported centers replace the existing clinics operated by local mental health associations and supported to some extent by contributions from local school systems and boards of health.

Massachusetts has never accepted the concept that there should be statutory or constitutional restrictions upon the levels of public spending by limits upon taxes such as percentages of valuation or fixed tax rates. Tax limitations are political and economic, rather than legal, but feelings change slowly about what ought to be spent and they vary markedly from one town or region to another. There are also external pressures in terms of competitive salary schedules or required state minimums, most notably for school teachers, and upon tax attractiveness (or the opposite) for business and industry. Indeed, one of the major arguments favoring adoption of a sales tax was that the heavy reliance upon the real estate tax for the ever-mounting costs of local government was a definite obstacle to attracting new industry and increasing employment in Massachusetts. In view of the strong pressure from various groups such as the parents of mentally retarded children, the local mental health associations, and the groups established throughout the state to plan for the future community mental health centers, and the general public belief that poor conditions in some of the state institutions need considerable improvement, it would appear that mental health expenditures will continue to increase.

It is not at all surprising that the Mental Health Planning Project recommended a statewide system of mental health centers that are to be integral parts of the Department of Mental Health, rather than locally established units aided by departmental funds as are the existing mental health clinics. To be sure, local interest might be stimulated by requiring substantial local contribution toward the cost of the proposed mental health centers, but this was hardly practical when budgets of three-quarters of a million dollars for each center were concerned. Furthermore, the community to be served by the new type of center would

e an aggregrate of persons in a collection of municipalities, rather than
socially defined community.

At the same time, the Mental Health Planning Project's recommen-
lation clearly recognized the necessity of an institutional link between
he proposed centers and the communities in which they would operate.
The *Report* urged that each center should have a community mental
ealth board with significant advisory functions. Members of these boards
vould be nominated by local agencies and appointed by the governor.
This procedure would qualify them as governmental agencies so they
vould be able to receive and expend voluntary and public funds.

It is difficult to determine the effect of political fragmentation on fi-
ancial support for mental health purposes. Once the state assumed the
ull responsibility for inpatient care of the mentally ill in a system of
tate hospitals and schools, political fragmentation had little effect. Had
nental health services remained a function of local governments, it is
ikely that some of the more affluent suburban areas would have invested
nore for community mental health services than is presently available.
However, the amount of such difference is conjectural, and if state-sup-
)orted centers are developed throughout the state, total expenditures
or mental health services will be greater than would have been the case
ad local mental health services been an optional matter of local initia-
ive.

STAFFING MENTAL HEALTH SERVICES

t might be supposed that if any metropolitan area among those studied
vas well supplied with trained manpower, it would be Boston. Greater
3oston is one of the major centers of the nation for research and train-
ng in psychiatry, in medicine generally, and in psychology and a host
)f related fields and concerns. There are also many notable training cen-
ers in other parts of Massachusetts. Consequently, the state ranks very
vell in comparison with the national average of professional personnel;
·elevant figures from a national survey are shown in Table 2. Thus, the
tate ranked from 50 per cent to more than 100 per cent above the na-
:ional average.

It is difficult to assess the total percentage of the state's manpower re-
;ources working in the Boston SMSA because of the likelihood that many

Table 2: Professional Manpower in Massachusetts
Compared with U.S. Average

	Massachusetts	U.S. Average
Physicians per 100 inpatients in state and county hospitals	1.27	0.90
Professional personnel per 100 inpatients in public mental hospitals	7.90	4.50
Full-time employees per 100 inpatients in public mental hospitals	45.00	36.00
American Psychiatric Association members per 100,000 population	12.30	6.70
Professional hours in outpatient clinics per 100,000 population	424.00	174.00

Source: U.S. Department of Health, Education and Welfare, Fifteen Indices for 1962.

reported as "part-time" are employed by more than one of the institutions or agencies reporting. A number of smaller clinics have part-time service of less than ten hours weekly by psychiatrists, psychologists, or both; this often was provided by more than one individual. The figures reported in the Boston SMSA for the full-time category alone suggest that approximately one-third of the psychiatrists and psychologists work in the metropolitan area. Such professional services are by no means confined to residents of the Boston SMSA, especially insofar as outpatient services and nonpublic hospitals are concerned because of the relatively sparse services provided in other parts of the state. Furthermore, many out-of-state residents utilize such services.

It has been noted that not only is the present organization for providing mental health care discouraging to many persons drawn from lower socioeconomic groups, but that the standard methods used in psychotherapy work much less effectively with many such clients. Thus it cannot be presumed that a given level of "need" in terms of the estimated numbers of persons affected can be directly translated into requirements for more of the same type of treatment, staff, and facilities. However, this still is a very significant component in the gross level of need in the Boston SMSA.

The second major component of unmet need is an increase in the quantity or quality of assistance being provided to those already being

served to some degree. A general lament of those involved in such serv-
ces is that resources are insufficient, even if a less demanding form of
help than "long-term, once-a-week, intensive psychotherapy" is found
to be sufficient in many cases. However, the substantial need on the part
of many thousands of persons in the Boston SMSA for services they now
lack is going to require a massive infusion of resources, as well as improvement of the quality and effectiveness in using resources now existing.

One approach to securing more definite figures on professional and
paraprofessional personnel is to utilize the average staffing forecasts for
the new centers. The staff needed merely for the high-priority nine community mental health centers proposed for the Boston area would constitute a major part of the entire existing resources of the area and would
allow nothing for the improvement of existing services and institutions
in the area or for the requirements for normal replacement of the present
staff. It should be clear that the personnel problem in the mental health
field in Massachusetts is of staggering proportions. This is especially
true of psychiatrists because of the very lengthy training and high dollar
investment currently required to train such persons.

While it may be hoped that vigorous development of alternative methods of treatment that are less demanding of skilled staff may produce
major innovations and that research into the causes of mental illness may
lead to significant results such as those felt in the mental hospitals after
introduction of the tranquilizing drugs, such a happy result cannot be
relied upon to solve the manpower problem. In consequence, it comes
as little surprise that the *Report* of the Mental Health Planning Project
begins its section on training and manpower as follows:

Manpower problems in mental health planning for Massachusetts are best
exemplified in one word—"need." In every profession which has come
under scrutiny—psychiatry, psychology, social work, nursing, occupational
therapy and others—the conclusion seems warranted that we are not meeting present manpower needs. As the contemplated new developments in
community mental health emerge, we will be in an even worse manpower
plight ten years from now. . . . Plans for mental health and training manpower personnel needs during the next ten years have been considered in
the context of an evolutionary thrust in the scope and magnitude of mental
health which is of almost revolutionary dimensions. . . . This increased
scope, which includes that total population and incorporates the public
health point of view, enormously increases the magnitude of the field of
mental health and of the problems of training and manpower.

This unambiguous definition of the personnel needs for Massachusetts can only lead to the conclusion that the problems faced by most of the other states in the country are even greater. The nation's needs are related to those in Massachusetts because of the traditional role of the state's institutions, in Greater Boston especially, as a major national training center. This means that any plan for manpower development here must take into account considerably more than the needs of Massachusetts alone, large as these may be.

The *Report* did not attempt to define specific numerical targets or give dates, even for the needs of Massachusetts alone, let alone demands upon Massachusetts training centers for assistance to meet the needs of other states engaged in similar programs. However, it urgently recommended a wide variety of actions.

In summary, the situation in Massachusetts in respect to personnel requirements in the mental health field is relatively good as compared with the average throughout the United States. However, it is very inadequate in the light of even those needs presently existing, let alone those envisaged as arising if the community mental health centers in Massachusetts are expanded by two or three each year, if other programs are improved and/or amplified, and if the demand from other states increases for graduates of Massachusetts training programs.

CONCLUSIONS

It may be argued that the nature of the community mental health program in the Boston SMSA was determined in large measure by the founders of the Massachusetts Bay Colony who reproduced the parish form of government found in Old England. This resulted in the development of parish-municipalities covering the whole area of the state. As new public functions were accepted, they tended either to be assigned to the town government—instead of to county governments—or else to be provided on a statewide basis.

This organization based on municipalities that were expected to provide all local services from their own tax revenue had a second effect in that there was less tendency to turn to the state government for assistance in meeting the costs of local government than in most states. Reciprocally there has been an aversion on the part of state leaders to advocate or to adopt new state taxes. As a consequence, the level of state aid to municipalities has been lower than in most states, most notably in respect to public education. In order to meet demands for improved local services, municipalities have raised real estate taxes to very high levels.

The third effect of the fragmentation of the state into several hundred cities and towns has been to shape both public and private organizations on a municipal basis. Even for those public services that required a larger unit, such as regional high schools, the component units are always two or more municipalities. Private social welfare agencies have varying sets of service areas, but they too utilize the local units of government in defining such areas. Similarly, the field areas of virtually all state agencies run along municipal boundaries. In Massachusetts, county governments generally have never emerged as more than areas of judicial organization. Thus municipal pride and independence, the custom of emphasizing reliance upon local real estate taxes, and traditional geographic and organizing patterns are three results of political fragmentation that are of key importance in the organization of modern mental health centers in Massachusetts.

The concept of the "community mental health center"—generally a regional unit rather than a true community unit in Massachusetts—was to a considerable extent formulated and experimented with in the state before the passage of the 1963 federal legislation. There is a substantial degree of consensus about the nature of community mental health centers. It seems agreed that these units should be relatively close to the population being served, that they should provide a broad spectrum of services, that they must have some ties with a wide variety of public, semipublic, and private agencies within their service area, and that they should be subject to a considerable measure of local control.

However, there has been a substantial flexibility in the proposed organization, depending upon the mental health resources available within their respective service areas. Some may be essentially autonomous units with some degree of linkage with the state mental hospitals serving the area; some may be operated on the grounds of state mental institutions and very closely related to the hospital organization; some may be operational segments of voluntary general hospitals, although still parts of the state Department of Mental Health and subject to a considerable measure of control by representatives of the area they serve.

Because of the long traditions of state responsibility for mental health services, the difficult local fiscal situation, and the marginal concern of community leaders in most municipalities with mental health, it seems unlikely that there will be much local debate over provision at public expense of community mental health services of the extensive sort envisaged by the 1963 Act. This is due to the vigorous local resistance to proposals that the cities and towns should assume significant fiscal responsibility for mental health services. Therefore, such services either will be financed by the state, hopefully with generous and continuing federal assistance, or they will not exist at all.

Consequently, the major policy decisions concerning local mental health services will continue to be made at the state level, and by relatively small groups of professionals in the state Department of Mental Health and state budget officials supported by a few interested citizens. It is possible that the governing councils, when they are established for the proposed thirty-seven community mental health centers which are the goal in Massachusetts, may become significant participants in the state's policy decisions concerning mental health services. However, if the absorption of the existing local mental health associations in the detailed affairs of their particular unit is a useful guide, the attention of the area councils will be centered primarily on the complex problems of meshing existing public and voluntary mental health and related services with the new centers for some time to come. The primary limiting factor to the establishment of centers would seem to be the availability of the staff, and this should be far less a problem in the Boston SMSA than in the more remote hinterland.

X: MINNEAPOLIS–ST. PAUL

CHARLES H. BACKSTROM

THE MINNEAPOLIS–ST. PAUL metropolitan area dominates the upper Midwest section of the United States. Economically the "Twin Cities" constitute the northwestern outpost of the economic heartland of the nation. To the west lie the northern plains, basically an agricultural region with sparse population, an area of slow growth or even declining population. To the north lie the northwoods, even more sparsely populated than the plains. This was a great lumber and iron producing area in the past, but today recreation appears to offer the greatest potential for growth.

ECOLOGY

The economy of the metropolitan area is well balanced among manufacturing, trade, and services. It is stable because growth within the metropolitan area itself has more than offset decline in the hinterland. On the edge of the national heartland, the area has not attracted heavy industry. Rather, in an earlier day the Twin Cities emphasized processing agricultural and timber products and wholesale trade, and served as a transportation and financial center. In more recent years, metals and machinery manufacturing—especially electronics—for national and international markets has grown rapidly. The desirability of the area as a place to live and the quality of the labor force are cited by industries as the main reasons for their location there.[1] A distinguished university, a first-rate symphony orchestra, two major art museums, the new but already famous Tyrone Guthrie Theater, a science museum, a zoo, and major league baseball and football combine to offer residents education and pleasure.

In 1960 the standard metropolitan statistical area (SMSA) had a

I wish to express my appreciation to Richard Murray, who, as research assistant, helped immeasurably in collecting the information upon which this study was based.

[1] Twin City Metropolitan Planning Commission, *Metropolitan Economic Study #5* (St. Paul: The Commission, 1960).

population of 1,482,030, making it the fourteenth largest in the country. This represented an increase of 331,000, or 28 per cent, since 1950, the equivalent of adding another city the size of St. Paul to the metropolitan area. This rate of expansion placed Minneapolis–St. Paul among the fastest growing metropolitan areas in the United States. Current estimates of the 1970 population in the five counties of the Minneapolis–St. Paul SMSA indicate an increase to almost 2,000,000. For 1980, the Twin Cities Metropolitan Planning Commission estimates stand at 2,500,000, about a 65 per cent growth in twenty years.[2]

Presently the metropolitan area consists of five counties—Hennepin (Minneapolis), Ramsey (St. Paul), Anoka, Dakota, and Washington—although for local planning purposes two additional counties on the fringe of the urbanized area to the southwest are often added. In the past, Minneapolis dominated the metropolitan area in size, but suburban areas within Hennepin county have now reached virtual parity with Minneapolis. The same can be said for all suburban areas when compared to both central cities together (see Table 1).

Both Minneapolis and St. Paul were surrounded at an early date by incorporated municipalities and neither has grown by annexation in recent years. Minneapolis actually lost 39,000 people during the decade before 1960, reducing the city's population to less than a half million. This astounded the local planners, who had apparently underestimated the continued exodus to the suburbs of younger families and the loss of residential areas to freeways and urban renewal. St. Paul's somewhat larger area of remaining open land became fully populated in the 1950s, however, and the city grew slightly to about 313,000.

The suburban areas, on the other hand, were booming during the fifties. This growth followed usual patterns: spilling over the boundaries of the city, filling up the inner ring of older suburbs, then beginning to occupy a new, outer ring, where the galloping subdivisions irregularly meet remaining farms and occasionally engulf smaller rural communities. By 1960 only 53 per cent of the metropolitan area's population lived in the central cities, as opposed to 72 per cent in 1950.

Certainly the most prominent feature of the metropolitan area is its bicentrism. The hyphen between Minneapolis and St. Paul in its name indicates the juxtaposition of two distinct political entities. The two cities

---

[2] Twin City Metropolitan Planning Commission, *4,000,000 by 2000!*, The Joint Program, Report No. 2 (St. Paul: The Commission, 1964).

Table 1: Population of Minneapolis–St. Paul Subdivisions

	1960 Population		% Growth 1950–1960
Minnesota	3,413,864		14.5
Mpls.–St. Paul SMSA	1,482,030		28.8
% of state total		(43.4)	
Hennepin	842,854		24.6
% of SMSA total		(56.9)	
Minneapolis	482,872		−7.4
% of SMSA total		(32.6)	
% of county total		(57.3)	
Ramsey	422,525		18.9
% of SMSA total		(28.5)	
St. Paul	313,411		0.7
% of SMSA total		(21.1)	
% of county total		(74.2)	
Anoka	85,916		141.5
% of SMSA total		(5.8)	
Dakota	78,303		59.7
% of SMSA total		(5.3)	
Washington	52,432		51.8
% of SMSA total		(3.5)	

Source: U.S., Bureau of the Census, *Final Report* PC(1)–25A, Number of Inhabitants, Minnesota (Washington: U.S. Government Printing Office, 1961).

obviously share the same physical region and have been drawn into close economic interaction. Yet, historical, demographic, and economic differences, encrusted with tradition and attitude, have kept the two parts distinct. They cannot be treated together as a single unit.

The Twin Cities are twins only in the fraternal sense that their embryos developed contemporaneously and in close proximity. Subsequent historic and economic events accelerated and perpetuated the division. Later the two cities were brought closer together physically by expanding toward each other. Very recently population mobility, the expansion of feasible commuting areas, common problems of environmental control, and a more mature, less jingoist attitude on the part of prominent residents have led citizens to develop a more cooperative spirit. But contrasts between the two cities are still striking. Journalist John Gunther characterized the distinction by describing St. Paul as "railroads, Irish, Catholic, and Democratic" and Minneapolis as "grain-milling, Scandinavian, and Republican," and spoke of their "virile rivalry." [3] There is some truth here, but there is more to the separatism than this.

At first St. Paul, serving as the state capital, was the dominant city. But after the railroad and lumber industries had reached their zenith, St. Paul's growth was limited in comparison to Minneapolis. Only a few hundred miles to the east are the fringes of the Milwaukee-Chicago urban outreach. It was easier for the distributing industries serving the Dakotas-Montana area to locate in Minneapolis, where they did not have to begin their transit with a long, cross-urban trip. Minneapolis' potential service area westward was unlimited for many hundreds of miles, bounded only by those of Spokane and Seattle to the northwest, and those of Omaha and Denver to the southwest. Thus Minneapolis had the greater opportunity to become a major regional service center and developed accordingly. Though the centers of the cities were only about ten miles apart, in an important sense they lay back to back, a position not conducive to intercourse. The division between the cities was reinforced by the pride and prejudices of political and civic leaders and the policy of each city's press not to impinge on the territory of the other in news coverage or in promoting circulation.

A palpable separatism developed, extending to things commercial, cultural, and civic. Thus, there are two separate downtown shopping centers with major hotels and convention facilities, separate financial institutions, separate airports and railroad terminals, and even separate sports facilities. Each city has its suburbs that are oriented primarily to itself in jobs, trade, and interest.

Since the metropolitan area is not a single-centered unit, the major governmental parts must be introduced separately. Hennepin county, on the western (Minneapolis) side, is geographically large—565 square miles. Furthermore, its land has been the most suitable for both mass subdivision and large-lot luxury suburban living. To the west and northwest lie relatively flat plains readily usable for tract housing; to the southwest is the more hilly, forested, lake area so attractive for distinctive, individually planned homesites.

The western Minneapolis suburbs are already cities with a history; most of the inner ring suburbs were in existence by 1900. These cities are not tiny space stations in orbit around the mother planet; they con-

[3] *Inside USA* (rev. ed.; New York: Harper, 1951), p. 323.

stitute large aggregations of people by themselves. Thus, in 1960, ten of the fifteen largest cities in Minnesota were in the metropolitan area. By 1980 Bloomington, to the south of Minneapolis, may well replace Duluth as Minnesota's third largest city.

Long-delayed legislative reapportionment kept the suburbs' voice unduly weak in any state-instituted metropolitan matter. From 1913 until 1962, Hennepin suburbs together had only one state senator and two representatives, which meant by 1960 a ratio of about six times as many people per member as in Minneapolis, despite the fact that the city was underrepresented in contrast to the rest of the state. Reapportionments in 1962 and again in 1966 gave suburban Hennepin seven senators and fourteen representatives. These new legislators, moreover, have rapidly developed sophistication in acquiring and handling power, so that in the 1965 session they often successfully challenged the established outstate and central city legislative veterans on important matters.

Essentially the same situation prevailed on the Hennepin county board. All of the suburban area was represented by one of the five county commissioners until 1963. Then redistricting extended three of the four city districts into suburban areas. According to some sources this was an attempt to preserve the seats of the city members. If so, it was not entirely successful since one new suburbanite was elected. Suburban control may be as close as the next election.

Minneapolis has a weak mayor-council government and the mayor has less formal power than in any large city in America. Operating under a home-rule charter, the citizens of Minneapolis have repeatedly turned down a charter revision that would provide for a city manager, or for any increase in the mayor's powers. The mayor does not have power to submit a city budget. His appointive and administrative powers are limited to the police force. He or his representative sits with a single vote on multifarious independent boards and commissions that run city activities, under only partial financial control by the city council or a separate Board of Estimates and Taxation. A mayor's influence depends on the extent to which he exhibits personal mass leadership or builds solid partisan backing among the aldermen. Hubert Humphrey (1945–1948) was the outstanding master of this skill.

Ramsey county, the eastern or St. Paul side of the metropolitan area, is the smallest county geographically in the state, occupying 180 square miles. St. Paul, with 74 per cent of the county's population, includes most of this area. Thus the suburban population in Ramsey county cannot out-strip St. Paul because most growth on that side of the area will of necessity take place in surrounding counties.

Relations between the central city and the suburbs in Ramsey county have not shown historic conflicts as in Hennepin. The overwhelming proportion of population in the central city, special governmental arrangements, and different attitudes of officials may explain this. First of all, the Ramsey county board, operating under a special law, has the mayor of St. Paul as chairman. City members of the county board are elected at large. Moreover, city-county functions have been more closely integrated than in Hennepin county. Further, the legislative delegation, at least until the reapportionment of 1966, had few purely suburban seats. Observers have claimed that the combination city-suburban districts restrained potential conflict. Others, however, including those who pushed successfully in 1965–1966 for separate suburban legislative districts, argued that suburban interests had merely been suppressed rather than resolved under the old arrangements, and that the worm was about to turn.

St. Paul itself is one of the few cities in the nation still operating under a commission form of government, that heritage from Galveston which, as one wag put it, has done more damage to American cities than the tidal wave did to Galveston. One modification of the classic model has been made in St. Paul: an independently elected comptroller receives budget estimates from the several departments. Electing all members of the city government at large has meant that individual councilmen who become popular through their pursuit of pet causes or those whose names become especially familiar to the public are virtually unbeatable. St. Paul votes heavily Democratic in state and national elections, but its mayor for three terms (1962–1966) was an assiduous independent in city elections who actively sought the Republican nomination for governor. As in Minneapolis, the St. Paul mayor's leadership is largely informal; he is the chairman of the council but heads no administrative department.

Dakota county lies to the south of St. Paul. The concentration of population, and—to some extent—of problems, in the northern part of Dakota county has led its commissioners to establish a subcourthouse there. Forecasts of urban growth project for Dakota the highest growth rate of any county in the area between now and 1980: almost one and a half times more people than its 1960 total of 78,000.

Washington county, east of St. Paul, has for its county seat Stillwater, one of the oldest communities in the state. The southern part of the county is rapidly acquiring working- and lower middle-class housing developments while the northern part houses the more affluent.

Anoka county occupies the northern part of the metropolitan area. The city of Anoka, the county seat, is presently at the edge of the contiguous urbanized area, although the entire county is within easy commuting distance of Minneapolis and St. Paul. The county's population is heavily working class with a lower than average family income level. The birthrate among the young families living there equals that in some Latin American countries. Their tract houses are built on a sand plain and have private wells and septic tanks. A state health department study showed almost 50 per cent of all suburban wells to be polluted, more than 10 per cent seriously.[4] Exceedingly rapid growth, and the fact that the county is not yet fully urbanized, have resulted in some conflict and alienation between the northern and southern parts of Anoka county.

This thumbnail description of individual counties constituting the metropolitan area points up the fact that the metropolitan area cannot be thought of simply as a unit. There are substantial differences among the counties, which themselves show internal differences. Yet each must be given some consideration as a discrete unit, for counties in Minnesota, while established initially as administrative sub-arms of state government, have acquired ever more attributes of local government, including significant policy-making authority and responsibility for providing local services.

The growth of county functions has given these units of government a new significance in the popular mind. Counties are the primary operating unit of state welfare programs. They have become land-use planning authorities. They are assuming responsibility for providing parks. These functions, with the traditional responsibility for law enforcement, highways, and agricultural development (county agents have become suburban-living advisers in metropolitan counties), make county government busy and important. In some localities in the metropolitan area lack of vigorous municipal government means that the county sheriff is the chief of local police, county highways are the principal streets of the settled areas, and county relief systems are the sole source of health and welfare aids.

[4] Twin City Metropolitan Planning Commission, *Metropolitan Water Study, Pt. II*, Metropolitan Planning Report No. 6 (St. Paul: The Commission, 1960).

Lest it be suspected that a sort of Los Angeles county service-providing arrangement may be developing, however, one should hasten to add that county governments are by no means alone, or even dominant, in providing local services. The burgeoning of municipalities and special districts has been the most remarkable development in postwar metropolitan growth. The five-county Minneapolis–St. Paul metropolitan area contained 261 units of government in 1962. Besides the 5 counties, there were 105 cities and villages, 86 school districts, 51 townships, and 14 special districts. Without major annexation by Minneapolis and St. Paul after 1890, urban growth resulted in many new incorporations, and twice as many villages have been created in the metropolitan area since 1945 as were formed from 1900 to 1945. By far the most common type of incorporation action has been simply to transform the old townships into villages.

Unlike New England towns, which initially at least had some geographic rationale, Minnesota's townships were the six-mile-square surveyor's townships, strictly a mapping convenience, following no natural features except major rivers or lakes, although none crossed county lines. Not only were the powers of townships too limited to meet urban service demands (although the legislature gave them special status as "urban towns" with most of the powers of villages), but also the direct democracy they practiced became impractical as the population grew. So incorporation to a representative form of government such as a village was obviously the thing to do.

School districts in Minnesota are independent units of government, each with its own popularly elected board and its own taxing and decision-making powers subject to increasingly close state regulation. In recent years school districts have been under considerable pressure from the state Department of Education to consolidate, so that by 1965 the seven-county metropolitan area had only 69 out of an original 252 school districts remaining. Two additional independent school districts were created, one for the city of Minneapolis and one for the city of St. Paul, to separate the schools from regular city government. In the densely settled suburbs near the cities, the independent districts are generally very large geographically. This gives the obvious advantages sought in consolidation; but since the district lines do not ordinarily follow municipal lines, one school district often encompasses several municipalities, and some municipalities are split among several districts.

While the separateness of the several components of the Minneapolis–St. Paul metropolitan area—major cities, counties, suburban municipalities, and school districts—deserves emphasis, there are some governmental jurisdictions overlying the other divisons and including more than one of the basic governmental units. These more nearly areawide governments include the Minneapolis–St. Paul Sanitary District, the Metropolitan Airports Commission, and the Metropolitan Mosquito Control District. Moreover, the Twin Cities Metropolitan Planning Commission, technically a state agency, had served the entire area. In addition, there is a less comprehensive regional district for hospital administration, one for sewage disposal in a few suburbs, as well as county soil conservation districts and one county park reserve district.

The principal special districts were created one by one by the legislature in response to insistent demands that a desired service be performed by a single agency. Thus, the Airports Commission was given control of all local airports and was able to raise funds by taxation to build one giant facility for the entire region.

Areawide civic associations grew hopeful in 1967 that the legislature would create a strong elected metropolitan council, or at least a coordinating committee for these many areawide functions. Unfortunately, a 1958 state constitutional amendment, in the guise of strengthening home rule, gave every municipality a veto over special legislation that affected it. This amendment had to be voided by the legislature in order to make metropolitan government undertakings possible. A metropolitan council appointed by the governor was established, which absorbed the Metropolitan Planning Commission and got certain veto powers over local actions with metropolitan implications.

In the absence of some such multi-purpose governmental unit, the legislative delegations from Hennepin and Ramsey counties have exercised what authority the state exerts over the parts of the area. These large delegations require near unanimity in their caucuses on local legislation. Minority rule has often stymied change in local governments, but when local legislators have agreed on a package of local alterations the legislature has willingly gone along.

State administrative agencies have the customary supervisory and report-requiring powers over their functional agents at county and municipal levels. In many instances, notably water pollution control, this authority has not been exercised vigorously.

To summarize, in the Minneapolis–St. Paul metropolitan area, the following appear to be the most significant facets of the demographic, economic, social, and political setting in which governmental organization for mental health is to be observed: (1) The area is growing rapidly in population. (2) Almost all recent growth has been in suburban areas. The central cities, formerly dominant in population, industry, and politics, now stand at no better than parity with the suburbs, and their position will continue to decline. (3) Minneapolis–St. Paul has a smaller nonwhite population than most metropolitan areas its size or larger. (4) The economic base of the area is steady—well diversified and growing, but handicapped because of a declining hinterland. (5) The area contains a vast multiplicity of government units, but the counties and the state have taken over a few functions formerly exercised by townships and municipalities. (6) The metropolitan area has been strongly bifurcated between its two central cities, and this fact affects every activity. (7) Governments of the cities and counties are not well organized for exertion of strong leadership.

FORMAL STRUCTURE AND OPERATIONS OF MENTAL HEALTH PROGRAMS

Minnesota operates seven state mental hospitals and two nursing homes. Each offers complete psychiatric care for a precisely defined area. Special alcoholic units, however, are operated at only two of the hospitals. One serves as the major medical and surgical unit for all patients in the state. In addition there is a special state security hospital for dangerous patients and a new intensive treatment center for adolescents located in the Minneapolis–St. Paul metropolitan area. Two of the regular state hospitals are located in counties now on the fringes of the urbanized area.

State officials claim that the Minnesota mental hospitals are not the stereotyped snakepits that modern doctrine seeks to eliminate. In the first place, patient population runs from only 695 to 1,820, with a total of 8,004 beds in all institutions. Furthermore, the primary emphasis of the hospitals is treatment, not mere custodial care. About 70 per cent of their space is now "open-door," that is, without restraint, and 50 per cent of the new admissions are voluntary. Occupancy has been reduced by a large-scale evacuation of senile patients to nursing homes in an attempt to allow the hospital staffs to concentrate upon treatment of the acutely ill. Patient population dropped from 11,300 in 1954 to 7,700 in 1964, where it has stabilized or increased slightly. The median length of hospitalization has remained at about ten years. Significantly larger numbers of patients are staying less than five years and more than twenty years, while the numbers staying five to twenty years have dropped substantially. State medical personnel believe that custodial functions cannot be completely ended because some place is needed for the schizophrenics until cure or prevention is possible, or until intensive rehabilitation guidance and long-term sheltered workshops are available for them.

Despite the progress in medical care that has been achieved, private professional observers describe conditions in the hospitals as "abysmal." The drop in average patient load, which some hoped would lessen the need for staff, actually has emphasized the shortage of trained personnel, because those patients who remain are in need of intensive care. State medical officials, while proud of the relative progress, recognize these needs and constantly press for more staff. They have begun a special program to combat depersonalization, hoping to create an attitude among the staff that will help a patient maintain his sense of individual dignity. Furthermore, they are reevaluating their patient work programs to ensure that all work assignments are therapeutic rather than exploitative.

In response to the critical need for more residential treatment facilities for children, the state legislature in 1963 authorized a Minnesota Residential Treatment Center at Lino Lakes on the northwestern fringe of the metropolitan area. It was proposed to the state legislature as a unit that would provide intensive treatment for emotionally disturbed or psychotic children. The large initial and operating expense of the center was justified on the basis that this intensive treatment would mean most of these children could be returned to the community after a few months and the state would be spared the cost of providing long-term custodial care.

The state maintains three major institutions for the mentally retarded. None of these is in the Minneapolis–St. Paul metropolitan area proper, although one is close to it. There are three state special schools for the retarded, two of which are in or near the metropolitan area. These institutions are large (up to 3,000 patients), dangerously overcrowded, have two-year waiting lists, and are critically understaffed. All of these state mental institutions are under the direction of the state Department of Welfare, Division of Medical Services.

In related fields, the Youth Conservation Division of the state Department of Corrections operates training centers for boys and girls and a diagnostic center at Lino Lakes in the metropolitan area. The latter institution is physically the other half of the Welfare Department's intensive treatment center for adolescents. All youthful offenders convicted of crime and juveniles judged delinquent are committed to the Youth Conservation Commission. The Lino Lakes facility is the intake unit, where a decision is made regarding the treatment and the facility that will be the most productive for each young person. It is not a treatment facility. The Adult Corrections Division operates the state prison and the men's and women's reformatories.

The state has an Advisory Board on Problems of Alcoholism and an alcoholism unit far down the hierarchy of the state Department of Health, which has no significant treatment program. However, two state mental hospitals have units for alcoholics. Another agency closely related to mental health is the Governor's Citizens Council on Aging in the Department of Welfare, a promotional group which operates no facilities.

A Vocational Rehabilitation and Special Education Division, part of the state Department of Education, supervises public school programs for the mentally retarded. Minnesota now requires that all school districts have a consultant in this area and one for the emotionally disturbed.

The concentration of mental health activities in the state Department of Welfare avoids some of the major departmental rivalry over the control of mental health activities typical elsewhere. Such separation as there is—welfare, corrections, rehabilitation—results from the problem of defining mental health, a difficulty that shows up at all levels. For example, what kinds of people should be dealt with by a mental hospital and what kinds by a prison? A former state corrections commissioner stated that approximately 30 per cent of all inmates of the state prison and reformatories should be treated by mental hospitals. Despite the efforts by the Minnesota criminal control agencies to emphasize rehabilitation and correction, relatively little is done for those who are mentally ill. Very severe cases are transferred to the state security hospital. The state prison offers some psychiatric services on a consultative basis.

The same problem of definition occurs with juveniles. One child internalizes his maladjustments and is treated for mental illness; another acts out his aggressions and gets into trouble with the law. The state training school for boys is not staffed for medical psychiatric care, although it has psychiatric social workers.

Similarly, the distinction between vocational rehabilitation and welfare activities on behalf of discharged mental patients is not easy to draw for administrative purposes. Giving the state Department of Education responsibility for vocational education, thus separating it from other aspects of treating the mentally ill, has both advantages and disadvantages. On the disadvantage side, welfare workers charge that vocational rehabilitation people are more concerned with numbers than with cure. Welfare workers often feel that the vocational rehabilitation counselors hesitate to invest their time in a client unless he has a high likelihood of becoming employable. They assert that the vocational rehabilitation people gladly skim off those former mental patients who are almost certain to be placed in a job, leaving to the welfare workers the hard cases they believe to be unemployable. The Hennepin county welfare mental health unit has assigned one person to find jobs for these marginal people. The success rate has been low, but finding jobs for even seven or eight per month of the seventy-five on the list is considered worthwhile.

On the other hand, the state Vocational Rehabilitation Division has a strong commitment to rehabilitating mental patients and has long had its counselors assigned to state mental hospitals on a part-time basis. The state hospitals have now become more rehabilitation conscious, although rehabilitation personnel believe planning must begin when the patient comes to the hospital, not immediately prior to discharge. The Vocational Rehabilitation Division pays for the evaluation of many mentally ill patients by private agencies such as the Minneapolis Rehabilitation Center. It originally helped to establish Circle F (a Minneapolis club for social rehabilitation of the mentally ill) and still buys services from private agencies.

The community mental health centers in Minnesota vary in the degree of vocational rehabilitation they attempt. The degree of coordination between a mental health center and the vocational rehabilitation agency seems to be dependent upon the outlook of the local medical and welfare personnel. Fragmentation of mental health care also arises from the attempt to distinguish mental retardation from mental illness. The public school programs for educable and trainable mentally retarded are administered from the state level by a part of the Vocational Rehabilitation and Special Education Division of the Department of Education. But the state institutions for the retarded are administered by the Department of Welfare's Medical Services Division.

In this latter instance, the state association for the mentally retarded feels its cause has been neglected by the medical people who run the mental health program, and most of the professionals and administrators admit that the feeling is justified. But psychiatrists insist that programs for the retarded should be kept under medical control. Programs for the retarded have not been given the attention or the funds that they need. Groups for the retarded, on the other hand, do not acknowledge any need for medical direction. They claim they will seek medical consultation for diagnosis and treatment when needed. State planning for the new federal mental health and mental retardation programs has been divided in Minnesota, but this has caused no debilitating controversy.

The Board of Health for a long time had the most to do with community mental health activities, since it was the state agency that dispensed Hill-Burton hospital construction funds. It supported additions of psychiatric wings to general hospitals that could demonstrate potential by having at least two psychiatrists available to use such facilities. All except one of the qualifying hospitals were located in the Twin Cities metropolitan area. Even with federal mental health center construction funds available, Hill-Burton grants would support less than comprehensive inpatient facilities. A happy bit of coordination came about when the executive officer of the state Board of Health was named chairman of the facilities committee of the state mental health planning committee. Then the facilities committee was designated to serve also as the group that screened applications for construction of mental health centers under the new program. Thus, the experience of the Board of Health in processing hospital construction applications was put to use, and conflicts were avoided.

The University of Minnesota is a separate public corporation, and although it is independent of direct state control it is dependent to a large extent upon state funds. The legislature elects the regents, who constitute the governing body of the university. A special appropriation is made to the university hospitals to provide medical care to the indigent, a service begun in 1913. Since for a long time this was the only direct service of the university to rural areas, it has been an important political asset to the university in its relations with the legislature. The medical staff of the university hospitals is periodically reminded that medical care of indigents is one of the principal services of the university. County welfare boards were established in 1937, and since 1950 funding for indigent medical care has been spread to other sources. But indigent psychiatric service is more valuable to counties than are the other medical specialties. If a county certifies that a mental patient is indigent, and if he is admitted to the university hospital, the university pays the entire cost, whereas the county must pay half for the other medical services. The reason for the exception is to enable the university to compete with state mental hospitals for patients for teaching purposes. For counties without mental health centers, or with inadequate centers, the university is virtually the only source of psychiatric care besides the state mental hospitals. For children, it has been the counties' only resource. But because it must serve the whole state it cannot handle all the needs of any single county.

A psychiatric unit was first established at the university in 1929 and the psychopathic hospital was established in 1945. Presently the psychiatric resources of the university include inpatient, outpatient, and child psychiatry departments, as well as a rehabilitation center. The facilities are available only on referral from doctors. The Psychiatry Department, unique within the hospital, controls its own admissions, again apparently for teaching reasons. This does not mean that only patients with unusual problems are desired; students need run-of-the-mill clients as well. The university claims to have a minimal waiting list, one day for adults and seven days for children. The admissions officers think the number refused is small, and probably random, yet county welfare officials talk about two-year waiting periods for child care. The present university psychiatric staff is intensely community-psychiatry and service oriented, and metropolitan health centers report no difficulty in referrals.

The University of Minnesota must also be considered a local resource for the metropolitan area. Located virtually in the center of the metropolitan area, the university is a part of the community in many ways. Its many specialists are as close as a local phone call for professional consultation. The medical, social service, and administrative staffs are available for service on community committees. Thus Community Health and Welfare Council mental health committees are often led by university faculty, and the head of the Psychiatry Department is on the Hennepin County Mental Health Center board.

A highly significant role of the university in the community is its control of staffing in all the public hospitals. The Dean's Committee (the heads of the Medical School departments) makes joint appointments in the university hospital and on the staffs of Hennepin County General Hospital, Ramsey County–St. Paul General Hospital, and the Veterans Administration Hospital in Minneapolis. In effect, the university committee is responsible for professional care at those other hospitals and all the residents and interns are supplied by the university. This relationship has a two-way importance. The university can assure its medical students competent instruction, and the hospitals benefit by being able to attract first-rate staff and being assured of a complete supply of qualified residents and interns.

Many St. Paul–Ramsey welfare leaders resent this "octupus stranglehold" on the public hospitals. They think the university is motivated only by the selfish desire to have its graduates trained at someone else's expense. The St. Paul people also believe the university doctors are too research-oriented and make unreasonable demands on records and facilities. Some local officeholders, expressing their resentment of the situation, and desiring more prestige for St. Paul (the university Medical School is, after all, in Minneapolis) started a movement for a separate medical school in St. Paul, based on their own cluster of private hospitals and several undergraduate colleges, of which the community is deservedly proud.

Some mental health services are provided for the metropolitan area by the federal government through the Veterans Administration. A local VA Hospital maintains a 102-bed psychiatric unit and provides inpatient psychiatric treatment primarily for acute, short-term cases. Cases not connected with the military are accepted, but according to these priorities: (1) emergency cases, (2) service-connected disability cases, and (3) non-service-connected disability cases. The hospital itself maintains an outpatient service for veterans with non-service-connected psychiatric illnesses, since they are not eligible for treatment from the VA's Mental Hygiene Clinic. The hospital treats about 800 patients annually, of which more than half are from the metropolitan area. Since psychiatric unit occupancy averages more than 98 per cent, there is frequently a waiting list for those who do not need immediate treatment. Long-term psychiatric care for the chronically ill veterans from the metropolitan area is provided by a large VA Psychiatric Hospital at St. Cloud, about seventy miles from the Twin Cities.

In general the Veterans Administration appears to provide its clients comparatively good psychiatric services, both inpatient and outpatient. The VA Hospitals spends about two and a half times as much per patient-day as do the Minnesota state hospitals, and the ratio is similar for the Mental Hygiene Clinic. Of course, the VA has the additional advantage of a well-defined patient population and a relatively constant demand.

The Veterans Administration mental health programs are distinct from other community mental health resources. There is little interchange of either information or clients, for example, between the VA Mental Hygiene Clinic and the community mental health centers in the metropolitan area. Still these closed system characteristics are mitigated somewhat by contacts among professionals on the staffs of the several facilities. Some VA mental health personnel hold faculty posts at the university and the VA outpatient clinic is affiliated with the university as a training center.

The principal local government mental health programs are conducted by the community mental health centers. Three of the five metropolitan area counties operated community centers in 1965. It is more difficult to identify the other mental health programs of local government departments, since they deal with aspects of behavior not generally thought of as solely mental health problems—antisocial behavior, dependency, family problems. The mental health activities of court services and welfare departments will be mentioned briefly later.

The Hennepin County Mental Health Center in Minneapolis comes the closest to being comprehensive of any center in Minnesota. But its own priorities are for clinical work, training, and research, in that order. The center offers inpatient, outpatient, day-care, night-care, and emergency service, and it carries on some research. It conducts regular consultation with teachers and with public health nurses. The staff initially rejected community education, in the sense of talking to groups about what they do. They felt such a role would be presumptuous, since the university specialists and mental health association spokesmen were so readily available. But in 1964 the Hennepin county center reported thirty such contacts. Another educational activity is an experiment in mental health guidance for parents of normal children, which is conducted on a voluntary, tuition basis, one day a week for twelve weeks.

The services of the Hennepin County Community Mental Health Center are generally regarded as excellent. The professional qualifications of the psychiatric staff are high, and the medical director is hyperactive in pursuit of ideas. Its teaching association with the University of Minnesota attracts the cream of interns from the area. The center is not, however, beyond criticism. For some time it had no facilities for adolescents and in off-hours interns are assigned to emergency services.

The Hennepin county center presents a special problem for overall hospital administration because it is at the same time both the psychiatric department of the county general hospital and an agency with broader responsibilities. Since the center receives some funds from the state, and because it has a specially constituted board to formulate policy, members of its staff feel they should have more independence in determining their own workload, in assigning and classifying their own personnel, and in evaluating their own accomplishments. As a result there have been frictions, culminating in a public dispute between the director of the center and the professional administrator of the hospital.

Ramsey county's mental health center was established much later than Hennepin's and is not as large. Yet it is a vast improvement over earlier facilities. Most social agencies in St. Paul are sympathetic toward its problems and charitable in their expressions about the operation of the new mental health center. There have been staffing difficulties and the center has lacked continuous strong leadership.

Like Hennepin, the Ramsey County Mental Health Center is the outpatient psychiatric facility of the county's general hospital. There is an inpatient service, but it must be kept administratively separate, since the state will not match expenses for inpatient service. It was feared that otherwise the centers might become small state hospitals without direct state control. However, the state restriction is a fiction which is largely budgetary and does not present insuperable obstacles medically. But when an outpatient of the center is admitted to the hospital, the separation can be annoying, because the same doctor is supposed to follow him and treat him. If an inpatient is put on outpatient status, the inpatient staff continues to treat him. The Ramsey Mental Health Center provides day-care only through one of the Amity Clubs, which are social or discussion groups for former patients. The center staff also works with school counselors and gives lectures to the staffs of voluntary agencies as well as consulting on individual cases.

One part of the county Welfare Boards' work that can be classified as mental health activity is providing aftercare for discharged mental patients, and the Ramsey County Welfare Board has such a unit. Much of the regular intake interviewing and supportive counseling by welfare workers also includes elements of mental health. As the former chairman of a local welfare board stated, "Most cases can be cured with money. If you had eight kids and $64 a month, you'd be mentally ill, too."

In Minnesota, court services operate under the state district court but are paid for by the county. They handle probation and parole, pre-sentence investigations, and supervision of divorce settlements. Hennepin county has a superb court service unit, deeply involved in mental health activities. It employs three part-time psychiatrists, three full-time psychologists, and various medical people. Fifty of its social workers have master's degrees. A detention home for juveniles is maintained but its thirty beds are not sufficient for the need.

One of the results of local government fragmentation is that the level of service in units bearing the same names is quite different. Community mental health centers in Minnesota, formed under the same law and given the same name, differ greatly in the kind and quality of services. This is partly by design since psychiatrists feel that different communities have widely different mental health needs. This may be true within a metropolitan area, because different kinds of people live in different parts of the suburban area. Dakota County Mental Health Center officials feel that their working-class people expect a much more directive approach. Such people do not want to hear about deep-seated origins of their behavior; they want a shot or a pill or to be told what to do. Such an approach might not work in a higher-class suburb, where people's ideas of psychiatry lean more to nondirective psychoanalysis for self-understanding.

Furthermore, mental health services of certain kinds may already be available in a community, or only one kind of service may be in short supply. Promoters of a new center may feel they could not gather sufficient support unless they could promise to meet critical needs and not duplicate existing services. For these reasons the first step in establishing a new center is to have a community study itself and determine what it wants in the way of additional mental health services.

At least the local mental health board should draw up a list of goals to submit to applicants for the directorship of their center so that they do not hire someone who will not satisfy their expectations.

Unfortunately in most instances, a community is not able to formulate a clear statement of what it wants. It is more likely that the psychiatrist they retain will be the one who convinces the board that his program is what they need. Especially in the rural areas of the state where there are few psychiatrists, the board has little choice. In effect a potential director may be able to say, "Take me or leave me; love me, love my doctrine." This is probably the best explanation for the founding of Minnesota's most radical mental health center, located in the northern part of the state. It is headed by a highly respected former University of Minnesota psychiatrist who chose the northwoods area because he liked to fish and hunt. He organized his center's program on the theory that the psychiatrist should not treat anybody but should spend all his time as a consultant to the other professionals and subprofessionals in the community—ministers, physicians, teachers, police—and they in turn should do whatever mental health work is done. This approach has been widely reported and generally applauded, although its effectiveness continues to be studied.

For all these reasons, the centers in Minnesota are vastly different and usually reflect the motivations of their director. The state medical services department does not seem to be worried about these differences, or it may realize that control of psychiatric services in any case would be difficult. Instead, the state has instituted rigorous standards of qualification for the staff of any center it supports.

The Hennepin County Mental Health Center in Minneapolis and the Ramsey County–St. Paul center are almost completely medically oriented. They treat the sick and only, they hope, acutely ill. Initially this was their only mission. Since their original establishment they have moved slowly toward a broader program of community services. It should be noted that they do not treat the long-term chronic cases, who may well constitute the most seriously ill.

This very lack of comprehensive approach opens the Hennepin center to criticism. It means that the center is doing only part of the mental health job in the community. Someone else—other local government agencies or private agencies—must pick up the remainder. But the existence of separate agencies emphasizes the need for coordination, and coordination is always less than perfect. Some of the private voluntary associations think the center is too medically oriented, that it does not have a broad enough concept of mental health. The Hennepin Mental Health Center, they charge, does not see the relation of family, job, and community pressures to mental illness. Outsiders think the center staff feel themselves superior because they are under medical direction. The center insists upon treating a referral as a new case and makes a new diagnosis, and sometimes the referring agency is not informed of the disposition of a case.

One of the consequences of fragmentation of services among local governments and between agencies is that several jurisdictions may each be dealing with a single problem of a mentally ill person. These contacts with different agencies not only may be ineffective, but at times contradictory. The Ramsey County Welfare Department has achieved some measure of fame with its "family-centered" approach. All contacts with a given family are coordinated through a single case worker and this approach is now the official policy of the state Welfare Department. Hennepin Community Mental Health Center is arranging family conferences including representatives from all agencies dealing with the individual, but much remains to be done before the system will be effective.

The public school system of the Twin Cities metropolitan area is highly fragmented. In 1965 sixty-nine independent school districts remained in the five-county metropolitan area, with Hennepin county alone divided into nearly forty districts. Enrollment ranges from 72,000 in Special District No. 1 (with the same boundaries as Minneapolis) to less than 500 in several of the districts in western Hennepin county. Since school services in the mental health field are provided essentially on a district-by-district basis, the tremendous population and financial resource disparities among the metropolitan districts results in great differences in the level of services available.

This fragmentation at the local level is further complicated by the fact that school districts occasionally cut across county lines. Since most local mental health services, such as community mental health centers, are provided by counties in Minnesota, inequities occur. For example, one of the most populous school districts in the metropolitan area includes parts of Hennepin and Anoka counties. Hennepin county had a community mental health center to which those children within the school district who resided in Hennepin county could be referred by the school authorities. Anoka county, however, was without a community mental health center, and thus children in the same school who were Anoka residents were not eligible for service. A similar situation exists in the southern end of the metropolitan area. The Dakota County Mental Health Center had established good relationships with the school counselors in a two-county district, only to have to refuse to serve some pupils because they happened to live in Carver county.

As with other social service agencies, it is difficult to determine the extent to which schools are providing mental health services. Presumably, school nurses, social workers, counselors, and visiting teachers are involved. School psychologists and consulting psychiatrists can quite clearly be classified as participants in treating mental illness.

In order for the schools legally to involve themselves in a mental illness case there must be a school problem, and normally this means the child must present some sort of behavior or learning problem to his teacher. The school's basic role in mental illness programs is one of finding cases. Particular school districts may provide limited psychiatric, psychological, or neurological services for emotionally or mentally disturbed students, but in cases where intensive or prolonged treatment is necessary the schools refer them to public or private agencies.

School districts in Minnesota bear the primary responsibility by law for educating mentally retarded children. Retardates are classified as trainable if their IQ is below 50. Those above this level are classified as educable and must, by law, be educated by the local district. Local school districts may choose whether to provide classes for the trainables.

Minneapolis' public school system was one of the first in the country to provide mental health services for students. A child study unit was established in 1924. Psychiatric, psychological, and neurological services for the one hundred separate schools in the district are channeled through this central department. Direct referral to Hennepin County Mental Health Center is made in more extreme cases.

Minneapolis community resources for mental illness have been found by school people to be generally adequate. Emergency help is always forthcoming. The Child Study Department feels that it has been most fortunate in obtaining good consulting specialists. The chief psychologist in the department noted that, although it pays its consultants minimum fees, it has no trouble in getting help. Establishment of the Hennepin

County Mental Health Center has been particularly helpful to the Minneapolis school programs, and private community agencies have also been used extensively by the schools. Cooperation is particularly close between the Washburn Clinic, an outpatient facility that specializes in the treatment of children with emotional and behavioral problems; the mental health facilities at the University of Minnesota are also used on occasion.

School authorities sometimes feel the mental health center does not continue treatment of children long enough and that it is frequently difficult to find hospital and residential treatment facilities. Diagnostic services generally seem adequate but there appears to be a shortage of community treatment services. The Child Study Department notes that case-finding has improved as individual teachers become more aware of the problems and their signs.

The St. Paul public school district provides similar services in the mental health area through referrals, a Child Study Department, and special classes for the retarded. The St. Paul schools are beginning to make use of the expanded mental health services available at the local level since the establishment of a Child Psychiatry Division in the Ramsey County Mental Health Center. Their major community resource, however, remains the Wilder Child Guidance Clinic, with which the schools have long maintained close relations. Wilder Clinic, however, is able to accept only about one half the referrals made by the schools. The University of Minnesota facilities remain an important secondary resource for St. Paul schools.

Some mention should be made of the fact that the mental health services provided by the public schools are not paralleled in the parochial systems. The public schools operate the only existing classes for retardates, and other than making referrals, the parochial schools provide no services for mentally ill students. Services of the Child Study Departments in Minneapolis and St. Paul, however, are available to parochial students.

In the numerous suburban districts, school mental health services vary greatly. There seems, however, to be an effort to increase services of this kind. A number of independent school districts are in the process of adding psychologists to their medical staffs. Almost every district's program for retarded children is undergoing expansion. Within the larger, wealthier suburban districts, mental health services seem to be on a par with, or better than, those found in the central cities. Edina-Morningside, for instance, employs three psychologists for a school population of less than 10,000, while Minneapolis employs nine psychologists for more than 70,000 students. Edina operates some six classes for retarded children and seems to utilize community mental health resources as much as does Minneapolis. This is to be contrasted with a poorer and more sparsely populated district like Blaine in Anoka county, which employs no psychologist.

Some effort has been made to overcome the fragmentation in school mental health programs that results from the existence of numerous independent districts. Informal cooperation among neighboring districts is fairly common. For example, if one district does not employ a psychologist while one nearby does, whenever the first needs the services of a psychologist it usually is able to contract for the second district's psychologist on a fee basis. Some outlying suburban districts contract with one of the two large urban districts for mental health services. The Education Research and Development Council at the university received a grant to establish an interdistrict program for the trainable retarded. The program, called the Cooperative School Rehabilitation Center, includes some thirty-eight districts and enables these districts to provide services which they would not otherwise be able to furnish, since there are seldom enough trainable retardates in a single suburban district to justify establishing a special class.

To some extent, fragmentation in public school mental health programs is overcome by the efforts of other agencies providing mental health services. The county community mental health centers, for example, have worked with public school staff personnel to increase their case-finding ability in order to facilitate referrals, and school nurses in most metropolitan school districts have been familiarized with the operations of the centers, but the existence of both public and private schools creates a problem in that public school nurses do not serve parochial school children. The public health nursing service, which is under the county, fills this responsibility.

Public school nurses are thought by some to have the best access to homes for initiating mental health treatment or referral. Families are accustomed to home visits by school nurses, whereas they might resent visits by school or county social workers or juvenile authorities.

Schools come in for some criticism for their failure to detect mental illness early. Juvenile officials charge, for example, that they are never called in until overt acts of violence or serious maladjustment are displayed. They believe if teachers were alert they could detect potential trouble earlier. It is charged that teachers, especially in the elementary grades, hesitate to call for assistance lest they be thought incompetent disciplinarians.

The extent to which general social service agencies are involved in mental health programs is difficult to assess, but taken together they represent a considerable community resource. More than one hundred social workers and counselors are employed and they annually see over ten thousand individuals in the metropolitan area. Agencies like the Family and Children's Service of Minneapolis and St. Paul and the various sectarian agencies offer a wide range of services that include family counseling, foster home care, homemaker services, and adoption services. Strictly defined, these agencies are only indirectly involved in mental health programs. They have neither the professional resources nor the desire to treat clients with severe psychological or emotional problems. They serve primarily as case-finders and referral agencies for community mental health facilities. On the other hand, it seems fairly obvious that in providing many of their regular services they are making some contributions in the mental health field. The state Welfare Department's study of problem families in Anoka county found that 21 per cent of the total caseload of social service agencies were also known to mental health agencies. More significantly, 58.4 per cent of the mental health agency cases were known to the social service agencies. One family counseling agency executive reported that at least 95 per cent of the people they see have psychological problems.

Voluntary hospital psychiatric services for the mentally ill are available from eight general hospitals in the Twin Cities in addition to Homewood, a small psychiatric hospital, and Glenwood Hills, which was formerly a 300-bed psychiatric hospital but now has converted some of its beds to general medical use. Most hospital psychiatric facilities are of recent origin. The state Board of Health encouraged the establishment of a number of these units with the aid of Hill-Burton funds. Units at Northwestern and Abbott Hospitals were added within the last two years and newly expanded units have been set up at Fairview,

St. Mary's, and St. Joseph's Hospitals. At present there are some 500 private psychiatric beds available in the Twin Cities. On the average, about 6,000 patients are treated annually.

The inpatient services available at these private hospitals consist of electro-shock therapy, medication, and occupational therapy. The only outpatient psychiatric service provided by the hospitals consists of electro-shock therapy. Most of the cases admitted to the private hospitals have neurotic or comparatively mild psychological symptoms. These hospitals are equipped to deal with only a small number of severe cases since few closed wards are available, although more are being added. The cost per day in a private psychiatric hospital averages about $35 to $40, and since most health insurance does not cover this type of illness, patients tend to be drawn from the more well-to-do classes. In view of this fact and the moderate nature of the illnesses of most private hospital psychiatric patients, the contribution made by the private hospitals in providing mental health services is probably less than one would have imagined. The state hospitals receive almost everyone who is seriously ill.

Until the recent establishment of the state facility at Lino Lakes, which has not appreciably fulfilled the metropolitan area's requirements for care of mentally ill children, virtually the only residential treatment units available were privately operated. Five such units are scattered about the metropolitan area. In all, they have a capacity of 170 children, which is woefully inadequate. Almost every private social service agency questioned mentioned the unavailability of residental treatment facilities for young people as a major problem. It is particularly difficult to place children who present severe behavior problems since most of these private units are equipped only to handle moderately disturbed children.

Three mental health clinics supplying public services are operated under private auspices in the Twin Cities. Each is supported in a small way by the state as a community mental health center. The Hamm Memorial Psychiatric Clinic in St. Paul provides individual, family, and group psychotherapy for adults with limited ability to pay. The Wilder Child Guidance Clinic, established in the 1920s, has grown into one of St. Paul's leading mental health resources.

The presence of two private clinics providing some services to the people in the community unable to pay for treatment is a possible explanation for St. Paul's tardiness in securing a public community mental health center. The directors of the private clinics, however, have consistently urged the establishment of a public treatment center, pointing out that their privately operated mental health programs were meeting only a fraction of the community's needs.

Washburn Memorial Clinic in Minneapolis provides outpatient psychiatric treatment for children. This clinic has a much smaller staff and caseload than the Wilder Clinic, and when one considers that its service area, the Minneapolis community, has almost twice as many people as does Wilder's service area, the proportional difference becomes even greater. Perhaps, then, the absence of anything approximating adequate private mental health clinic facilities in Minneapolis contributed to the relatively early establishment of a community mental health center for Hennepin county.

There are a number of privately financed social rehabilitation programs in the Twin Cities. Among the agencies with such programs are Circle F, the Minneapolis Rehabilitation Center, the Rehabilitation Center and Workshop of Greater St. Paul, the Kenny Institute, and the Minneapolis Curative Workshop. To some extent, all of them deal with mental health problems.

The basic sociopolitical division of the metropolitan area into two substantially distinct areas is reflected in those mental health programs operated under private auspices. Separate "Greater" United Fund organizations exist—one in Minneapolis and one in St. Paul, which include their proximate suburbs. Fragmentation of services between the two cities is obvious. For example, the Catholic and the Jewish family agencies in Minneapolis provide services related to mental health that are virtually identical with those provided by another Catholic agency and another Jewish agency in St. Paul. Of the three privately operated mental health clinics in the Twin Cities, the two in St. Paul, Wilder and Hamm, do not accept clients from Minneapolis and its suburbs, while the Washburn Clinic in Minneapolis accepts very few residents from Ramsey county. Little coordination exists between most Minneapolis and St. Paul agencies engaged in similar mental health programs. For example, both the Wilder and Washburn Clinics treat emotionally disturbed children but there is virtually no contact, either formal or informal, between them.

In addition to this basic split between private mental health programs in Minneapolis and St. Paul, further fragmentation occurs within the two cities. Family services programs are duplicated internally by various sectarian agencies and nonsectarian agencies. In Minneapolis persons with identical problems may seek help from the Catholic Welfare (if a Catholic), from the Lutheran Social Service (if he is a member of one of several synods), from the Jewish Family Service (whether or not Jewish), or from the Family and Children's Service (if he is a resident of Hennepin county). Eight Twin Cities' private general hospitals operate small psychiatric units and five small privately operated residual treatment units for children are located in the area.

Formal coordination among various agencies providing mental health services is limited. Informal coordination by means of cross referrals, splitting cases, and the like is more frequently the case. An agency like Family Service in St. Paul may refer a client to the Hamm Clinic for certain problems but Family Service will remain active in other aspects of the case.

The social service agencies themselves seem to feel there is some informal coordination, at least within their city, St. Paulites in particular. The director of the Wilder Child Guidance Clinic believes a close interrelationship exists between members of his staff and other groups and boards of directors in the community. He has served on many boards such as the Community Chest, United Jewish Council, Children's Council, and has found a good deal of interplay. The Wilder Clinic seems to serve as a principal coordinator for St. Paul mental health programs because it has some connection with almost every private social service agency in the city and can function as an important information source. Something of the same web of informal communication and coordination exists in Minneapolis but it is apparently much weaker. For one thing, no private agency is involved deeply enough with most other private mental health resources to serve as a central coordinator.

Most observers have been critical of interagency relationships. Few workers are in a position to see more than their own agency. Supervisors of Community Information and Referral Services are in the best position to judge, and in both cities these people stressed the serious lack of information and coordination among agencies. Staff at the Referral Services estimate that they spend 25 per cent of their time on inquiries from other agencies about who provides certain services.

The Community Health and Welfare Council of Hennepin county is the principal coordinating force. Once the research arm of the United Fund agency, it is now officially separate, though the United Fund relies on it exclusively for recommendations on which agencies should be admitted to the Fund, and how contributions should be divided. The council was separated from the Fund so that it could participate in government health and welfare programs, which spend ten times more than do the private agencies. The council operates through committees that survey areas of need and recommend programs to answer the needs. The committees are broadly based in the community, drawing heavily upon professional and technical people from the University of Minnesota Medical School or School of Social Work as well as prominent lay citizens. Each committee is staffed by a professional employee of the council. The whole operation is supervised by a dynamic, persuasive, and tenacious organizer, who participates in most community decisions within his area of interest. Thus, under Health and Welfare Council direction the need for improved psychiatric services for children and adolescents was assessed, documented, and decided. In addition to urging facilities for young people in the mental health center, the director persuaded a Catholic orphanage to become a residence for disturbed boys when its original function was no longer needed.

In addition to community research, the Health and Welfare Council serves as entrepreneur for some action programs. It has received a federal grant for juvenile delinquency control, as well as one in the poverty program. The council administers these projects but operates them through the Board of Education, the Welfare Department, and the Family and Children's Services. The council has influenced community action by supplying imaginative ideas to public leaders. Then its officials help to persuade other formal government decision makers to accept these proposals, which someone else appears to be initiating. In every instance in this study where a public figure was identified as the originator or sponsor of a program in mental health or related fields, the Community Health and Welfare Council director was found to be involved also. In St. Paul the planning agency is still a part of the United Fund. The director must divide his time between the fund-raising activities and planning. Only recently have the planning staffs of Minneapolis and St. Paul United Funds had formal liaison with each other, even to the extent of having lunch together once a week. Under a former administration, members of the St. Paul staff were forbidden to have contact with their Minneapolis counterparts.

A formal coordinating body for community agencies has been established in each city to serve as an information and referral service. Its purpose is not to tell the several private and public agencies what to do, but to find some agency to provide services needed for a patient at a particular time. In Hennepin county, the information and referral service is a branch of the Community Health and Welfare Council. The referral service has published a useful reference manual of services available from the many agencies, including a list of eligibility requirements. Typical inquiries come from agencies that feel they cannot help someone who has applied to them. Since the voluntary agencies offer services, not cash, this often means referring the person in need to the county Welfare Department for assistance.

In St. Paul the referral service is operated by the public health nurses. These referral directors, as might be expected, are more conscious of unfilled gaps in community services than other workers in the agencies. They report that all too frequently patients are shunted from agency to agency either because they are nonresidents, have multiple problems, do not fit existing categories for treatment, or are personally obnoxious.

One of the most difficult problems in the Minneapolis–St. Paul metropolitan area is coordinating the operations of private hospitals. Hospital costs to the patient are among the highest in the nation. Yet, it is said that present patient charges are high in order to provide capital for more buildings. The hospitals are engaged in fierce competition to build satellite units in the suburban areas. Most health professionals believe hospitals are overbuilt for the present population and immediate future growth, and thus that the surplus rooms can only increase per patient costs. In each central city, and for the metropolitan area as a whole, hospital coordinating committees have been established to survey needs, and to approve new building projects. But not all hospitals have joined these committees, wishing like true imperialists to complete their own expansion before joining to hold down the expansion of others.

This lack of planning has become critical; Hennepin County General Hospital is now so outmoded that it must either be closed or replaced. If the voluntary general hospitals would share in the care of indigents there might be no need for a public general hospital. Plenty of facilities are available just now, even psychiatric facilities, but the private hospitals are reluctant to accept indigents unless money is available to pay costs. A recent study committee recommended that General Hospital continue to operate and that new buildings be constructed for it. This recommendation is precipitating considerable political discussion, but no organized opposition has been heard. Most arguments ultimately will revolve around the site and, of course, how the costs are to be shared, rather than the need for the hospital. The university is in the forefront of those who insist that Hennepin General's teaching function be continued, but it has refused to take it over. The direction of development of the federal medicare program may in the long run determine what is done.

During the past decade Ramsey county and St. Paul went through these same arguments about the need for a county general hospital and finally decided to build a new facility, which is now in operation. At one point in the discussion someone suggested that the two cities and counties might better support one public institution, located between the cities. Readers of this account need not be told how this suggestion fared.

A series of new coordinating agencies, hailed initially by participants as the most favorable development they have experienced, has been undertaken by the state Department of Welfare to bring together all mental health agencies—state, local, public, and private. The new groups are the regional coordinating committees, intended to be established in each of the collecting regions of the state mental hospitals. Meeting once a month, these coordinating committees include state hospital personnel, county welfare boards, local general hospitals, community mental health centers, and private mental health institutions. The chief value of the coordinating committees seems to be that they offer people a chance to talk to their counterparts in the other agencies. Most of them had never met before the first meeting of the coordinating committee.

The welfare coordinating committes did nothing to overcome the main division in the Minneapolis–St.Paul metropolitan area, because two separate coordinating committees were planned, one in each region of the two metropolitan area state hospitals. In fact, the proposed west metropolitan (Hennepin-Minneapolis) committee never got off the ground. The Department of Public Welfare may have missed an opportunity to create a needed unit for rational mental health planning in the whole metropolitan area when it did nothing to encourage joint planning but merely accepted the historic bicentrism.

MENTAL HEALTH INTEREST GROUPS

The Minnesota Association for Mental Health is the principal interest group in the field. It was created in 1954 by the merger of two existing organizations: the Mental Hygiene Society, dating from 1939 and consisting mostly of professional people interested in prevention; and the Citizens' Committee for Mental Health, a legislative and social action group created by Governor Luther Youngdahl in the late 1940s to help promote his program. The association's origins are reflected in some remaining tension between the professionals and the social activists.

With an executive committee which meets monthly and a state staff of twelve persons, the Association for Mental Health is a highly centralized organization. At first it had only individual members, but later it conducted intensive organizing drives and by 1965 had chapters in half of the state's counties. The association seeks to enroll prominent community leaders as members and a county chapter is formed when at least forty members are enrolled. All funds collected locally are sent to state headquarters, with some allocated back for approved projects. The association also receives contributions from the Minneapolis and St. Paul United Funds.

The Minnesota Association for Mental Health sponsors fifty projects. The principal purpose is education of its own members, who in turn are expected to educate their communities about mental health. Occasionally large statewide conferences are held. These may induce other interest groups, such as the American Legion Auxiliary, to make mental health an item in their programs. County members are trained for volunteer work in the community and the association has sponsored various experimental and demonstration projects. It has an elaborate procedure for developing a legislative program, and prepares attractive printed materials for the legislators and the public.

The association lobbied actively for community mental health centers legislation long before the 1963 Act was passed and has repeatedly urged large state allocations for the centers. While it is difficult to assess the impact of an association on public policy, appropriations have indeed risen rapidly; and the association can probably claim some credit for the sophisticated approach to mental health programs on the part of Minnesota legislative leaders.

The growth and effectiveness of the Mental Health Association has been limited in recent years by conflicts over the executive directorship. The first director was an imaginative leader who cultivated prominent benefactors and had great influence at the state capitol. Upon his death, his assistant was elevated to the directorship over the opposition of some of the other leaders, and the resulting factionalism diminished the ability of the organization to move ahead. Another change of leadership occurred in 1966.

The other principal interest group in this broad field is the Minnesota Association for Retarded Children (MARC). Unlike the Mental Health Association, the Association for Retarded Children is highly decentralized. The state association employs three field men, but local organizations, countywide or multi-county, are independent. The local groups raise money for their own use but also send 35 per cent to state and national associations. The total group includes about 4,000 members, of whom perhaps 80 per cent are parents of retarded children. The executive director was an able lobbyist who had also developed considerable political sophistication among his members. Each local unit has a government affairs chairman, who brings its needs and projects to the attention of county board members and legislators. The effectiveness of the Minnesota Association for Retarded Children is shown by the fact that even in years of budget austerity community day-care centers for the retarded received substantial increases in legislative appropriations.

Few other groups in the mental health field seem to be active. A Minnesota Association of Psychiatry has only recently been organized, but private practitioners among its members generally have not involved themselves in public policy disputes. In general, psychiatrists trained at the University of Minnesota or at the Mayo Clinic in Rochester are strongly oriented toward community psychiatry, and work with community mental health centers.

The Minnesota Medical Association has not opposed community mental health centers, perhaps because the long-time chairman of its mental health committee is a psychiatrist who served many years as superintendent of a state mental hospital before returning to private practice. He has the confidence of both private and public practitioners. While the chairman has strongly supported the community mental health centers program, he has insisted always that the community programs be for the indigent only. He believes that the application of a means test for

subsidized psychiatric service silences any opposition that might otherwise arise among doctors. In only one section of the state has there been
opposition to the establishment of a community mental health center
from the medical profession.

A few right-wing organizations exist in the Minneapolis–St. Paul
metropolitan area, which might be expected to be opposed to mental
health activities. But they have been more concerned about communism
and free love at the university than threats of mass brain washing through
psychiatry, and consequently they have been no handicap to the development of community mental health programs.

Fragmentation of government obviously affects the organization of
interest groups. The Minnesota Association for Mental Health had to
organize local associations by counties when it was decided that community health centers should be organized by counties. Moreover, since
most legislative districts include one or more whole counties, lobbying
is easier when chapters can concentrate on a single legislator. Both Minneapolis (MARC) and St. Paul (SPARC) have their own chapters of
the Association for Retarded Children. In both instances there are
enough clients to fill several day-care centers and workshops.

INFLUENCE PATTERNS

Governmental decisions in Minneapolis are in the hands of the city
council.[5] The mayor has no formal powers over general administration
of the city except for the police. His staff is small; and aldermen, jealous
of their power, have kept the loyalties of city department heads. As a
result, the mayor finds it difficult to get information about what is going
on and complains he has to read the newspapers to find out anything.
Typically, Minneapolis mayors have not tried to exert influence beyond
their limited formal powers, contenting themselves with ceremonial functions. When a mayor attempts to exert influence on policy making in the
city, the city council generally regards him as a usurper.

The council itself does not act as a unit. Most important, each alder-
man supervises administration in his own ward. A citywide viewpoint or
policy seldom emerges in the council. Political organizations could

[5] A rigorous study of community power has yet to be made in Minneapolis and
St. Paul. As a result, the following account of influences in the area is im-
pressionistic. Alan Altshuler described Minneapolis and St. Paul in 1959 for the
Joint Center for Urban Studies.

bridge these gaps, but do not. The council is divided into caucuses, called by the press "liberal" and "independent" (or conservative). Liberals are those generally endorsed by the ward and city conventions of the Democratic-Farmer Labor Party. The Republicans for the first time in 1965 formally endorsed candidates for aldermen in most wards, although they had supported some candidates more or less openly for a number of years.

Neither party, however, is always able to control its caucus members. Several of the liberals have gained election without the endorsement of the DFL Party. Others were endorsed only because the party knew they could win a primary contest with or without endorsement. Incumbents frequently dominate their party ward clubs and therefore are powers in their own right and need bear no allegiance to central party spokesmen. The Democratic-Farmer Labor Party in the city is severely factionalized into groups roughly identified as "labor" and an "intellectual" group referred to by their opponents as the "university crowd." The current mayor is leader of the "intellectual" group and is considered highly suspect by the "labor" element, who contested his first nomination. Thus, the DFL party provides very little unifying force in the city government.

Some of the Independents are closely identified with the Republican Party, others are merely anti-Democrat. The council has been divided 7–6 one way or the other in recent years. Regardless of formal control, a clique of conservative aldermen from each group has tended to dominate the important committees such as Ways and Means. In 1963 this group was sufficiently cohesive so that its members voted together to organize the city council when the liberals who were in the majority could not agree on how to divide the committee positions.

The Independent group was led by a veteran of twenty-two years, a shrewd, capable, and domineering personality. Called "the uncrowned king of Minneapolis," he was openly contemptuous of any mayor, the metropolitan press, and the suburbs. His principal accomplishment has been careful management of the city's spending and debt, so that the city now boasts an AAA credit rating and therefore can borrow at low rates. To accomplish this, his critics say, city services are also held at low levels.

Downtown businessmen are thought to be the prime influence on city decisions in Minneapolis. An extensive downtown urban redevelopment, claimed to be the largest contiguous area of renewal in the nation, was conceived and managed politically by this group. Their formal organization is known as the Downtown Council. Its principal members include a vice president of one of the two major banks, downtown real estate owners and managers, and executives of the largest department store, a locally owned enterprise. The Downtown Council has taken a vigorous stand against decay of the downtown shopping center. In addition to promoting public outlays and private redevelopment, their own enterprises are making huge commitments of improvement capital to buildings, parking facilities, and beautification programs. The Chamber of Commerce, the Board of Realtors, Small Retail Grocers' Association, and liquor interests are less in the foreground on government decisions but are thought to be influential with councilmen on individual decisions that affect their interests.

Hennepin county operates under the standard Minnesota form of county government: five commissioners who administer virtually all major functions of county government. Technically the commissioners act through their own committees and their membership on other functional county boards and committees which include outsiders. But the Hennepin County Welfare Board is composed of the same five men who serve as county commissioners. For a number of years the county board was city-dominated by a DFL majority of 3–2, although county officials like city officials are elected on a nonpartisan ballot. The minority Republican members and the other two majority members left day-to-day administration essentially to the chairman of the board, and since administration is not easily separable from policy, this meant he was the key policymaker. He was a trained public administrator, and in political philosophy he was devoted to expanding the services of the county. He hired competent administrators for the county departments and gave them full support. As a result, Hennepin county gained a reputation for superb welfare, probation, and highway work. Decried as a dictator by the opposition, and resisted in his attempts to centralize personnel, accounting, and data processing by the elected county auditor and treasurer, he was nonetheless unassailable until the DFL lost control of the county board in the 1964 election. Then he lost all his formal positions of decision making.

Loss by one party implies gain by the other, and this is true for the Republican Party in county affairs. While formerly the Republican members were not active in their party, the newly elected members are, and the most prominent among them became chairman of the county commissioners. Dedicated Republicans also won several aldermanic races in the Minneapolis city elections in 1965. Consequently, the area may be witnessing the rise of the Republican Party as a responsible governing group.

Another influential organization is the Citizens League. This is a research, study, and recommending group of several hundred. Formerly confined to Minneapolis and Hennepin county, it became areawide in 1966. It is reform-oriented, supporting city charter revision to centralize administrative power under the mayor, tax reform, and consolidation of services under broader metropolitan area governmental authorities. Competently run, the Citizens League has had increasing success in getting its recommendations adopted by the legislature.

The area's delegations to the state Senate and the House of Representatives are an important part of the power structure in Minneapolis and Hennepin county. Because the local governments are limited to the powers expressly granted by the state, new or modified functions require state statutory authorization. Also new regional authorities must be established by the legislature.

Hennepin county had sixteen state senators and thirty-three representatives in 1967. Republicans held thirteen of the Senate seats and twenty-four of the House seats. While technically nonpartisan, Minnesota's legislature divides into caucuses largely along party lines. In the metropolitan areas, all conservatives are openly endorsed by the Republican Party although not all feel loyalty to party programs and leaders. The county legislative delegations act as a unit in most instances on local bills. This means that the delegation must be united in its support if a local bill is to have a good chance of passing. Generally this agreement comes only through excruciating compromise and log-rolling, and only a few major bills each session can secure such action. The transfer of Minneapolis General Hospital to Hennepin county control came about as a result of a compromise involving creation also of an integrated municipal court system for Hennepin county in which suburban interests and judges were protected.

Since salaries and allowances of all city and county officials are fixed by the legislature, legislators exert considerable influence upon local city and county government officials. Thus a legislator who becomes dedicated to a cause can be the instrument through which some new or expanded activity is made possible. For example, the dedication of the cochairman of the Hennepin House delegation in 1963 to the cause of mental health clearly facilitated favorable mental health legislation, especially since he was named chairman of the welfare appropriations subcommittee. It also induced county and city officials to support the center program.

Essentially the same importance accrues to the Ramsey county legislative delegation. Somewhat smaller (eight senators and sixteen representatives) and until recently heavily dominated by members of the Democratic-Farmer Labor Party, it has exhibited more unity of purpose, while practicing an even tighter unit rule. No doubt a more unified front by the city and county governments in dealing with their legislative delegation has much to do with Ramsey's historically greater success in achieving its goals.

In St. Paul, the Chamber of Commerce is far more influential in local affairs than its counterpart in Minneapolis. It has received national recognition for the large proportion of middle management it has put through the group's political action course. The chamber's observer is said to sit in on council and budget meetings and participate in approval or disapproval of spending decisions. The long-time city comptroller —the independently elected budget officer—is a dedicated conservative who expresses the dominant mood of the city. Prominent industrialists are likely to be mentioned as city influentials in St. Paul much more than in Minneapolis. In Minneapolis most of the big corporation heads do not live in the city, and their business interests are more nationally oriented than are St. Paul industries.

The DFL Party has nominally had a majority in St. Paul elections, but its great pluralities may have kept it from becoming a fighting organization. It has been low-key, controlled mostly by nonideological organization men. Some mayors and county board chairmen have advocated more welfare, public housing, and urban redevelopment. The Trades and Labor Assembly is a conservative central body that generally has looked upon the DFL Party as its subordinate political action partner but has not been notably successful in recent years in getting its candidates into office. The Republican Party has only recently come to life in parts of St. Paul to help elect a number of legislators and a mayor and is still nonexistent in other parts of the city.

The press in both cities is important politically. In St. Paul, as in

Minneapolis, both morning and evening papers are published by a single company. The St. Paul papers' editorial policy is considerably more conservative than that of the Minneapolis papers, but the St. Paul papers have supported welfare activities. The Minneapolis papers are reform-oriented, supporting charter revision and endorsing reform-type candidates from either party for local office.

On the statewide level, clearly the most influential governmental decision makers are the department heads of the state government and their professional staffs. The legislature has practically no staff but relies upon direct contact with department personnel and lobbyists for information. Department heads are appointed by the governor, but their terms do not coincide with his. Since the merit system of civil service extends high enough in the departments to include the deputy commissioners, patronage is not much of a force in unifying policy making under a political leader. The governor, therefore, is something of an interloper when he attempts to interpose himself between the departments and the legislature in their submissions to that body. Department heads may resent even being asked to send the governor periodic reports of what they are doing. The governor does have the important budgetary power and through his agent, the commissioner of administration, sets what will be in all likelihood the ceiling of the legislative appropriation. Usually appropriations are slightly less than the governor's budget.

A governor, if he is popular and leads a disciplined party that can elect a majority to the legislature, can bring an informal unity to otherwise divided government. Recent governors have not been notably successful in this. The long-time leaders of the state Senate have been almost pathologically antigovernor regardless of party. On some issues, however, notably mental health and mental retardation, governors traditionally have been quite effective.

In summary, general influence patterns in the Minneapolis–St. Paul metropolitan area indicate that political leaders, usually but not necessarily party leaders, are prominent in informal as well as formal decision making. A recent study identified public officeholders as foremost among opinion leaders in local and metropolitan government matters.[6] Commercial and industrial interests, the former more typical of Min-

---

[6] Gerald D. Hursh, "A Study of the Communication Behavior of Members of Voluntary Associations," Ph.D. dissertation, University of Minnesota, 1966.

neapolis and the latter of St. Paul, have much to say on matters that concern them. Labor is oriented toward bread-and-butter issues. Civic groups are active, and their role in supplying ideas and providing arguments for candidates should not be underestimated. Political party activity rather than old-family background or interest-group membership is the main channel for recruiting leaders. Long-time officeholders have acquired great power, although several of these giants have been toppled in recent elections.

Contrary to the characteristic evolution of services—from private to local governmental, to state, then to federal—mental health programs in Minnesota began at the state level. Typically, the impetus for transferring responsibilities from one level to another has come from private interest groups hoping to broaden the financial base of their operation or to encourage higher standards through centrally directed criteria. Yet the impetus for decentralizing mental health programs from state to local communities and private agencies comes from professionals in the field, mostly in federal and state government service.

The term "vertical dispersal" in mental health is peculiarly apt in that it connotes a dynamic tendency that is still going on. Minnesota has made a firm policy decision to transfer part of the responsibility for the care of mentally ill from the state to the local units and is proceeding accordingly. Moving patients out of the state hospitals into nursing homes is more than merely a transfer of location. Since the state operates only two nursing homes, with a total of 569 beds, someone else has had to assume this responsibility. While counties and municipalities presumably could build and operate nursing homes themselves, most of the homes are privately operated. Some are voluntary nonprofit or charitable operations by church groups while others are proprietary operations on the part of individuals or corporations. As of 1967 Minnesota had a total of 24,545 beds in nursing homes and boarding care homes.

The removal of state hospital patients to nursing homes has not always been a social victory, to say nothing of a welcomed political development. Although the state Board of Health licenses nursing homes, the board has not been staffed adequately to enforce rigorous standards. More than one-fifth of the beds are classified by the state as "unsuitable." Minneapolis and St. Paul, whose health departments formerly inspected nursing homes prior to licensing, were forbidden to continue this practice by a state statute, sponsored by a senator who himself allegedly operated substandard nursing homes. This is said to be Minnesota's classic example of conflict of interest. The law has, however, been by-passed by the executive of the state Board of Health who deputized the municipal commissioners of health to inspect for him. But demand for reasonably priced facilities has been so great that the authorities continue to allow undesirable homes to operate. As a result, in some homes the inmates have no planned program of activity. Occasionally a relative will petition the county welfare departments to have the patient read-mitted to a state hospital so he can get better care.

The financial burden of mental health care has also been dispersed vertically. While counties are supposed to pay for indigent persons committed to state mental hospitals, the charge is only $10 a month. To keep the same patient in a nursing home may well cost $85 a month. County welfare boards have not always been happy to accept this added fiscal load, although programs of medical assistance to the aged may lessen the burden.

Minnesota's experience with dispersal of mental health activities to communities antedates the federal act making community centers a goal of national policy. In the early 1950s the state set up three clinics, associated with state mental hospitals for aftercare of patients discharged from state mental hospitals, and one of these was in Minneapolis. The clinics were not comprehensive. They provided no outpatient care except for former patients, who did not use the clinics; they obviously were not satisfactory.

In 1953, state law assigned responsibility for aftercare of released mental patients to the county welfare departments. They still have this responsibility. This constituted the first attempt to devolve formal responsibility for a mental health program on the local community. It did not shift the burden, but rather offered a new service, since, except for the abortive state clinics, no one had been doing anything about former patients. The county welfare departments were not prepared for the new responsibility either by training or by increased support, and the response has been spotty. Some counties have developed an organization and personnel to do a complete job; others have done little or nothing.

A gap in coordination resulting from this vertical dispersal of responsibility is seen in the relationships between the state hospitals and the county welfare boards. According to regulations, the state hospital is supposed to notify the county welfare department of a patient's residence when he is released. But whether this is done depends upon the particular hospital and the particular doctor who has charge of the case. Some physicians resent the idea of turning their patients over to anyone and sometimes county welfare departments are not notified of the release of patients. Usually the welfare department does not seek out released patients but assists them if they appear. Some departments believe that the patients' relatives have the real responsibility for their care and will act only if no one else will.

A committed mental patient is given a provisional discharge from the state hospital for one year. After that year, an evaluation of his progress is supposed to determine if the discharge can be made final. If so, the patient can be returned to the hospital only through new commitment procedures. The county welfare department makes this evaluation.

Hennepin county has a special division, consisting of two sections of psychiatric social workers, to handle aftercare cases. In Ramsey county some 300 aftercare cases needing prescriptions filled or renewed constitute the principal workload of the mental health center. The Ramsey County Welfare Department supervises these charges in other matters, such as in their family life adjustment. There is no contact between the mental health center and the welfare people on these cases; on neither side do the workers have time and the two agencies are physically separated. The new county hospital building is only six or seven blocks instead of several miles from the welfare headquarters, and both sides think contact may be more likely after the move. Without coordination, the prescribing physician is handicapped by lack of contact, because he has no information about the patient's adjustment progress. Consequently he may be unable to determine whether he should change his prescription for the patient.

Differences in levels of service among the several governments in the metropolitan area is apparent. The Dakota County Welfare Department in 1965 had only one professionally qualified case worker with a master of social work degree on its staff of thirteen. In this county, aftercare is the responsibility of public health nurses. Anoka county had no specialists for aftercare. One intake worker was psychiatrically trained, but the patients were handled by a general overflow team.

The next major dispersal of mental health activities from state to local governments came about in 1957 when the legislature passed the Community Mental Health Centers Act. It provided that the state would pay

50 per cent of the cost of operating an outpatient mental health service, provided state standards for professional training were met.

Centers could be governmental or private. In the first instance, a mental health board is appointed by the county commissioners upon recommendation of a selection committee. The private nonprofit corporation alternative was made available to permit state support for existing mental health facilities as a means of providing centers where the county was unwilling to do it and to make employees eligible for social security. There was, however, some legal question as to whether local taxes could be levied for the benefit of a nonprofit corporation.

Counties rather than cities were chosen by the state as the instrumentality because the state Welfare Department operated through counties. Also, the state Welfare Department is primarily oriented to out-state, that is, the area outside the Twin Cities. This nonmetropolitan, or even antimetropolitan, viewpoint is clear in all state officials' discussions about the mental health center program. First of all they are interested primarily in physical coverage, a kind of map viewpoint, where they aim to get whole areas colored in on a map as an indication of service available. The metropolitan areas may seem less significant to the map makers because they look small on the map. Furthermore, the legislative power structure, to which the department must be finely attuned, has been until recent reapportionments strongly rurally oriented. Prominent members of the welfare committees have usually been from nonmetropolitan areas.

Further, the state Welfare Department sees its programs as performing some equalization of services. Officials frequently declare that the metropolitan counties can take care of themselves. Virtually all of Minnesota's private psychologists practice in the Twin Cities area. Per capita wealth and the sophistication of potential patients in seeking psychiatric help are greater. But the need for mental health services may be greater also. Some psychiatrists claim the pressures of urban life result in more mental breakdowns.

At first, state Welfare Department staff members went through the rural parts of the state preaching the need for county centers in order to encourage their establishment. Later, the department had second thoughts about the wisdom of the procedure, fearing that several centers were premature because more solid support should have been built in the community first, especially among members of the County Board, which would have to provide the financing. Some of the centers are now in a precarious condition.

The voluntary associations similarly concentrated on the out-state areas. Members of the Minnesota Association for Mental Health were drawn at first largely from the Twin Cities and primarily from Minneapolis. Consequently, association leaders thought it would be unnecessary to set up a separate local office, since the state office could provide for Twin City needs. Finally, a Minneapolis chapter group organized, but the absence of such a group at an early date may have delayed establishment of a Hennepin county center. There is no St. Paul chapter. Generally St. Paul leaders regard the association as a Minneapolis outfit, a disastrous image given St. Paulites' sensitivity about domination by Minneapolis.

Perhaps the best way to illustrate how things happen in the field of mental health in the Minneapolis–St. Paul metropolitan area is through a few short case studies of the establishment of county mental health centers.

Minneapolis had a limited inpatient psychiatric department located in the city's general hospital, which was used as a diagnostic and holding station for possible commitments. In 1955 twenty beds were added for short-term treatment facilities but a critical need for outpatient services remained. The Community Health and Welfare Council pointed to this need in survey after survey. The director advocated an outpatient facility for ten years before it was finally created. Countless meetings were held at which resolutions were passed supporting the idea, but action was stymied by the problem of obtaining the initial $100,000 to get started. The Minneapolis Welfare Board and the City Council had a miserly attitude toward existing welfare programs, even without considering new undertakings.

When the state act for sharing operating costs of outpatient mental health centers was passed in 1957, the Health and Welfare Council director wanted to apply for a grant. But the hospital administrator was unwilling to support the proposal and the matter was dropped. The appointment of a new hospital administrator and of a new head of the Psychiatry Department and the election of a new mayor eager to find a popular cause at last provided a convergence of sufficient forces to get the city to apply for a grant.

But the state Welfare Department wanted the center to be countywide. The mental health authority was changed therefore into a private corporation, appointed partly by the City Council and partly by the County Board. The city's financial contribution was the value of the space in the general hospital, which the Mental Health Board "rented" from it, plus that part of the staff time devoted to outpatient work. The county paid nothing at first; individual suburbanites who used the facility were supposed to pay one-half of the cost and presumably the state paid the rest.

By 1962 the County Board had taken over local funding for outpatients but not for inpatient facilities toward which the state would pay nothing. More money was then available for the whole center because Minneapolis was required to pay only for inpatient care. When the county's contributions reached more than $250,000 the County Board insisted on abolishing the private corporation board and operating the center itself as a part of the hospital. The standing hospital advisory committee was enlarged by four to comply with the state requirements of nine members on the Mental Health Board.

It is important to note that the role of the director of the Health and Welfare Council was to prod politicians and administrators into acting. The role of the County Board chairman was to devise paper transactions about the value of the Minneapolis contribution in order to rapidly shift the financial load to the county. The Mental Health Board was carefully selected so that its membership included all the people who would have to make decisions about the center. These included the leader of the Minneapolis City Council; the chairman of the county legislative delegation, who was willing to be led by mental health professionals; the County Board chairman, who became treasurer of the Mental Health Board; the head of psychiatry at the university, who insisted that the mental health center be tied closely to the existing general hospital; plus prominent local citizens who had long been interested in mental health projects.

In Ramsey county and St. Paul, an even longer time elapsed after the Act was passed before a mental health center was established, although professionals, including the present and past directors of county welfare, had been pointing out the need for many years. In Ramsey county the Welfare Board, which operates the public general hospital, is once removed from elected officeholders since it is appointed partly by the City Council and partly by the County Board. The Welfare Board's budget is screened by a fact-finding committee composed of members of the city and county boards. When the two governing boards have approved it, the sum needed to finance the board is apportioned between the city and county governments according to a ratio fixed by statute.

People concerned with welfare in St. Paul argue that this is a better arrangement than the Minneapolis one where the county commissioners constitute the Welfare Board. Hennepin county is equally satisfied with its arrangement because the county commissioners do not have to justify their budget to anyone. There is much dissatisfaction in Hennepin, however, with the township relief system, which means a separate Welfare Board is necessary for Minneapolis and for individual suburbs to handle relief payments. Ramsey county handles all relief as well as traditional categorical aid programs through one agency. But the separation between the Welfare Board and city and county elected officials in St. Paul means that three sets of officials rather than one have to be consulted on any innovations. In the planning stage of the mental health center it was hard for the welfare-oriented professionals and voluntary association people to interest city and county politicians in a mental health facility they would not run. It was still harder to explain and justify the requirement of establishing yet another board—a mental health board—to purchase outpatient psychiatric services from the Welfare Board that ran the hospital. There were lengthy and continual arguments with the mayor and the city and county attorneys before action was finally approved. Once this occurred, new money had to be found to match the state's grant, and this was even more difficult to do given the St. Paul climate of opinion.

In the Ramsey county case there were notable communication failures and a conspicuous absence of the ingenious devices for neutralizing objectors and co-opting decision makers. Some Ramsey officials liked the idea of having a different set of people on the Mental Health Board because it got more people involved. But they were not the decision makers on policy and money and had responsibility without authority. As in Hennepin at first, the Ramsey hospital administrator did not wish to fight for the new mental health service, leaving a crucial breach in the ranks of agitators. Political officeholders may support an administrator in something he strongly desires, but they are unlikely to push a project that has political risks unless he supports it.

The establishment of a mental health center in Dakota county—the next in point of time in the metropolitan area—must set some kind of record for efficiency and ease in getting a favorable decision. Behind this appearance, however, lay flawless groundwork.

The state Welfare Department was active in stimulating Dakota county people to try to get a center. But the prime mover in Dakota county was the head of the county Mental Health Association. She spent almost five years in preparing for the final push. Support was garnered from every source of influence. These included prominent members of the association equally distributed among every county commissioner's district; strong professional encouragement from the county welfare director; the county auditor, who was the informal executive of the County Board; members of the Junior Chamber of Commerce, which had adopted mental health as a project; a union official from the dominant meat packers' union, who was personally committed to the cause; the county probation officer; the Ministerial Association, which was interested in family counseling; and a prominent local physician who had recently specialized in psychiatry.

With this preparation, it was not surprising that the hearings produced not a single word of testimony against establishment of a center. It was approved by the county commissioners forthwith, as have been all subsequent budget requests. The Mental Health Association leaders obviously understood the influence structure in the county and were able to make enthusiastic supporters of everyone with a legitimate stake in the decision.

The delay in establishing a mental health center in Anoka county provides another case study. The Mental Health Association leadership there was highly committed, but high-pressured in its demands, and apparently more vocal than action-oriented. The county welfare director was skeptical of the benefits of a mental health center and thought that it would deal only with the unhappy and the neurotic who could better be treated by existing agencies. He felt strongly that the county did not need another case-finding operation. If welfare professionals do not favor a program, the political leaders will not act. Finally in 1966 Anoka county moved to adopt the comprehensive mental health center concept, without trying to establish a single facility to meet all needs. An executive director was appointed to coordinate the several services that would be provided by different existing agencies.

The state Department of Welfare contains the most important mental health decision makers in the state. The incumbent commissioner of welfare, while a political appointee of the governor, is not an active partisan. As a professional with a national reputation, he has had the confidence of several administrations of both parties. He is also well regarded in the legislature.

The Medical Services Division, which operates all state institutions for mentally ill and handicapped, also has had strong professional leadership. The former director, the leading force in the enactment of the state Community Mental Health Centers Act, moved to the national stage, where he has helped shape national legislation in the same field. His successor is an able psychiatrist with a flair for crusading. He, too, is acquiring a national reputation by asking hard questions about the effect of federal regulations and challenging the hierarchy-approved doctrinal assumptions. For example, he believes that a neighborhood mental health center that is not devoted to handling major mental illness could quickly be buried by ambulatory neurotics, or "unhappy middle-class housewives."

The best illustration of the state Welfare Department in operation is the recent preparation of a state plan for mental health. Most of the people concerned with the plan were unhappy about the way in which it was prepared. Granting their competence, officials in the Minnesota mental health hierarchy are supremely confident about the way they run their affairs. More objective observers, however, believe that a few other states have carried new psychiatric concepts further and better than Minnesota. The attitude of smugness in the state department made it resentful of the federal planning concept. There were plans enough in the hopper to carry the department forward for many years. Also the new definition of adequacy for mental health centers was resented, because the department thought it was progressing as fast as possible in setting up the kind and the number of centers that could reasonably be maintained with existing and foreseeable resources.

Most of all, the Minnesota executives resented the necessity of opening the department's planning process to a large number of outsiders. The federal planning grants were welcomed because they provided more staff for the state department, which could also carry on other planning and research projects awaiting action. Since a planning council was required, the department wanted to use the planning process to cultivate a wide understanding and support for mental health activities among organizations with even remote concerns for mental health. About sixty-five people were asked to join the planning council. Eight committees were established. Then they were left pretty much on their own to prepare recommendations. In the meantime, tentative plans from the "planning for planning" stage had to be submitted to get the major federal planning grant. These were largely drawn up in the department by the medical advisory committee. They were then put before the full planning council, but deadlines left no alternative to the giving of formal approval.

Several prominent professional and voluntary leaders resigned from the planning council when they concluded they were wasting their time in window dressing for the department. Others, equally dissatisfied, loyally stuck with the council and tried to make some worthwhile suggestions for long-term and intermediate planning.

The facilities committee actually became an administrative committee to apply the criteria for awarding federal construction money to community mental health centers. This was the most significant immediate result of the planning effort, and perhaps an unanticipated consequence.

State Welfare Department people insisted that Minnesota would not allow itself to be rushed in its planning. They predicted that the state would forego the first distribution of federal money if it meant unrealistic changes in the Minnesota organization. These protests against overstrict and unrealistic regulations may have helped to make the new federal program more flexible. But at the same time, Minnesota administrators under pressure from local centers and the mental health association were becoming less resistant to the new federal demands. County centers began to adopt their own construction plans and applied for funds in anticipation of availability. Actually this meant that centers already in operation got top priority. If the Act was meant to build mental centers where there were none, it failed in Minnesota, at least on the first time around.

The state planning council was not continued after the state plan was completed. Continued planning was expected to be done by the local community mental health center boards. Any statewide coordination that might become necessary would be provided by the existing state agency, with the assistance of a newly formed citizens' community mental health advisory committee.

Clearly the existing state mental health bureaucracy dominated the

state planning process. The great difficulty of organizing diverse groups
to produce specific results and recommendations is apparent. Intensive
specialized staff work with well-formulated alternatives is necessary to
elicit criticism from specialists, for this is how specialists and interest
group leaders work best.

The state planning process illustrates the unavoidable conflicts arising
from the problem of defining mental health. The planning council had
one committee on "nonmedical problems," but the chairman claimed he
had to force his way onto the planning council in the first place, since
the medical definition of mental health fixed by the department's orientation would have excluded him.

Planning for mental retardation was done apart from the general mental health plan. Entirely different methods were used. The planning group
was limited to twenty-five, small enough to fit around a single table, and
only representatives of closely identified interests were included. A full-
time specialist in community organization planning was hired as staff.
Close liaison was maintained with the governor's staff and the governor's
name was used freely to lend prestige to service on the committees. Professionals from several departments were vice chairmen of task forces,
and they had enough time to prepare their reports carefully.

Despite their lack of formal powers, Minnesota governors have had
great impact on the mental health field. Governor Luther Youngdahl
(Republican, 1948–1951) is credited with beginning leadership in the
area of mental health. He endeavored to improve the state's mental
health programs with every personal, political, and publicity device available. Newspapers exposed conditions in the mental institutions. Restraints were publicly burned. The result was public response strong
enough to force the conservative legislature to increase drastically state
appropriations.

The lesson of Youngdahl's success was not lost on subsequent candidates for the governorship of Minnesota. Every governor since that
time has put major emphasis on further development of mental health.
One recent Republican governor had initially made his name in the state
as the leader in the state Senate of programs to improve mental health.
His DFL successor pushed mental health programs, this time for the
retarded, far ahead of any other item among his legislative priorities.
And the legislature outdid him in appropriating for new staff beyond his
request.

Most interesting has been the gradual conversion of several more fiscally conservative members of the legislature to supporting mental health programs. Some of these legislators probably saw the light because of voter approval of what the governors requested. But others admit to being overcome by facts. They were induced to visit the mental institutions on tours arranged by the interest groups and the governor, and they found it difficult to continue to oppose spending to improve treatment, care, and research for the mentally ill or handicapped.

MANPOWER

Lack of qualified personnel is the single most critical problem facing Minnesota's state mental hospitals and community centers. Nine of Minnesota's twenty-one public mental health centers were without a psychiatrist as medical director in 1965. Centers are finding it increasingly difficult to hire psychologists. Where no psychiatrist is available, the position of medical director is filled by a nonpsychiatrist M.D., and a social worker is the program director. Out-state centers without a psychiatrist in residence often employ a consultant from the Twin Cities area for one day a week.

Some psychiatric positions at state mental hospitals also remain unfilled. The Lino Lakes intensive treatment center for adolescents had to use part-time consultants from Anoka State Hospital during the first two years of its existence. None of the private general hospitals in Minneapolis or St. Paul have a psychiatric resident to care for patients in their new psychiatric wings.

Community mental health centers are not under the restrictions of the state personnel classification system in paying their psychiatrists. In fact, some observers believe a real impetus toward the community mental health centers came from the desire to escape the low pay scale for professional people in state hospitals. Local mental health boards, on which some businessmen are likely to serve, were not shocked by the necessity of paying $22,000 for a medical director. The state will match "within reason" any pay for a psychiatrist who has board certification. A psychologist, to have advanced standing, must be a diplomate in his association, have a Ph.D., and four years' experience. He can earn up to $15,000. A social worker has advanced standing with a M.S.W. degree, five years' experience or one year additional professional training. An

M.S.W. with four years' experience can earn $10,000. There is no official recognition of a specialist or psychiatric social worker.

Another problem in obtaining staff may be the location of facilities. Minnesota state hospitals, in accord with doctrine and community attitudes of the time, were established well outside the urbanized areas where most of the medically trained people live. Any attempt to cover the state with readily accessible community mental health centers runs into the same problem of attracting psychiatrists to some areas. To be sure, some psychiatrists have been attracted to the northern part of the state because of its fine recreational features, but it is sometimes said that psychiatry is an urban profession. At least cities generate enough business to keep private psychiatrists busy without cultivating clients.

Even within the metropolitan area, however, the publicly employed mental health staff are unevenly distributed. Hennepin county pay scales have been high, and well-trained social workers are drawn here from the other counties and municipalities in the metropolitan area. Anoka and Dakota counties have fewer qualified social workers. State-supported community mental health centers throughout the state employed sixty-four social workers, of which about half were in the six metropolitan centers.

Community mental health center boards complain that state standards for personnel in the mental health centers are unreasonably high. Some of the mental health center boards would like to have the state establish a category of probationary psychiatrist, one who is still completing his residency. This would enable a local physician interested in psychiatry to do further course work and return to the community to finish his requirements while working at the centers. State administrators, however, believe that more intensive recruiting efforts and continued increases in salary will attract staff more effectively than reducing requirements. The state enforces its personnel requirements by refusing to match local expenditures for less than qualified personnel.

A few professional observers believe that a continuing obstacle to obtaining personnel for community mental health centers is lack of prestige. Psychiatrists as a class, to be sure, do not suffer from lack of prestige in medical circles in Minnesota, as may be true in some areas of the country. In pay and status, psychiatrists are at or near the top among physicians in the state. A psychiatrist at a state hospital has the lowest status and those at a community mental health center the second lowest. The prestige drops even lower if the psychiatrist is not the director.

This explains the resistance on the part of some psychiatrists to separating the job of the medical director from administrator or program director of a center. The psychiatrist may feel he is retained only to sign prescriptions.

To overcome these frictions, the University of Minnesota Medical School has begun to train its graduates in team concepts of community psychiatry, where the social worker, the psychologist, and the psychiatrist work together in handling cases, with regular consultation to share suggestions. Instructors report that, even at the student level, the psychiatrists-to-be resist any indication that they are not the sole boss.

It is difficult to determine the total number of professional mental health personnel in the Minneapolis—St. Paul area because of inadequate records. Approximately 140 psychiatrists belong to the Minnesota Psychiatric Society, but not all of these are board certified. Most are concentrated in the metropolitan area, with a high percentage in Minneapolis. The University of Minnesota has about 27 psychiatric residents.

At the present time there are about 400 psychologists with an M.A. or Ph.D. living in Minnesota. About 70 students currently are enrolled in the University of Minnesota's doctoral program in clinical psychology. Its psychology program is heavily oriented toward medicine, as opposed to counseling, although 50 students are in counseling psychology with another 30 in school psychology. In all, there are some 250 graduate students in the Psychology Department.

The counseling psychologists believe the training of their people in Minnesota is neglected by NIMH, which will not support more than one kind of program at a single institution. The counseling psychologists believe that they have an important identification and early treatment function in combating mental illness because their location in educational institutions or industry brings them in contact with people with mental problems at an early stage, and they reason that they are likely to be more readily accepted by a person in need of mental help. The number of counseling and guidance personnel in the state has increased rapidly in recent years under the stimulus of the National Defense Education Act.

In addition to other manpower shortages, Minnesota needs more registered nurses to care for the mentally ill. The situation is critical at the state hospitals, where some twenty-seven registered nurses' positions were vacant in 1965. The university has recently established an M.A.

program in psychiatric nursing. At present only six Minnesota nurses caring for the mentally ill are classified as psychiatric nurses.

The staff requirements for a comprehensive community mental health center as envisioned in the 1963 federal Act are the principal reason state officials have found it hard to accept this concept as a realistic program for the state. Therefore, they do not envision many "federal-type" mental health centers being established. Instead, the three-man team—psychiatrist, psychologist, and social worker, or multiples of the latter two members—is likely to man most Minnesota centers in the near future.

FINANCING MENTAL HEALTH ACTIVITIES

As elsewhere in the country, the lion's share of public financing of mental health activities in Minnesota is borne by the state government. State spending for mental health programs has increased rapidly in recent years. Expenditures for state hospitals rose from $12.6 million in 1955 to $18.3 million in 1963, an increase of 48.1 per cent in nine years, while the resident population of the hospitals was declining from 11,300 to 7,466, a decrease of 33.8 per cent. The state spent $4.6 million for institutions for the mentally retarded in 1955 and $10.3 million in 1963, an increase of 166.7 per cent. The state's matching appropriations for community mental health centers rose from $170,000 in 1958 (the first year of the state program) to $750,000 in 1963, and the appropriation for 1966 is $1.2 million. Nursing home expenditures rose from nothing in 1960 to $2.8 million in 1963, while residential treatment facilities for children cost $250,000 in 1962 and 1963; the appropriation for the newly completed Lino Lakes facility was $750,000 for the 1964–1965 fiscal year. Including administrative costs and other mental health services, such as those provided by the University of Minnesota, state expenditures for mental health activities rose from the neighborhood of $20 million in 1953 to about $35 million in 1963.

In addition to the recent planning grants for mental retardation and mental health studies provided by the federal government, some federal financing of particular mental health activities in Minnesota has occurred. Most of the private hospital psychiatric units recently constructed in the Twin Cities were built with the help of Hill-Burton funds.

Until recently, local government financing of mental health activities was primarily through county welfare departments, which assumed part of the cost of services for indigent county residents committed to state mental hospitals. In addition, the county welfare departments were legally responsible for providing aftercare services to former mental patients needing assistance. In both these areas, the counties have not always met their legal responsibilities, in part because the state Welfare Department has not tried to enforce the regulations strictly, in part because many of the poorer out-state counties could not afford the financial burden, and also because sometimes the county of residence was difficult to determine. The more affluent metropolitan area counties have assumed more of the mental hospital and aftercare costs incurred by their residents than have the rural counties. Certain incidental expenditures, such as the cost of psychiatric examinations in commitment cases, must also be assumed by the committing county.

The Minnesota Community Mental Health Centers Act of 1957 led to the assumption of direct responsibility by counties for financing some mental health activities. Local government appropriations for community centers in the Minneapolis—St. Paul metropolitan area rose from $77,000 in 1961–1962 to an estimated $489,000 in 1965–1966, a figure that excludes the cost of inpatient psychiatric care in the county general hospitals. The state does not match inpatient operating costs, so technically only the outpatient department is part of the mental health center.

County welfare departments also purchase some mental health services from privately operated agencies or institutions. For example, the expensive annual fees that privately operated residential treatment facilities for children charge are usually paid by welfare departments. The limited mental health programs in the public schools are financed solely by the local school districts. The state Vocational Rehabilitation Agency also buys local services.

Financial support for a number of mental health activities in the Minneapolis—St. Paul metropolitan area is drawn from the private sector. The three privately operated mental health clinics (Hamm, Wilder, and Washburn) receive over two-thirds of their operating budgets, which totaled more than $400,000 in 1964–1965, from parent foundations. The United Fund contributes about $40,000 a year to the support of two of the five residential treatment centers for children in the Twin Cities and gives more than $1 million annually to service agencies indirectly involved in mental health activities. Psychiatric units in eight metropolitan area voluntary hospitals were partially constructed with funds from a privately subscribed hospital building fund.

It is difficult to assess the extent to which individual patients pay for mental health activities. Clearly most of the cost of services for private inpatient psychiatric services (which range from three to four million dollars per year in the Twin Cities) are met by individual patients or their families. The voluntary hospitals generally accept only those charity cases not eligible for services from publicly operated psychiatric inpatient facilities. Nor are the county welfare departments eager to pay $35 to $40 a day for private inpatient psychiatric services. On the other hand, the mental health centers and clinics reported that only a small proportion of their cost was met from individual fees. The state anticipates that many center clients will not be able to pay anything, and as a matter of fact will reduce the state grant proportionately if fees exceed 20 per cent of local funds.

Technically clients of social services agencies pay according to ability, but the agencies collect only a small percentage of their budgets from client fees. The private residential treatment facilities collect a substantial proportion of their budgets from fees, but these are almost always paid by county welfare departments or private social service agencies. The cost of mental health services provided by centers, clinics, and social service agencies are seldom passed on to the individual client.

Minnesota community mental health centers are supposed to treat only the needy. State regulations define the fee schedule. It is based upon 1 per cent of the family's yearly federal income tax payment per visit. If a person's federal income tax is more than $1,200 annually, his fee would amount to more than $12, which would mean that he is not eligible for treatment. How rigorously these standards are applied is unknown. The state holds, and at least some of the community mental health centers concur, that the income limitation does not preclude anybody from receiving an initial diagnosis, but it may keep the higher income groups from lengthy treatment. Some of the mental health centers have reacted by extending the diagnosis period.

Some workers in the field who dislike the income limitation speak of a concept of "psychiatric indigence." By psychiatric indigence they mean that some people who are not so poor as to need public assistance and who could pay ordinary medical bills would suffer financial hardships if faced with lengthy, expensive psychiatric treatment. Social workers taking this position believe that the government should pay for psychiatric care for anyone who needs it, regardless of income, unless the person chooses otherwise. This view is opposed by others who think that almost anyone can afford diagnosis and a few treatments if they take the same responsibility for caring for their mental health as for other aspects of life.

To make a judgment about the adequacy of spending for mental health activities in the Minneapolis–St. Paul area is difficult. Most of the political officials think the amount spent is fair considering mental health needs against other government programs. This is not surprising since they approved the budgets. State expenditures for mental health have risen faster than most other government expenditures as a result of the decision by legislators that this kind of expenditure is popular in the eyes of constituents. State department heads in the welfare field realize that the legislature must make basic factual and value choices among competing demands. By the time the legislature decides, of course, they will have done everything possible through public educational devices to create a favorable climate for mental health programs.

Counties have been designated by the state as the local governments that are permitted to operate mental health centers, although some centers are under private control. The state limits its matching to $.50 per capita for this purpose, but this is a fairly generous sum. Using 1960 population, Hennepin county, for example, could spend $420,000 and be fully matched, while it actually spent only slightly over $300,000 in the 1965–1966 fiscal year. According to one County Board member, if the doctors in the Mental Health Center thought the county should spend more, the board probably would go along. While the county is limited to a one mill tax levy to pay its share, for Hennepin this would have amounted to about $600,000 in 1965.

In Ramsey county, on the other hand, money has not been so readily available. The detailed review of the Mental Health Center budget by the Welfare Board, the joint city-county review committee, and the parent bodies have made it hard to get new functions funded. Ramsey's maximum matching grant would be about $210,000, but it spent only $130,-000 in local funds on the outpatient center in 1965–1966.

Adequacy of spending can ultimately be measured only in terms of need. Here is where the definition of mental illness is important. If government is going to assume responsibility for dispelling all unhappiness and emotional conflicts then the financial need is unlimited. The prospect of this magnitude of spending usually results in a hasty retreat to defining governmental mental health responsibilities as treating only major illness. Minnesota observers believe that the demand for public mental health services will increase. Experience has shown that when a new psychiatric service becomes available, demand grows quickly to outdistance the level of service provided, thus proving Parkinson's law.

CONCLUSIONS

A number of serious problems for mental health programs result from fragmented government in Minnesota. In the first place, resources available to local governments that are dealing with the mental health problems are unequal. Generally, in public programs, equalization has been achieved by moving them up from local to state to national, so that more resources can be tapped and expenditures made where they are needed. The fact that the state pays 50 per cent of the operating costs of a center may mean that those communities with the most local resources get most of the available money from the state. At least the richest communities will get the services first; the poorer communities will have to make a hard choice between services of different kinds, and they will experience serious budget distortions if they try to raise matching funds to get grants. Inequality of resources is illustrated most clearly by the situation in Hennepin and Anoka counties. Most Anoka workers have jobs in Hennepin or Ramsey, but their mental health problems will have to be dealt with where they reside. Choosing a "community" smaller than a problem area and expecting it to pay for a function of government will create inequities.

The choice of the governmental unit to operate the mental health center will affect the result. The county may not be the most efficient or effective unit to operate the system. In a county like Hennepin, which will soon have a population of a million people, a single county mental health center may be too large to service suburban areas and city alike. The federal regulations seem to say clearly that this would be too large. And yet the center was established on a county basis, even when the base hospital was still solely a city operation, because of the desire to seek a larger tax base for the mental health facility and to serve a whole area equally. Dividing the county for mental health services, if attempted, will create new inequities.

The requirement that a mental health governing board must be established in the same size area that the mental health center will service appears to be unwise and perhaps dysfunctional. This is like saying that a school board should operate only one school. Rationally, the area covered by a single board should be large enough to ensure an adequate tax base and a good supply of professional and political leadership. There is no reason why a board could not operate several mental health centers if the population served is too big for a single one. Thus, the choice of the county as a Mental Health Board area in Minnesota can be justified because it is the largest local unit of general government. Where the counties are big and prosperous, this works out fairly well. Where they are small enough to combine, it may also prove satisfactory, although a board serving two counties is not as clearly accountable to the people for the operation of the center and may not have the political support necessary to make it viable.

At least there should not be more than one board in an area, as in St. Paul, where there are three, one for each center. Moreover, boards need not be special boards; an existing government board such as a county or a welfare board could ensure sound support for the centers. A mental health activity committee could be appointed to handle professional policy questions.

Consideration should be given to having a single metropolitanwide operation, either as a single function special district, or as one function of a multi-function metropolitan government. Why should new functions be organized in such a way as to perpetuate old divisions in a metropolitan area?

A larger area for a single board does raise the question of possible conflict with the desirability of having grassroots support for the mental health center in other than financial ways. However, the more basic question is whether it is necessary for a community or governmental unit to have some money of its own involved in a program before it gives loyal support. How close to the people they serve must a professional staff be? Is it a peculiar function of psychiatry that requires successful practice to be carried on only at the neighborhood level?

Still another fragmentation problem is that the jurisdictions of the agencies concerned with mental health activities in the Minneapolis–St. Paul metropolitan area do not coincide. The voluntary associations do not coincide with the counties that are operating the mental health facilities. United Funds are established more on a work-area basis. Southern Anoka county is included in the Hennepin county fund drive. Northern Dakota and western Washington are in on the Ramsey county fund drive. Yet southern Anoka probably does not get its share of United Fund services because it is not convenient for Anoka clients to come to the Minneapolis headquarters of the agencies supported by United Fund. If the mental health center is to use some of the facilities of the voluntary agencies for referrals, they will be using some of the funds of residents of another county. Or, if the center accepts a referral from a voluntary agency, the patient might be from another county and ineligible to be served.

The boundaries of school districts do not coincide with the boundaries of the municipalities or the counties. A similar problem of residence requirements occurs. Cross-charges could be arranged if the counties concerned would agree.

Some inefficiencies are bound to result from the duplication of services available from similar agencies in the same area. At first blush, it might appear that the need for mental health services is so great that there could be no real duplication. Thus, if Catholic Welfare takes care of some families and Lutheran Service helps others, fewer families will wait for service from the general Family and Children's Service. Also, sometimes private agencies that appear to be duplicating services really serve different (by sex and degree of illness) clients. The programs may complement each other and therefore help fill gaps caused by fragmentation of programs among government departments or units. But surely there must be waste in overhead items such as rentals, or from administrative talent used on too small a unit. Worst of all, fragmentation of services results in clients' being referred from one agency to another and often means a loss of the clients themselves. Many persons who need help will not make the effort to go from one agency to another. It may prove difficult or impossible for them to explain their problem again and again to new people. One respondent hypothesized a "cube rule," describing the increasingly high rate at which clients disappeared if they had to be referred beyond a second agency. Rather than risk a third disappointment, they gave up their search for treatment.

THREE: PITFALLS AND PROBLEMS

XI: COMPETING CONCEPTS OF
MENTAL HEALTH

"WE HAVE PASSED the point of no return in our long journey from a helter-skelter system of mental health services divorced from community life"—this is the conclusion reached by Robert H. Felix, the chief architect of the community mental health program. But the point of no return is not the point of no problems. Although it may be true that "whatever difficulties we shall face in the future cannot be more difficult than those of the past," as Dr. Felix asserts, yet some of the problems of the future stem from the same sources that raised difficulties in the past. One of these sources is the conflict and confusion existing within the mental health profession itself. What is the nature of this conflict and confusion, and what are the implications for the future of the community mental health program?

There remains, first of all, considerable controversy over the nature of mental health and mental illness. Secondly, and of particular importance, professional opinion is divided as to the nature and scope of "community mental health." There are, of course, other points of difference within the mental health profession, especially on questions relating to the administration of the program. But the two areas of conflict revolving about the definition of mental health generally and of community mental health in particular represent areas within the peculiar province of the mental health profession itself. Inability of the profession to resolve these questions will certainly complicate the massive effort to commit the country to the community approach on a nationwide basis. Competing definitions, of course, are to some extent a professional disease found in most occupational groups.

Neither the 1963 legislation nor the official pronouncements regarding the new community mental health program provided a clear definition of "mental health," which evidently was assumed to be a desirable absence of mental illness. Even psychiatrists differ about definitions of mental health and mental illness. To be sure, recent works on the question are helpful, but fundamental differences in approach make agreement difficult. [1]

Some understanding of these basic concepts and conflicts is necessary in order to understand the terms of reference within which mental health programs operate and new programs are suggested. The first concern is mental illness; the second, mental health. While mental disorders do not lend themselves to precise definition since they include a great variety of disturbances with many overlapping features, nevertheless, in layman's terms, at least two categories can be identified. These are neuroses and psychoses, which Dr. Francis Braceland and Father Michael Stock in their *Modern Psychiatry* have described as follows:

Neuroses are emotional maladaptations due to unresolved unconscious conflicts. Psychoses are severe emotional illnesses in which there is a departure from normal patterns of thinking, feeling, or acting. A certain degree of personality disorganization appears in the neuroses, and it is more extensive in the psychoses, but, in fact, the intra-psychic forces at work are the ones by which everyone is in some way affected. Every person is subject to anxiety, to changing moods difficult to explain, and at times to distortive and even primitive thinking. Each has available to him the same types of defense reactions and the same range of behavioral reactions, and it is now believed that anxiety lies at the core of most emotional disorders.[2]

The American Psychiatric Association, somewhat more precisely, has classified mental and emotional disorders in three overall groups: "1) Disorders Associated with Impairment of Brain Tissue Functions; 2) Mental Deficiencies, Primarily of Familial Origin and Existing Since Birth; and 3) that great category subsumed under the term 'Disorders of Psychogenic Origin Without Clearly Defined Physical Cause or Structural Change in the Brain.' "[3] "Mental deficiencies" in the sense used here would include mental retardation, elsewhere defined to mean "subaverage intellectual functioning which originates during the developmental period and is associated with impairment in adaptive behavior." Even these definitions may become outmoded in the light of advancing re-

---

[1] See especially Leopold Bellak (ed.), *Handbook of Community Psychiatry and Community Mental Health* (Washington: Grune and Stratton, 1964); Gerald Caplan, *Principles of Preventive Psychiatry* (New York: Basic Books, 1964); Marie Jahoda, *Current Concepts of Positive Mental Health* (New York: Basic Books, 1958); Karl Menninger, *The Vital Balance* (New York: Viking Press, 1963); Francis J. Braceland, M.D., and Michael Stock, O.P., *Modern Psychiatry* (Garden City: Doubleday Image Books, 1963).

[2] Braceland and Stock, *Modern Psychiatry*, p. 90.

[3] *Modern Psychiatry,* Diagnostic Manual of the American Psychiatric Association (Washington: APA, 1965), p. 93.

search, which has begun to yield data on changes in brain tissues accompanying mental illness.

These classifications of mental and emotional disorder have considerable usefulness, but even when they are accepted the question still remains—what are the characteristics of a mentally healthy person? Marie Jahoda noted in an earlier work that the greatest handicap to the systematic study of social conditions conducive to mental health is the very elusive nature of that concept. According to Dr. Jahoda:

As far as we can discover, there exists no psychologically meaningful and, from the point of view of research, operationally useful description of what is commonly understood to constitute mental health. Yet the establishment of some criteria by which the degree of mental health of an individual can be judged is essential if one wishes to identify social conditions conducive to the attainment of mental health.[4]

In Dr. Jahoda's view, there are two basic ways of answering the question of what mental health is. On the one hand, there is the response of the medical profession in general, which usually thinks of mental health as the absence of mental disease. On the other hand, psychologists and psychoanalysts are more inclined to regard mental health in positive terms as the presence of certain psychological characteristics that enable one to live a full and satisfactory life. A major difficulty with the first answer is that there is no general agreement on what constitutes mental disorder. To be sure, one can distinguish types of disorders; and it is possible to recognize severe forms of mental illness. But with less severe disturbance it is not easy to say whether a person is ill or not. As Dr. Jahoda put it in her report on mental health concepts for the Joint Commission in 1958, "To regard the absence of mental disease as a criterion [of mental health] has proved to be an insufficient indication in view of the difficulty of defining disease. Normality, in one connotation, is but a synonym for mental health; in another sense it was found to be unspecific and bare of psychological content." [5] To regard mental health in positive terms as the presence of certain qualities avoids this particular difficulty, but this approach too is beset by the problem of defining "positive" mental health.

Dr. Jahoda pointed to the emphasis on certain personal qualities, on

---

[4] In Ruth Kotinsky and Helen L. Witmer (eds.), *Community Programs for Mental Health* (Cambridge: Harvard University Press, 1955), p. 298.
[5] *Current Concepts of Positive Mental Health*, p. 22.

one's attitude about the "self," as one theme that constantly recurred in the professional literature concerning good mental health.

The mentally healthy attitude toward the self is described by terms such as self-acceptance, self-confidence, or self-reliance, each with slightly different connotations. Self-acceptance implies that a person has learned to live with himself, accepting both the limitations and possibilities he may find in himself. Self-confidence, self-esteem, and self-respect have a more positive slant; they express the judgment that in balance the self is "good, capable, and strong." [6]

But, she reported, there are numerous other criteria as well, such as the individual's reality orientation and the success of his efforts at mastering his environment. Adaptation and environmental mastery are emphasized in the literature and are grouped in a rough order of importance from ability to love and adequacy in love, work, and play, to capacity for adaptation and judgment, and efficiency in problem solving. The individual's ability to respond to situations that place him under emotional stress may be viewed as offering even more specific criteria than the more general concept of integration. In this regard Dr. Jahoda quotes Dr. Jack Ewalt's definition of mental health: "A kind of resilience of character or ego strength permitting an individual, as nearly as possible, to find in his world those elements he needs to satisfy his basic impulses in a way that is acceptable to his fellows, or failing this, to find a suitable sublimation for them."

To other psychiatrists, however, self-determination, self-expression, and the desire for autonomy as measures of mental health seem time-bound and culture-bound.[7] These concerns, they argue, are an American preoccupation; Europeans could maintain that acceptance of inter-dependency between individuals is a much better test of good mental health. "A reasonable dependence on others is one of the recognizable characteristics of emotional maturity just as excessive dependence can be characteristic of the immature person." [8]

However varied the many definitions of positive mental health may be, in Dr. Jahoda's view the qualities viewed as necessary "basically . . .

[6] *Ibid.*, p. 24.
[7] See Elaine Cumming, "Allocation of Care to the Mentally Ill, American Style," in *Sociology as Policy Science: Essays on Social Welfare Problems,* ed. Mayer N. Zald (not yet published).
[8] Ebbe Curtis Hoff, "Dependence," *Encyclopedia of Mental Health* (New York: Franklin Watts, 1963), II, 451.

can be reduced to two major areas: the relation of the individual to himself and the relation of an individual to the world around him." [9]

These two primary aspects of the mental situation of the individual are reflected in diverse institutional emphases in public mental health activities. Society's attitude toward the individual who suffers from mental illness was first expressed in provisions for segregating those "madmen" who might harm themselves or others. As more concern was felt for individuals who were mentally ill, this was expressed in efforts to help cure their illness through improved care in mental hospitals. The most recent major thrust of the thought and practice of mental health has been to consider the environment of the person who is mentally ill and—for the "frontier thinkers"—the environment of those who might become mentally ill in the future. This general concept is denoted by the term "community psychiatry," which Dr. Leopold Bellak thinks might well be considered a third major revolution in the history of psychiatry or, at the very least, a major evolutionary stage.[10] He holds that the first phase of psychiatry as an independent science began at the end of the eighteenth century in Western Europe; the period following the Age of Reason marked the passing of the era of demonology and the development of a new sympathetic attitude toward mental illness, with an increasing concern for the mentally ill and a desire to improve their lot. Clinical interest focused on the search for causes and for more effective treatment methods. Sociological aspects of mental disease came to be considered and theories of the psychogenic causes began to be discussed.

The second phase, in Dr. Bellak's view, was initiated about one hundred years later as the result of the development of psychoanalysis by Sigmund Freud. Not only did psychoanalysis gradually gain recognition as the first rational treatment method for psychiatric disorders, but it has given us added insight into the functioning of the human mind, its application to physical illness has enabled increased understanding of the emotional aspects of physical illness, and its application to the social sciences has helped us to understand the world in which we live and its effect on our behavior.

Community psychiatry is the third phase, which has multiple and varied roots.

[9] "Mental Health," *Encyclopedia of Mental Health,* III, 1067–68.
[10] See Leopold Bellak, "Community Psychiatry: The Third Psychiatric Revolution," in *Handbook of Community Psychiatry and Community Mental Health.*

It may be considered a truly evolutionary phenomenon in that it is largely a synthesis of the two phases in the development of psychiatry which preceded it. . . . it reflects the concern for the welfare of the psychiatric patient, which was previously characteristic of the Age of Reason. This concern was able to gather further momentum, primarily as the result of the increased insight into the nature and treatment of mental illness afforded by psychoanalytic hypotheses.[11]

Community psychiatry contains ingredients arising from the marriage of social and behavioral science—psychiatry and psychology, sociology and anthropology, and social work and physical medicine. Advances in public health and in epidemiology have also made contributions. Bellak believes that community psychiatry "can best be defined as the resolve to view the individual's psychiatric problems within the frame of reference of the community and *vice versa.*"

Once it is accepted that it is insufficient to merely wait for persons thought to be mentally ill to be delivered at the door of large, and usually isolated, institutions for treatment, then new patterns of action and organization are required. What are the practical implications of the vague term "community psychiatry"?

Such concerns can have two major thrusts: the first is still basically concerned with the individual who is mentally ill—or at least not in a state of full mental health—within the broad context of his family, work, and community; the second is concerned with the community environment itself. Both approaches envisage a major extension of mental health services outside the familiar mode of treatment in large mental hospitals, and both may be comprehended within the term "community mental health"; however, they are quite distinct and require separate treatment.

The initial meaning of "community mental health" was to extend the area of treatment from the isolated mental hospital to the areas in which patients live and work, which has led to gradual development of mental health units scattered throughout a state or county. Furthermore, it has been increasingly appreciated that community psychiatry will embrace a variety of resources, not merely a single center. Coupled with the belief that the use of such services will encourage the consideration of the total environment of particular persons who are mentally ill is the hope that having such facilities at hand will provide help much earlier in the course of the illness.

While there were small beginnings in these directions several decades

[11] *Ibid.*

ago, such action has increased since the end of the Second World War and has been vastly stimulated by the enactment of the 1963 federal legislation. As this major change was succinctly defined by Dr. Leonard Duhl,

prior to World War II . . . much of psychiatry was hospital oriented. After the war, psychiatrists became primarily patient-oriented. . . . The era we are now completing has experienced a reawakening in two directions: increased interest in the biologic aspect of mental illness, and a socio-psychological concern with family, the hospital and the broader community.[12]

In this period of transition, it has been obvious that there is not a single agreed-upon meaning of the term "community psychiatry."

John Cumming, then director of the Syracuse Psychiatric Hospital and chief of the New York State Mental Health Research Unit, freely admitted, "I do not know what community psychiatry is. Community psychiatry is the name that will be applied to what we will do in the next ten years . . . we can expect the words 'community psychiatry' to cover a multitude of different programs." [13] Will community psychiatry improve mental health services? Dr. Cumming wonders. While it is hard to deny the necessity of taking care of a patient in the mental hospital, he argues, it may be easy to forget about the same person if he is invisible in the community. Are we trying to remedy the neglect of the mentally ill in our large hospitals by simply moving them into the community? Will an answer to the problem be found simply by geography? After all, the *sine qua non* of community psychiatry is the replacement of large state hospitals by wards in general hospitals or by small hospitals in each community.

There are aspects of the trend toward community psychiatry, however, that Dr. Cumming found hopeful. Full psychiatric care for circumscribed groups of people may be provided by a psychiatric ward of a hospital, the psychiatric department of a medical center, or perhaps one of the proposed community mental health centers. "One of the great weaknesses in current psychiatric services," Dr. Cumming thinks, "is that they are provided by a network of unorganized medical and social services each with its own policies regarding selection of clients. Scarcely any attention is given to providing an effective referral service."

[12] Leonard Duhl, *The Urban Condition* (New York: Basic Books, 1963), p. 65.
[13] John Cumming, M.D., "What Is Community Psychiatry," paper read at Syracuse Psychiatric Hospital, June 1963.

An overall type of responsibility is built into the concept of the community mental health center. While there may be difficulties in maintaining the quality of services, any improvement in coordination would have much to commend it.

The second major aspect arises because it is quite clear that modern psychiatry, in the view of many of its practitioners, encompasses more than treatment of those afflicted with mental illness. Karl Menninger calls mental illness "personality disfunction and living impairment," and argues that "psychiatry should . . . provide a better understanding of human beings in trouble—yes, and human beings out of trouble—without pejoratively labeling them." [14] But greater understanding, or even cure, is not enough. The goals of psychiatry must extend further—to prevention.

With this emphasis, psychiatry becomes deeply involved in the well and the sick, in social structure, mores, attitudes, and values. A broad appraisal of the health continuum in that context also has implications for the goals of treatment. Those need no longer be confined to a reinstatement of the status quo ante (recovery in the popular sense), but might well push forward the development of new potentialities and transcendence of previous levels of vital balance to a state of being "weller than well." [15]

Menninger views human beings as "in a constant process of adaptation, subject to occasional major derailments. Estimating the severity and reversibility of these derailments . . . and determining how and why they occur, might enable us to plan logical and effective intervention."

Gerald Caplan in his *Principles of Preventive Psychiatry* describes preventive psychiatry as that "body of professional knowledge, both theoretical and practical, which may be utilized to plan and carry out programs for reducing (1) the incidence of mental disorders of all types in a community (primary prevention), (2) the duration of a significant number of those disorders which do occur (secondary prevention), and (3) the impairment which may result from those disorders (tertiary prevention)." In outlining a program of primary prevention, he states that it

would focus on identifying current harmful influence, the environmental forces which support individuals in resisting them, and those environmental forces which influence the resistance of the population to future pathogenic experience. This approach is based on the assumption that many mental

[14] Menninger, *The Vital Balance,* p. 5.
[15] *Ibid.,* p. 401.

disorders result from maladaptation and maladjustment and that, by altering the balance of forces, a healthy adaptation and adjustment is possible.[16]

Thus, primary prevention involves logistic and community planning issues that look beyond the individual to the total community picture. To be effective there must be a considerable measure of mental health education for a wide variety of community leaders and frequent consultation concerning day-to-day problems. In order to function effectively in this conception of his role, the "preventive" psychiatrist must be not only a competent medical specialist, but—beyond that—he

must also learn to coordinate his activities with those of many other professional and non-professional workers who are actively involved in dealing with the health, education, and legal and social aspects of the community problems posed by the mentally ill, and the mentally retarded and with community programs in allied fields. . . . it follows that preventive psychiatry is a branch of psychiatry, but it is also part of a wide community endeavor in which psychiatrists make their own specialized contributions to a larger whole.[17]

Menninger has graphically pictured the role of the psychiatrist of tomorrow as follows:

leaving the hospital . . . he visits the church, the factory, the medical clinic, and the general hospital. He stops in the nursery school and the grade school and the high school. He visits the prison and the detention home. In each case he makes his call and his suggestions and takes his leave—a kind of twentieth-century general practitioner who has awakened from a long sleep and gotten busy helping his neighbors, having given up his childhood dialect and learned to speak English.[18]

As has been sketched above, the terms "mental health" and "mental illness" are hardly models of clarity, and this is also true of "community mental health." This slogan was inscribed on the banners of those who succeeded in having the landmark 1963 federal legislation enacted, and obviously it served its purpose well. The term is suggestive of many good things, yet it is imprecise and flexible.

It is of interest to note some of the major components of the arguments favoring this movement in general. The primary component has been set forth above—that it was essential to consider the mentally ill person within the context of his total personal and social environment, rather than merely as an isolated human being incarcerated in a large

[16] Caplan, *Principles of Preventive Psychiatry*, pp. 27–28.
[17] *Ibid.*, p. 17.
[18] Menninger, *The Vital Balance*, p. 8.

institution. Related to this was the belief that it would be highly advantageous to provide services to persons with mental difficulties within their own communities, because it would be more likely that they would seek or be provided with care earlier than if the only source of help required hospitalization. Furthermore, it was believed that many persons with relatively limited problems could remain in their own community if help was available there during part of the day, or in times of particular stress. Not only was this far better for the individual, but also it would relieve the ever-mounting pressure on the mental hospitals. Thus, it was asserted that the investment of resources within the community[19] would forestall much larger investments of both capital and operating funds in expansion of the state and other hospitals for the mentally ill. Indeed, the more exuberant supporters of community-based mental health services seemed to believe that by the combination of the new tranquilizing drugs and the spread of community mental health centers the large mental hospitals will wither away not too long hence.

These were plausible arguments, and evidently they were persuasive to the United States Congress that enacted the 1963 legislation and has continued to provide funds to begin the programs developed with the planning monies provided to the states. Yet, as Dr. John Cumming has noted, the success of these plans rests upon a series of assumptions, none of which is so firmly established as to be considered axiomatic. In 1963, when the basic legislation was being considered, Dr. Cumming noted: "There are at the moment, as far as I know, no American studies that demonstrate that, when the quality of care is held constant, community-based treatment facilities function any better than those located in large hospitals." If this remarkable statement is valid, it would appear that the nature of mental health services and the investment of hundreds of millions of dollars throughout the country was substantially shaped for decades to come on the basis of firmly held and persuasively argued beliefs that lacked a substantial empirical base.

This point has been reiterated by a diverse set of opponents in the succeeding years. Some such opposition doubtless is entirely disinterested and merely concerned with improving mental health services generally. Another large segment of professionals who share the same sentiments, even though often they may suffer in silence, are those associated with

[19] The term "community" has been used with great facility but with extremely varied meaning in respect to mental health, as is examined in Chapter XII.

the large mental hospitals. They certainly disagree with the view that the large hospitals are about to wither away, and with the implication that the community mental health centers can provide a total replacement for them.

It may be tempting to envisage a dichotomy between the "disease" concept of mental illness associated with hospitalization, and the "environmental" concept of such illness associated with community mental health services and a broader view of the role of psychiatry. However, such a simplified concept is in error. The totality of community mental health services and the larger hospitals serving broader areas and meeting specialized needs should be viewed as providing an extensive continuum and variety of services. The great merit of such planned community services is that those public and private resources existing heretofore are linked in a coordinated way, and augmented by services provided in the new community centers. Yet even the most extensive system of such localized services will not supplant the large mental hospitals, although it may go far to relieve their overload.

Associated with this point is another substantial division of opinion among professionals in the mental health field. The advocates of the community approach strongly implied that such centers would enable the detection and successful treatment in their own communities of large numbers of persons who otherwise would wind up in the mental hospitals. Many of those associated with the hospitals believe that while the proposed community centers will indeed have some impact, most of their patients will be those who have never sought—or at least have not received —formal treatment before. In other words, substantial new categories of the "mentally ill" will be discovered and will absorb much of the energies of the new centers. Certainly the penchant of many community-oriented persons for implying, at least, that the centers will treat all comers suggests that this will be a real problem. Yet as William Ryan suggested in his study of services for the mentally ill in Boston, such an attitude is based upon "a hidden assumption . . . that all persons who are handicapped by emotional disturbance are entitled to service to lessen their handicap. In practice, society has made no such commitment and there is no mechanism for providing such services to all who need them, or even to all who request them." [20] As the complex of mental

[20] William Ryan, *Distress in the City* (Boston: United Community Services, 1965), p. 49.

health services and allied institutions becomes better established, the question of how far society's commitment extends may well become central; for the present, there must be careful study of how much the community centers do in fact intercept perceptible numbers of those who otherwise would have been sent to the large hospitals.

On the basis of the metropolitan studies, there seems to be relatively little criticism of the community mental health center concept as such. In most areas, there are at least some outspoken advocates of this approach to providing for the mentally ill, and there are relatively few within the profession who openly attack it. One of the exceptions is Dr. Thomas Szasz, professor of psychiatry, Upstate Medical College, State University of New York. Proceeding from his libertarian and antimedical position on "the myth of mental illness," Dr. Szasz perceives community psychiatry as a political effort at moral manipulation "to collectivize American society." [21] Though the Syracuse study (Chapter VIII) alludes to the influence of Dr. Szasz in that metropolitan area and in New York state psychiatric circles, it may be presumed that he has some followers in all the areas considered here, although not many within the profession.

On the whole, as the field studies demonstrate, there is a considerable degree of consensus on most aspects of the proposed community mental health activity, including the following points:

1. Public authorities are still and should be primarily responsible for dealing with the problems of mental disorder.

2. Mental illness is basically a medical problem and falls within the domain of medicine, though nonmedical professions and disciplines have their contributions to make to the mental health team and teamwork.

3. Voluntary (as against coerced) participation by patients in the experiences of diagnosis and therapy enhances the effectiveness of treatment.

4. "Community" is perceived geographically rather than sociologically, as an area in which the patient conveniently receives services close to "home" or "family" in lieu of the distant and "impersonal" setting of a state hospital.

[21] Thomas Szasz, "The Mental Health Ethic," *National Review*, XVII, No. 24 (June 14, 1966), 570. Relevant publications by Dr. Szasz include *The Myth of Mental Illness* (New York: Hoeber-Harper, 1961) and *Law, Liberty, and Psychiatry* (New York: Macmillan, 1963).

5. "Community" is also perceived administratively as a "participant" in the overall system for the care of the mentally ill, contributing financially and managing various facilities or centers.

6. The population to be served is the entire population of the community rather than the indigent or welfare segment alone.

7. Continuity of care is accepted as a cornerstone of the "bold new approach," with the understanding that it requires and envisages liaison between local centers and state hospitals, psychiatric and nonpsychiatric services, and public programs and private practice.

8. Comprehensive services include emergency, short-term, intermediate term, and long-term services in various treatment settings to meet diverse needs of diverse populations, as set forth in Public Law 88–164.

9. The continuum of functions for "community mental health programs" is being broadened to embrace all functions from prevention at the one end to restoration of the individual to a full role in society at the other, including early detection, primary and secondary treatment, recovery, and rehabilitation.

10. A mental health center is a physical facility and staff, but not that alone; it may be in another guise an administrative arrangement among various public and private facilities, or both.

It goes without saying that each of these aspects of the community psychiatry concept has special shades of meaning for particular localities. On this point the field studies shed little illumination; they do not even indicate the relative importance of each or the particular emphasis each has attracted in the various communities. In part, this is because the development of the proposed centers has rarely moved sufficiently far to provide evidence on such points. It would seem that the community psychiatry concept asserts or adheres to no definition of mental illness of its own but as a practical matter remains neutral on this issue, thus leaving it to the communities and states to identify their mentally ill population by criteria of their own choice.

Another conclusion inferred from the field studies is that community mental health as currently conceived in the SMSA's is by no means antithetical either to state mental health operations or the private practice of psychiatry. It accords recognition to the realities of both, reaching out to them for partnerships. If its champions have criticized state governments for the shocking physical conditions and dubious practices of state hospitals, they have made no effort to deprive the states of their mental health responsibilities or drive them out of the field altogether, but rather they have looked to reform under the leadership of state officials. They have welcomed the construction of new state facilities within their localities as contributions to community psychiatry, proposing at the same time that the states and local authorities and agencies work out their mutual problems of management and direction in order to ensure practical cooperation and continuity of care for the patients. Furthermore, they have urged the state authorities in charge of mental hospitals to modernize these institutions and reorient them toward direct involvement in community mental health programs. No one has argued for the complete disengagement of the state from the mental health field on the ground that its continued participation is incompatible with the basic tenets of community mental health.

Nor has there evolved a serious public or professional confrontation between community mental health versus the private practice of psychiatry. In theory the former neither sets up restrictions on the freedom of the latter nor does it invade its market place. Actually the federal Act specifies that the private practitioner is to retain management of his cases where his patient utilizes the facilities of the community mental health center. Many local organizations entitled to financial assistance are retaining practicing psychiatrists as consultants for referrals. County medical societies and psychiatric association chapters have openly endorsed the principles of community mental health or have simply remained silent on this subject, except in Massachusetts, where the medical society at one time recommended that the state disengage itself from local mental health programs. (In 1963 the American Medical Association headquarters did exploit its influence in political circles in opposition to the inclusion in the federal Act of specific provisions for federal financial support for the operation of community mental health centers. However, the 1963 Act has since been amended to authorize this type of support.) Some psychiatrists may have in their own mind associated government sponsorship of community mental health with the advance of socialized medicine, but the practical effect of such sentiments has been negligible. The profession has endured and cooperated with the state hospital systems for generations, though some members may feel that community-based programs under public control brings state intervention in medicine "closer to home."

Thus, on the whole, the concept of community mental health seems to have been accepted with varying degrees of enthusiasm; some indeed have become true believers, while others are at least willing to give the idea a fair trial. Furthermore, it may be presumed that some potential opposition has been stilled because the ability to secure available substantial federal funds in the general interests of mental health requires at least a symbolic acceptance of the concepts embodied in the federal legislation of 1963. Furthermore, the plans developed in the several states with federal planning grants had to meet minimum requirements that called for a considerable move toward the presumed goals of the community mental health campaign if the centers were to be eligible for more substantial federal funding in the future. There is no evidence in the field studies of such unyielding hostility to the whole concept of community mental health services that the entire project was rejected out of hand, although certainly not every aspect has been completely accepted.

However, the basic conflicts that occurred in several of the states over which agency was to be in charge of what was evidently to become a substantial federally funded activity were in some cases more than mere power struggles. They reflected the attempts of the older, hospital-oriented groups to retain control and to relegate the new centers to the status of satellites of the mental hospitals. The Seattle study develops comparatively the respective community psychiatry philosophies of the Department of Health and the Department of Institutions' Division of Mental Health. The State Health Director and the Supervisor of the Division of Mental Health of Institutions indeed had areas of disagreement. The two major differences in their approach rested on (a) the difference between a public health, epidemiological approach and a psychiatric perception of program and (b) an inter-agency difference as to the unit best qualified to carry out the job. In Syracuse, the county commissioner of mental health, a firm proponent of community programs, has kept up a barrage of criticism against the state Department of Mental Hygiene in regard to its interpretation of community mental health. In his thinking the commissioner assigns a high priority to "localness" and local management in community mental health programs, perceiving the state programs as wedded almost inseparably to the hospitals under state control. This view of the state approach was not far from the mark. However, the Department of Mental Hygiene in Albany has been able to alter its image, changing as it commits itself to the construction of hospitals in the under-served urban areas, arrogating to itself a major role in community mental health programs in these localities.

While it might be held that there is no serious opposition to the idea of community mental health *centers,* community mental health itself is such an amorphous concept that it only gains reality in respect to a given and concrete situation. The doubts or hostility toward the realization of the more long-term objectives of the community mental health movement will become apparent in the inevitable contests over the allocation of state funds to one or another aspect of mental health services. However, the availability of federal funds certainly strengthened the position of the advocates of community mental health activities; as such services are established, they should create a much more potent clientele group than the state hospitals ever would have. Consequently, the long-term struggle—in those states where there still is sufficient hostility to fuel such a fight—probably will be won by the community service groups. It seems unlikely that future conflicts over the allocation of growing resources will erupt into a full-fledged ideological battle between state mental hospitals on the one hand and the community services on the other; the occasion for such a direct confrontation has already passed, leaving deep scars in some of the states and no perceptible effect in others. The battles of the future are likely to resemble the quiet though deadly warfare of submarines far beneath the surface of the sea; probably they will be struggles for resources or influence largely within the state mental health bureaucracies.

Of course, as mental health programs become more community oriented, the probability of conflicts with educational, welfare, and other related bureaucracies is increased. Community mental health is such an undeveloped concept that administrative implementation involves a kind of empire building that logically requires taking over functions now performed in other empires and jealously guarded. Thus community mental health as a governmental program may appear to others as an octopus whose grasping tentacles extend in all directions.

The scope of any governmental service is inevitably a compromise between what enthusiastic advocates urge and what less sanguine souls are willing to accept and pay for. Aspects of a new governmental program, which at its early stages evoked almost religious fervor, often seem primitive and even misdirected after only a few years. As the function gains acceptance or as the problems become more complex, the accompanying accommodation to competitive political reality forces experimentation, and important changes in approach follow.

The provision of mental health services resembles this general model in many respects, but at the same time it seems to have certain distinctive attributes of quite a remarkable character—particularly in respect to current stages of development and what may lie ahead. In the first place, there remains considerable controversy over the nature of mental health and mental illness. In consequence, debate over the nature of public programs needed and over the scope of such programs continues unabated. And, of particular importance, professional opinion is divided as to the nature and scope of "community mental health," and experience concerning the effectiveness of efforts in this vein is relatively limited.

To establish a new governmental program, or a major expansion of an existing one, it is usually necessary to secure and maintain broad institutional and popular enthusiasm and support. In the case of the community mental health program embodied in the 1963 legislation, this effort acquired something of the character of a crusade with the development of an attendant ideology. The effect was to commit the federal government to an approach which is the subject of considerable, though usually muffled, professional and organizational controversy. Yet the concepts underlying this extensive program of public action are sufficiently unclear that implementation in particular states might vary substantially in order to accommodate varying attitudes or historical and institutional factors. This conceptual vagueness leaves the future development of the community mental health enterprise subject to an unusual degree of potential experimentation, which may be viewed as either advantageous or hazardous depending upon one's perspective.

Intriguing and deserving of research and experimentation as these far-reaching suggestions may be, there is nothing to indicate that they have been accepted or even seriously considered as policy guidelines— let alone translated into action—in the metropolitan areas of this study. Those involved in the development of community mental health services were still primarily in the planning stage, tackling the knotty legal, financial, diplomatic, and operational problems that had to be solved before any kind of expanded operation could get under way. Consequently, the prospect that the United States will soon see the glorious beginnings of community psychiatrists functioning as social engineers, as some might hope, or, on the other hand, the machinations of a group of self-anointed philosopher-kings bent on the collectivization of American society, as some obviously fear, seems distant indeed.

XII: THE SEARCH FOR COMMUNITY

THE CENTRAL THRUST of the federal government's 1963 attempt to change and markedly expand mental health services is the development of a network of community mental health centers (CMHC). What was intended by "community" is not altogether clear, and that confusion has serious implications for the successful implementation of the program. Some kind of community involvement in the establishment and operation of these centers was contemplated, and each facility was supposed to service some kind of community. The involvement idea reflects a sociological view of community while the service approach implies geographic catchment areas stemming from administrative concerns. Both are problematical and raise serious questions regarding the future of the program.

The circumstances surrounding the development and passage of the 1963 legislation suggest that the community idea stemmed largely from concepts of care calling for an interweaving of mental health services into the very fabric of the local society. Four basic concerns were expressed by the principal advocates of the community centers program: first, the therapeutic concern for the mentally ill persons; second, the functional concern with how the centers might operate; third, the concern about organizing and financing the centers; and fourth, concern over the "load factor" of the growing number of potential mental patients and the consequent strain upon the large mental hospitals.

The view that the medical staff ought to be thoroughly familiar with the mental patient's environment, his "therapeutic community," and that this is best accomplished by providing mental health centers "close to home" [1] is so central to the federal program that it might seem

---

[1] For example, see statement of Secretary Anthony J. Celebrezze during the hearings prior to passage of the 1963 Act: U.S., Congress, Senate, Subcommittee on Health of the Committee on Labor and Public Welfare, *Hearings on S. 755 and 756,* 88th Cong., 1st Sess., 1963, pp. 17–18; statement of Dr. Francis J. Braceland, pp. 60–61; and statement of Mr. Frank Proctor, p. 91.

self-evident that this goal, at least, can be attained. Yet like many self-evident ideas, this goal of the CMHC program is not necessarily self-achieving. It may be substantially valid for CMHC's in dense urban areas, although even here the medical staffs' depth of understanding of conditions in the seamier parts of the urban complex may be questioned. However, if the CMHC serves an extensive hinterland as well as the urban center in which it is situated, the medical staff is not likely to understand the particular environment of their patients from such outlying areas any better than the state hospital staff. Furthermore, since even the most optimistic advocates of community mental health centers do not forecast the immediate withering away of the state hospital systems, there would continue to be many mental patients whose "therapeutic community" would be no better understood than before.

The functional concept of the community mental health center reflects the basic commitment of its advocates to comprehensive care and positive mental health. Since almost every mental patient has a network of family, friendship, and neighborhood relationships where he lives, a community-based facility would be much better situated to work with this set of relations of the patient than would a distant hospital staff. Further, much of the secondary defense against mental illness must be provided by existing local agencies since formal mental health resources are grossly insufficient to meet all needs. Moreover, existing local agencies and individuals can be of great help in matching up the various needs for service and the agencies that can provide them.[2]

The concern with the functional community of the mental patient is the positive side of the concept of his therapeutic community. The staff of the CMHC can utilize the patient's family, church, neighborhood organization, social organizations, and place of work to strengthen him and avoid hospitalization or to ease the return to relative mental equilibrium if he has been hospitalized. Beyond the functional community of the individual patient is a larger network of social organizations and agencies which may be of assistance in maintaining or regaining mental health. This group of agencies might be termed the "contingent functional community."

[2] See statements of Dr. Francis J. Braceland during the hearings prior to passage of the 1963 Act, *ibid.*, p. 61; statement of Mr. Mike Gorman, pp. 48–49; and statement of Mr. Boisfeuillet Jones, U.S., Congress, House, Subcommittee of the Committee on Interstate and Foreign Commerce (Mental Health Supplemental), *Hearings*, 88th Cong., 1st Sess., 1963, pp. 19–20.

From the perspective of the individual patient, all such resources would be strengthened and their activities would be coordinated with the developing community mental health program. The CMHC staffs would work with such organizations to care for many persons who otherwise might require service from the center itself.

A third idea underlying the commitment to the community center concept has been a kind of localism resembling ideas of grassroots virtue permeating the American political tradition. Many mental health advocates have concluded that local mental health facilities ought to be integral parts of the communities they serve because of the need for some local financial support and the network of functional relationships described above. These partisans feel that awareness of the need for better mental health services must be developed in the local communities. It is crucial, therefore, that an opportunity be provided for appropriate groups and individuals in the community to participate in the policy direction of the centers.[3]

Finally, the advocates of community mental health centers have stressed the very practical consideration of the strain on mental hospital facilities presented by the increasing need for services. Many people believe that by providing prompt service in a local setting for persons in distress, and by providing outpatient service and day and night care, community mental health centers can substantially reduce the pressure upon state mental hospitals.[4]

Evident in the discussion of the relationships of the new community mental health centers and their "communities" is the ideal of the New England town of the nineteenth century. No doubt this ideal retains a sentimental significance in American thinking but does it fit the facts of urban America today? Can urbanized areas, where most Americans live, be equated with "communities" in the old sense, where some citizens, at least, felt responsible for all? Scott Greer, in *The Emerging City,* has concluded that the freedom of individual location and action

---

[3] See statement of Dr. V. Terrell Davis during the hearings prior to passage of the 1963 Act, Senate subcommittee hearings, p. 141; and see Arthur C.K. Hallock and Warren T. Vaughn, Jr., "Community Organization—A Dynamic Component of Community Mental Health Practice," *American Journal of Orthopsychiatry,* XXVI (Oct. 1956), 691.

[4] See statement of Dr. Robert Felix during the hearings prior to passage of the 1963 Act, Senate subcommittee hearings, pp. 190–91; statement of Dr. Blain, pp. 121–23; and see President Kennedy's message, reprinted on pp. 23–32, esp. p. 25.

in large-scale society makes this impossible. Exceptions occur in only a few instances. He says:

The local area is not a community in any sense in the highly urbanized areas of the city; it is a community of "limited liability" in the suburbs. Communication and participation are as apt to be segmental as in any formal organization that is extraterritorial. And many [persons] are utterly uninvolved, even in the strongest spatially defined community.[5]

On the other hand, while the nature of "community" in large cities is unclear, people do engage in community activities. Despite the anonymity and mobility of urban living, probably very few people are completely decommunitized. Perhaps we just do not yet know the structure of the real community in modern urbanized areas.

Using the vague term "community" may have provided a workable way of starting the effort to obtain local mental health services, but what real effect has this concept had on the new program? Is there any significant sense of "community" in large metropolitan areas? Do proposed service areas of CMHC's have any relationship to existing communities, and, if so, what? To what extent will a belief in local decision making as an ideal be allowed to obstruct the development of what is viewed as a vitally needed public service? The case studies suggest some of the answers.

There is little evidence in the case studies that the metropolitan areas as such had any significant consciousness of being "communities." The sole exception seemed to be that in all cases charitable fund raising has been centralized and is conducted through some sort of "community chest" drive, while the continuing coordination of supported services is carried out by a "united community services" type of unit. Possibly in certain areas, baseball or other professional athletic teams spark some degree of metropolitan consciousness from time to time, although they are primarily associated with the central city from which they hail. In most other respects, however, in the areas studied here there was far more conflict than harmony between central city and suburbs, between city and county governments, between urban areas and rural hinterland, between local governments and the state, and between clashing personalities at all levels. These are significant portents for the would-be coordinator of the mental health resources of a metropolitan area.

Furthermore, even if there were more sense of metropolitan com-

[5] Scott Greer, *The Emerging City* (New York: The Free Press, 1962), p. 103.

munity in evidence than was reported, the areas studied were in all cases far too large for a single CMHC to serve adequately. Some will need two or three, others will need perhaps four or five, while metropolitan Boston may well require upwards of fifteen. Whether mental health center "communities" can be used to help overcome present divisions such as central city–suburban hostility or whether they will have to be designed to parallel present lines of social cleavage remains to be seen.

The 1963 Act, as passed, is not very helpful as to the kind of center/locality relationship intended. The Secretary of Health, Education, and Welfare was authorized to grant funds for local centers when he found "that the services to be provided . . . will be part of a program providing principally for persons residing in a particular community or communities in or near which such center is to be situated . . . essential elements of comprehensive mental health services." This wording suggests a localized concept of "community" appropriate for urbanized areas, providing no relationship other than geographic proximity is envisioned; but it has little usefulness when applied to the more rural areas of the United States. The regulations issued to govern the administration of the law, however, are more specific, perhaps reflecting a confrontation of the community ideal with the practical realities of population and geography in the United States. While community mental health center is defined in words that parrot the legislation, the following two statements are more revealing:

(b) "Area" means the geographic territory which includes one or more communities served or to be served by existing or proposed community mental health facilities, the delineation of which is based on such factors as population distribution, natural geographic boundaries, and transportation accessibility.

(c) "Community" means an area or that portion of an area served or to be served by a program providing at least the essential elements of comprehensive mental health services.[6]

Thus, the tautology: a community mental health center is a facility offering comprehensive mental health services for persons residing in a particular community or communities, and a community is a geographic area which is offered comprehensive mental health services by a

[6] *Community Mental Health Centers Act of 1963, Title II of Public Law 88-164, Regulations,* Part 54.201 (b) and (c), in U.S., *Federal Register,* May 6, 1964, p. 5951.

community mental health center. According to the regulations, then, a "community" is simply the service or "catchment" area of the mental health facility.

A service area interpretation presents problems. Though some latitude was allowed for particular cases, the regulations directed that each state plan provide for mental health centers serving populations ranging from 75,000 to 200,000. Moreover, the regulations specifically required that the centers be "so located as to be near and readily accessible to the community and populations to be served, taking into account both political and geographical boundaries."

Some general principles about service areas for facilities of all kinds are quite firmly established.[7] Their size, both in terms of population and geographic area, depends on variables defined by environing conditions such as population density, per capita demand for service, transportation facilities, and the nature of other services distributed from the same location. These considerations suggest that the size of populations to be served by a mental health facility must be itself quite a flexible variable.

In heavily urbanized areas, it will not be difficult to define sectors with the required population. In more sparsely settled locales outside the metropolises, however, a large geographic area may be required in order to provide the minimal population base for a mental health center. If facilities so placed could satisfactorily perform the functions for which they are intended, why not ignore the population standard in the urbanized areas and concentrate wholly on optimal service efficiency?

Emphasis on a catchment area concept of community leads to a denial of the view—fundamental to the community mental health center idea—that community integration is crucial to service efficiency. At the same time, too great an emphasis on the involvement concept of community tends to obscure service efficiency. Either could well result in a frustration of the purposes of the federal program. The "idea of community" is therefore crucial to the implementation of the 1963 Act.

If mental health care is to be community-based, the question becomes, what is a community? Sociologists have defined communities as broadly

---

[7] For a general theory see August Losch, *The Economics of Location* (New Haven: Yale University Press, 1954), esp. Chapter II. For specific studies pertaining to the medical services areas see Brian J. L. Berry and Allen Pred, *Central Studies: A Bibliography of Theory and Application*, Section VIII, "Medical Service Areas" (Philadelphia: Regional Science Research Institute, 1961), pp. 87–88.

as international communities and as specifically as those of single organizations or institutions. Economists have seen the community in market and service terms. Political scientists have considered community in the context of influence and decision making within defined governmental areas as these relate to social structure, stratified or otherwise. The obfuscation is summed up by Charles R. Adrian as follows:

The term, community, is confusing and inconsistent, both as it is generally used in social science writing and as it exists in the minds of citizens when they discuss their own problems. . . . To the citizen, the concept of community may simultaneously include an area both larger and smaller than a given city. For example, it differs for purposes of water supply, community chest campaigns, retail trading, educational facilities, hospital service, religious worship, police protection, and other activities.[8]

American sociologists originally derived the idea of community from the study of ecological areas.[9] A modern concept of the metropolitan community in the United States probably dates from the writings of N. S. B. Gras, who contended that at each stage of technological development there arose a unique kind of community appropriate for utilizing the new methods of wresting a livelihood from the environment. The most recent form of economic organization, metropolitan economy, "has risen in national states and is based upon the union of a great commercial city as a nucleus and a large hinterland" which are mutually dependent.[10] R. D. McKenzie extended Gras's notion of the metropolitan community, basing its genesis on the development of motor transportation.[11] A fairly elaborate picture of metropolitan organization was provided in Donald J. Bogue's *The Structure of the Metropolitan Community.*[12]

More recently, Talcott Parsons employed an analytical scheme for discussing community, while maintaining territoriality as an organizing

[8] "The Community Setting," in *Social Science and Community Action,* ed. Charles R. Adrian (East Lansing, Mich.: The Institute for Community Development and Services, Continuing Education Service, Michigan State University, 1960), p. 3.

[9] See especially Amos H. Hawley, *Human Ecology: A Theory of Community Structure* (New York: Ronald Press, 1950); Robert M. MacIver, *Community: A Sociological Study* (3d ed.; London: Macmillan, 1924); R. D. McKenzie, *The Metropolitan Community* (New York and London: McGraw Hill, 1933); and Robert E. Park and Ernest W. Burgess, *Introduction to the Science of Sociology* (2d ed.; Chicago: University of Chicago Press, 1924).

[10] N. S. B. Gras, *An Introduction to Economic History* (New York: Harper, 1926), p. 183.

[11] See McKenzie, *The Metropolitan Community.*

[12] Ann Arbor, Mich.: University of Michigan Press, 1949.

principle. He defined community as "that aspect of the structure of social systems which is referrable to the territorial location of persons and their activities." [13] He specifically chose the word "referrable" and avoided the word "determinant" because although territoriality sets limits on action and influences its course, it does not, as a rule, totally deter-mine it. Indeed, man's ingenuity has steadily reduced the intractability of geography and distance.

Parsons proposed four different aspects of the influence of territorial-ity on social action. They were: first, the location of all of the social processes to do with family, that is, residence and neighborhood; second, the location of work; third, the nature of the systems of communication and transportation that are developed to facilitate social life; and fourth, governmental boundaries.

All four of these aspects of community are relevant to the distribution of any kind of service because they reflect the everyday patterns of social behavior, but some of them seem to be more natural organizing principles than others. Of the four, that of residence and neighborhood probably has the most common-sense relationship to the idea of com-munity, and the concept of a catchment area is essentially a notion based upon giving services to everyone who resides within a delimited geo-graphical area. An even more common organizing principle is the use of governmental boundaries such as school and hospital districts or wel-fare zones. Both of these familiar bases for organizing services can be used to cover all of the people living within an area and seem to have been the primary, if not the sole, aspects of community considered in the drafting of the regulations and in the planning efforts. Each, how-ever, presents difficulties, which will be discussed in greater detail below.

Less familiar as organizing principles for community care are work-place and communication pattern. Nevertheless, both are rational alterna-tives. Many health services are already occupationally based, as in the well-known Kaiser plan and the various health programs of the United Automobile Workers in Detroit. Workplace does present technical dis-advantages because it is hard to imagine how the principle of inclusive-ness could be made to cover all of the people who are not in the labor market. Workplace is, however, a possible basis for organizing sub-systems of distribution where decentralization is desired.

[13] *Structure and Process in Modern Societies* (Glencoe, Ill.: The Free Press, 1960).

Finally, the patterns whereby people relate the various geographically separated parts of their lives and reaffirm their communal ties might be used to plan and distribute services. Major access roads, marketing centers, churches, and especially emergency rooms of general hospitals, to which more and more people are turning, could all feasibly be used as bases for distributing or decentralizing services. Indeed, because psychiatry as a speciality is not markedly dependent upon expensive equipment and facilities it is more free to use natural points of social interaction than perhaps any other major speciality of medicine.

While more helpful than many, Parsons' definition of community is not easy to turn into criteria for establishing the boundaries of a community, or a way to determine whether an area belongs to one or another community. Yet the community approach to mental health problems, with the apparent aim of using the institutions and processes of the community for therapeutic and preventive purposes, seems to demand that such criteria be established, and that a community encompassing the major facets of the daily lives of the persons served be delimited. But the everyday patterns of social behavior involve links and chains of links among people, organizations, and institutions in the provision of the daily requirements of life.

Viewing community in terms of the interrelatedness and integration of daily life has led many social scientists in the United States to think of large areas encircling a great city as the "natural" communities within our country. Included within such an area are many large and small towns and hamlets, as well as open country. Clearly the metropolis is not a unit to which people necessarily respond with sentiment or even recognition. However, evidence amassed over the years suggests that within a large and modern nation a smaller area will not have the kind of independent internal organization and integration necessary to justify the name community.

The pattern of development of community mental health facilities is likely to be influenced by the existence of metropolitan communities in a number of ways. First, the dominance of the large central city as a beginning point for the diffusion of new ideas and practices suggests that it is more likely to develop plans necessary to implement the 1963 Act than its rural hinterland. In most instances central city plans will probably be completed more rapidly than those for the rest of the metropolitan community, and central cities are likely to have facilities

in operation before the rest of the area. It seems likely that these facili
ties will be reasonably well integrated with other important institution
in the central city. Not only are they likely to have formal entrée inte
the school system and the social services community, but in all prob
ability they will also be integrated into the informal organization of th
metropolitan medical community. Knowledge about these facilities wil
spread throughout the metropolitan community via both formal anc
informal networks of communication.

These hypotheses are confirmed by the six field studies. The locatior
of large medical complexes in the central cities of the metropolitan area
surveyed explain why they furnished a disproportionate number o
members of planning committees. Better integration into both the forma
and informal structure of the central cities than in the outlying area
was also reported.

The early development of central city services would reinforce the
long-standing propensity of hinterland people to seek specialized service
within the city. This is certainly true in Minneapolis, Syracuse, Boston
and Seattle, where central city facilities serve a large hinterland. Will the
location of centers in the hinterland reverse the very strong tendency o
psychiatrists to locate in the densely populated urban centers anc
close-in, upper middle-class suburbs? If not, the present uneven distribu
tion of mental health services across the large metropolitan communit
will be continued.

In order for a facility to provide a given mix of services efficiently
there is a minimum number of clients it must serve. Given a per capita
demand for the services offered by the facility, acquiring the necessary
minimum clientele probably depends on population density and the
maximum distance people are willing to travel. Population density withir
the metropolitan community declines, at first rapidly and then more
slowly, as the distance from the center is increased. Consequently, the
geographic size of catchment areas would increase with distance from
the center of the metropolis.

To be sure, one might argue that travel distance and population
density are irrelevant because in the absence of other facilities a patien
seeking treatment simply will travel as far as required—he has no choice
Given the scarcity of mental health services, the person needing them
is faced with an inelastic supply. This position, however, assumes tha
persons needing help will recognize that fact and, further, that they wil

seek help where available. This is highly dubious, and a contrary assumption appears to lie at the very heart of the new community centers program. If utilization of professional services at early stages of developing illness is a major concern of the community mental health movement, then distance and accessibility become crucially important. After all, the potential client does have a choice, the ultimate choice of whether to seek or not to seek help.

It will be impossible to compensate entirely for the basic problems of sparse populations in very large parts of the United States. Community mental health centers will simply have to cover large areas in many states such as West Virginia in order to obtain anywhere near the required minimum population. Thus, community, in the sociological sense of social relationships, will have to be sacrificed in the interest of obtaining a large enough geographic catchment area.

Mental health resources are unevenly distributed across the metropolitan community. The core of the area is the location for many activities cognate to mental health services. Large hospitals and medical schools are located there and mental health workers, doctors, public administrators, and many teachers are concentrated there. Access to the personnel, facilities, and other resources of related institutions is an important advantage for community mental health centers located in the central city. Referral of a patient for elaborate neurological examination or long-term rehabilitation, for instance, would be considerably easier to arrange within the central city than elsewhere.

Because of the concentration of resources in the central core of a metropolitan area, the idea of numerous out-lying mental health centers each offering comprehensive services for catchment areas limited to 200,000 population will not work. Indeed, whether the network of basically similar comprehensive centers apparently envisioned by the community mental health advocates ought to be developed in metropolitan areas is highly questionable. The goal should be the development of a web of limited satellite or neighborhood clinics related to a comprehensive regional center in much the same way as the general practitioner family physician is to the hospital-based specialist.

There may well be a need for specialized agencies serving an entire metropolitan area as well as a large hinterland. Often only by these methods can economies of scale be achieved and existing resources used most efficiently. The neat concept of a community mental health center for every community offering the same services, simply does not fit the facts of life in the larger metropolitan areas. Indeed, the nature of community suggests, not homogeneity, but a diversity of functions related in such a way as to form a whole. The basic problem in the implementation of the Community Mental Health Centers Act of 1963, then, is not how to provide a grid of similar facilities in homogeneous locales, but how to provide a differentiated array of services organized and articulated over the whole of the variegated metropolitan community.

The large central city is an amazingly tightly integrated system in itself. Frequently, work is located in one place, home in another, school in a third place, shopping in yet a fourth. To isolate a single, self-contained neighborhood as a subcommunity within the central city seems an extremely difficult task.

Yet, a major characteristic of the metropolitan core is segregation. While the pattern may be changing, different groups of people do reside in different parts of the city; and this residential differentiation is important in locating mental health facilities. A series of detailed studies has demonstrated conclusively that cities are segregated not only on the basis of race and ethnic origin, but also on the basis of occupational status, educational attainment, religion, and even age.[14]

When confronted with the problem of choosing medical or paramedical services all manner of extraneous and nonrational considerations enter into the individual's decision process. It is quite clear that when a layman is faced with the problem of evaluating a service whose realistic adequacy is difficult to judge, the racial and ethnic background of the providers of the service may influence his decision. The importance of ethnic group membership as a factor in medical practice has been stressed in several studies.[15]

The distrust and resentment of the white man by large groups of Blacks, reflected in the violence of recent years, suggests the importance

[14] For a relatively recent review of much of this material see Beverly Duncan "Variables in Urban Morphology," in *Contributions to Urban Sociology*, ed Ernest W. Burgess and Donald H. Bogue (Chicago: University of Chicago Press 1964), pp. 17–30.

[15] See, for example, Oswald Hall, "The Informal Organization of Medical Practice in an American City," Ph.D. dissertation, University of Chicago, 1944 David N. Soloman, "Career Contingencies of Chicago Physicians," Ph.D. dissertation, University of Chicago, 1952; Josephine J. Williams, "Patients and Prejudice Lay Attitudes toward Women Physicians," *American Journal of Sociology*, Vol 51 (Jan. 1946), pp. 283–387.

of a compatible racial background of service personnel in guaranteeing acceptance and effective utilization of mental health services. Although it is certainly true that the scarcity of medical personnel will prevent the selection of psychiatrists on the basis of ethnic origin, it might prove advantageous to select major contact personnel, be they secretaries or social workers, on the basis of ethnic, racial, or even social status. In some places, without some conscious adaptation in this direction, it is quite possible that, to the local residents, mental health facilities might appear to be foreign agencies to be regarded with considerable suspicion.

While ethnic, social, and economic homogeneity of particular neighborhoods in many cities may bear on the prospects for local acceptance of a mental health center, most identifiable residential areas fall short of the self-conscious interdependence of the community ideal. To be sure, community activity and organizational life are not wholly absent. Well-marked informal communities are found all over—with centers in bars, coffee shops, grocery stores, barber shops, and the like. Whether communities so defined are relevant for the purposes of the mental health centers program, however, is questionable. Are identifiable residential areas of appropriate size, and do they possess the capacity for co-ordinated action assumed by the community centers program? Taking such communities into account might require using a small area base for the service area of the mental health facility. The primary market would then probably be the local residential population, and the clientele homogeneous. As a consequence, it might prove necessary for the local center to design its program to meet the particular needs of its local service area. But would this be possible without significantly constricting the range of services which could be provided economically?

Under the regulations governing the administration of the federal program, planning for the community mental health centers must take cognizance of "other health planning and planning in such areas as urban development, welfare services, and related facilities." [16] The close relationship among other health and welfare services, and the desirability of coordinating mental health activities with them, is undeniable. But service districts for these related activities, where clearly defined, have been drawn with particular purposes and needs in mind, and as a consequence they rarely coincide. Moreover, in most instances such districts were not designed to serve some predefined "community" and

[16] *Regulations,* Part 54.203 (d) (2), *U.S. Federal Register,* May 6, 1964, p. 5952.

commonly have little present significance or rationale other than as catchment areas. Nor are these catchment areas for different services likely to be of the same size, much less conform to the population standards of the mental health centers program. Thus, rather than providing a convenient basis for locating community mental health centers, the service districts of related health and welfare activities are more likely to exacerbate the problem of coordinating services if either the community ideal or population standards are rigidly adhered to.

These then are some of the problems attending the idea of community when applied to the present-day metropolitan central city. Even in the tightly knit metropolitan core there are likely to be residential subcommunities with significant identities. In some instances these may have important relevance to the aims of the program, both in mobilizing support for expanding locally based mental health services and in integrating those services into the fabric of local society. Yet it is also clear that such communities will vary greatly in size and in many instances may be small residential neighborhoods owing much of their identity to ethnic, racial, or economic homogeneity. Achieving acceptance of services demands deliberate adjustment to such residential variations, yet very often such neighborhoods are likely to prove far too small to provide the service population necessary to support anything more than a very limited kind of facility. Furthermore, it is quite unlikely that these identifiable residential communities will correspond with the administrative districts employed by the various health and welfare services.

In short, the ideas of community integration, a limited service population, and coordination with related health and welfare services that have shaped the development of the mental health centers program push in contradictory directions. The realities of big-city living in the mid-twentieth century suggest that rigidity of approach to the community idea, whether thought of in catchment area or local involvement terms, will hamper the development of an effective program. The catchment area concept, given the population standard of the regulations, will require in many instances that variations from one residential area to another be ignored, variations that may lie at the heart of community identity. On the other hand, insistence on local involvement in the operations of a particular facility assumes a degree of community identity which is usually lacking. Moreover, since the service districts of other health and welfare activities will not usually be coterminous nor developed on the basis of a "community" idea, an insistence on any rigid definition of community would pose a very real threat to the possibility of achieving meaningful coordination of related services.

But a rigid insistence on one aspect of community is precisely what is developing under the community centers program. The ideals of community integration and local involvement, however ill defined they may seem, have yielded to the administrative precision of the residential catchment area. Not only are the workplace and the communication pattern aspects of community being ignored, but rigid insistence that the service areas of the centers fit the population standards of the regulations makes it unlikely that those catchment areas will bear any significant resemblance to real residential communities. Moreover, in much of the United States, relating centers with catchment areas of this size to local governments will be difficult because of governmental fragmentation and dispersion.

Yet, what justification is there for the population size insisted upon by the federal administrators unless community integration and involvement are the goals? Certainly a service population of 75,000 to 200,000 does not assure maximum economy in providing services, nor even optimal accessibility. Something appears to have been lost since the community centers program was initiated. The "bold new approach" of 1963 shows great promise of becoming merely an expensive expansion of decentralized facilities closely resembling the outpatient clinics predating its adoption.

XIII: GOVERNMENTAL
FRAGMENTATION AND DISPERSION

THE 1963 COMMUNITY MENTAL HEALTH CENTERS ACT represents a national commitment to grassroots-supported, easily accessible, comprehensive mental health centers. This national commitment has sweeping implications. A mental health facility handy to its clientele and able to provide comprehensive care has one implication. A mental health facility deeply involved in community life for referral and support carries other implications. Control by local officials adds a third, and local financing yet a fourth. If the first goal were the only one sought, it could be achieved by state action alone, merely by locating state facilities in cities. Indeed, the state of Louisiana has done just about that. But many supporters of community mental health believe that success requires responsible local involvement. They acknowledge that some centers could be operated by voluntary general hospitals under local private auspices. But they go further. They argue that the community mental health center must be controlled and financed by the community. For the programing of locally controlled mental health centers in metropolitan areas, governmental fragmentation poses a number of specific problems.

THE RESPONSIBLE LOCAL UNIT

Given the premise of responsible community control, a first problem encountered in fragmented metropolitan areas is which of the many existing governmental units should assume responsibility for operating mental health centers. Should it be the city, the county, or some special-purpose authority? In New Orleans, the state has continued to provide the public centers in the area. In Boston, the state and the towns combine to provide operating responsibility. In Minneapolis–St. Paul, the county plays the predominant role. In Seattle, a consolidated city-county health department has entered the field, but major responsibility still rests with state agencies. It is patent that no single definitive answer as to the proper local unit has emerged. Indeed, if there is any consistent pattern, it is that of state involvement.

Furthermore, experience since 1963 suggests that governmental fragmentation is not the sole factor determining progress in programing mental health in metropolitan areas. Seattle has a highly fragmented government and its progress in establishing community mental health centers has been slow. On the other hand, Minneapolis–St. Paul, equally fragmented, has moved swiftly to implement its program. Boston, with a complex government and a tradition of much private activity as well, is adapting readily to the new concept. But Houston, with a relatively uncomplicated array of local governments, is lagging in regard to mental health services. New Orleans, however, the least fragmented, has a variety of community type services.

There is another metropolitan area dimension besides fragmentation that affects local involvement. The mere existence of a multitude of governmental units within a metropolitan area does not indicate whether or not the bulk of the area's population resides within the boundaries of a single local authority fully able to provide unified government for its citizenry. The extent to which the metropolitan population in the United States was concentrated in the largest city in each area in 1960 ranged from 11.3 per cent in San Bernadino–Riverside–Ontario to 88.1 per cent in El Paso. In well over half of the metropolitan areas less than half the people resided in any single city. In only nine did the largest city of the area contain as much as two-thirds of the metropolitan population. In the metropolitan areas surveyed in the field studies, the range was from 75 per cent in the city of Houston to 27 per cent in Boston. In short, adding the factor of population concentration to the number of governmental units does not alter the conclusion that American metropolitan communities, in the great majority of cases, fall far short of achieving unified government.

Concentration of population appears, in fact, to present some special problems for mental health programing. Concentration of an area's people within two cities with well-developed independent identities (Minneapolis–St. Paul provides an example) breeds problems of coordination that are more difficult to resolve than those of another metropolis where approximately the same percentage of the population lives outside the largest municipality but is distributed among a number of relatively small satellite communities, as with Syracuse. In a twin cities situation, not only may actual unification be impossible, or at least highly unlikely, but civic pride and intercity rivalry may hamper recognition of a community of interest and the desirability of cooperative effort in attacking common problems. But concentration of population in a single governmental unit does not necessarily mean that that unit will undertake to sponsor a community mental health program. New Orleans, for example, contains the bulk of the area's population and has the greatest base of financial resources. Yet the city does not spend a cent on community mental health. In short, concentration of population may provide a clue as to local units with the resources to be financially responsible. But being financially able is not the same thing as being politically willing.

Governmental fragmentation may also compound the problems of political inertia. Existing governmental units prefer to handle new functions in the same way as they treat present services. They would assign the new function to an existing department or create a new one to provide the new service to the people in the same area who are receiving other government services. Public officials prefer to budget for the new service within their existing program structure, hopefully with some new source of revenue or at least permission to expand their present sources to pay for it. Such an arrangement obviously would least disturb current operations. Proponents of a new service may prefer to have it handled in a separate, clearly identifiable way, particularly if they had been frustrated in earlier attempts to receive the service from the existing government. Some kind of leverage may be necessary to move independent local units to provide the service.

In Minneapolis–St. Paul the county, for example, initially was designated the unit of government to establish mental health centers. As a consequence, the rest of the area is more or less compelled to divide by counties or combinations thereof, since the state will wish to deal with equivalent units. In Boston, centers were established by towns or groups of towns. In some instances, state administrators will not think innovatively about areas of service; that is, they will tend to organize mental health in the same way they handle other matters. On the other hand, in New Orleans, state officials have contributed heavily to advances in the area's mental health services.

There is another problem posed by fragmentation. Existing political units, be they counties, cities, towns, or whatever, are unlikely to coincide with an ideal area that might be drawn for given services. Local units of government were originally established to provide the minimal services. Units convenient in a horse-and-buggy era cannot be expected to be the most convenient or efficient in the automobile or post-automobile age. As more services are performed by local governments, the ideal area is harder to define because the area of convenience, economy, or even physical necessity differs for each activity. Most local units are today too small for efficient or rational service areas.

Specifying a given level of government as the host or the building block for mental health center areas immediately results in inequalities of size. Counties in the Minneapolis–St. Paul metropolitan area range from a million to a few thousand. If all local units beyond a certain size were allowed to have their own mental health centers, the smaller remaining units would not always cluster into the right size, no matter how logical their geographical combination might seem, nor would they necessarily be compatible. In the Boston area, for example, the state authorities wanted to allow local initiative to suggest the combinations of municipalities that could work together in establishing a single center. But then a few separated municipalities were left with no place to go. The same situation applies in Minnesota, where counties are the building blocks. The state agency's map will show that every county is theoretically in a mental health center area, but this does not represent actual participation. Presumably, some of the combined counties could break off and form their own mental health center at some later time when resources and need warranted.

The rational optimum for meeting local needs might well be to have single-district governments for each separate service. Such an alternative has been rejected in doctrine principally because noncontiguous, overlapping layers of governmental units are difficult to control through democratic elections.

Supposedly, a very large unit of government, such as most states, could handle all services, each through a series of purely administrative service districts. Many present state services typically are provided in this way. Yet the service administrators may be frustrated to the point of demanding common regions to make supervision of the several field staffs more economical and better coordinated.

Complicating the task of defining areas of service, the regulations spelled out that a community mental health center should serve a population between 75,000 and 200,000 population. Trying to fit the actual units of government into the population limits, except for those which fortuitously fall within them, requires one or more of the following adaptations: (1) Some kind of agglomeration of existing smaller governmental units would have to be organized to make a center feasible. (2) In the case of units already larger than the limit, some kind of subdivisions would be required. (3) A new special-district government of the requisite size could be created with powers to construct and operate a mental health center. Or (4) the limitations could be ignored or administrative changes sought. Early experiences under the Act show many of these adaptations.

In Minneapolis–St. Paul the decision to use the county as a unit for community mental health centers was made by the state Welfare Department, the designated mental health authority. The Welfare Department had always dealt solely with counties in their categorical welfare program; therefore, the state agency promoted the county as a logical unit for mental health centers. No thought apparently was ever given to doing it any other way, despite the quite well-accepted view among governmental officials and political scientists that the counties in Minnesota, as elsewhere, were noted neither for their administrative organization nor their ability to perform services efficiently.

In the Boston metropolitan area, municipalities have been encouraged by the state to band together for mental health center support. No alternative to this cooperation presents itself, for there are no "higher level" units of general local government that amount to anything in Massachusetts.

In other areas, logic seemed to point to the county, an existing general government unit considerably closer to encompassing the entire metropolis than were the municipalities. If only counties are considered, the problem of multiplicity of government units shrinks drastically. In fact, the Houston metropolitan area consisted until recently of only one county, and Seattle has a slight population spillover into a second county. Syracuse and Minneapolis–St. Paul show three and five counties respectively. Supplying a service throughout the metropolitan area could thus be simplified if counties were to take on the function of mental health, but still it is not a matter of a single decision.

Designating the county as the unit to sponsor a community mental health center does not obviate the imperative for coordination within the metropolitan area. Many of the standard functions of the municipalities and school districts are related to mental health and will have to be fostered, or pulled together, by the county mental health agency.

Moreover, it would be inaccurate to think of the county as a superior unit to the municipality; although in almost every state the city is inside as well as outside it, the functions of the county do not, in fact, appreciably overlap those of the city. More generally, accommodation is made to share responsibilities. Thus, the city may have a public health department, so the county public health department handles these duties only outside the city. The sheriff usually is the chief law enforcing officer only outside of the domain of the city chief of police, and so on. When city and county departments are consolidated to provide joint facilities and services, arguments about cost sharing have been known to arise; this has been shown in the Houston–Harris county hospital dispute.

The unit that is too large to have a single center, as defined in the regulations, runs into another problem. No subdivision that might be made would have separate taxing powers without special legislation or possibly constitutional revision. There is no evidence that the drafters of the federal regulations wished to allow or provide for a single administration, say for a large county, while providing a number of mental health centers under a single board. Presumably, the doctrine that to be effective a center must be locally controlled with implications of a neighborhood type of control would preclude this.

If this is indeed the requirement, the population limit for a community mental health center is unrealistic. The guiding principle should be not size, but that the governmental unit sponsoring it be a viable one in terms of an adequate tax base and leadership supply. The unit must have a present political reality. Harris county, Texas; Hennepin county, Minnesota; and King county, Washington, are good examples of suitable units for control. Once overall control is established, the actual organization of services to be offered could be worked out flexibly. Sub-centers (with neighborhood advisory committees if that is desirable), feeder clinics, such as New York's store-front circuit clinics, or Seattle's Community and Eastside Community Psychiatric Clinics, could be closely tied to central facilities. Besides relating better to the political and governmental reality, this suggestion might be the only one practicable during a time of staff shortage.

The service arrangement should take into account existing private facilities that might make the need for public facilities smaller. Factors such as physical space available or driving time to the center are useful to consider. Two hours' driving time, even in Texas, seems to be too long. One hour is probably a maximum in metropolitan areas. Research should be undertaken as to how convenient a center must be to serve the need. In lower-class areas, facilities should be handier to avoid expense of transportation and to preclude the chance that travel would discourage the poor who are rooted or trapped in small areas and for whom travel is strange. The physical location of a center can also create neighborhood political problems, as the strenuous resistance of the residents of a New Orleans neighborhood to a proposed outpatient facility in their "front yards" attests.

Formerly a rarity, but now a common necessity resulting from United States Supreme Court decisions since 1962, reapportionment of state legislatures may have significant effects not only on state-local government relations, but also on intrametropolitan relations. Universally the metropolitan areas of states have gained by reapportionment. However, the effects on policy of the shift of legislators from rural to suburban and sometimes to central city areas are as yet unclear. Hypothesizing must suffice for the moment. A further fragmentation of government might take place as a result of legislative reapportionment. Only relatively narrow deviations in population among districts are permitted (from less than 1 per cent in some court-imposed plans to perhaps 10–20 per cent where legislatures have been allowed to draw at least a temporary plan). These restrictions are so close that traditional districts, which included whole counties or cities, have had to give way to artificial legislative districts that violate municipal and county boundaries. This result has been strongly fought by legislators in rural areas, where legislative districts and county lines themselves had some psychological reality in terms of traditional community feelings. In the metropolitan areas, municipal boundaries are not so meaningful. Greater mobility of the population and the relative newness of many suburban jurisdictions, or the changing of city boundaries through annexation in some parts of the country, have prevented the traditional patterns from developing so deeply, although municipal officials who are trying to build a civic consciousness as well as ensure their own jobs resist splitting their city among legislative districts. If a new division is made every year, legislators may be less tied to traditional units and more ready to impose areawide solutions to metropolitan problems.

In sum, governmental fragmentation presents the problem of the appropriate unit for responsible operation and control of the community mental health center. Experience since 1963 indicates that there is not likely to be a single definitive answer to this problem. Experience further indicates that where there is a local will to have a community program a way will be found through the maze of fragmentation. Also suggested is the possibility that there may be no local will. In that case, state action will be necessary.

URBAN CONSOLIDATION

Urban consolidation is a radical solution to the problem of fragmentation that is often endorsed by political scientists. No doubt structural improvement in our metropolises is possible, but the limitations of major organizational change as a means for eliminating governmental fragmentation are readily apparent. Extending the jurisdiction of the central city by annexing adjacent unincorporated territory, particularly in the South and West, is still useful in preventing an expanding urban population from splintering into a number of separate and independent entities. But in most metropolises the addition to the city of unincorporated fringe areas is no answer, for the typical pattern is more and more that of a central city surrounded by a number of incorporated suburbs or even two or three central cities each with its bedroom satellites. In most states the annexation of incorporated places requires popular approval by referendum vote in each affected governmental unit, an approval which is usually very difficult to obtain.

It is hardly surprising that bedroom suburbs should resist annexations. Some of them predate the metropolitan explosion that rendered them suburban, while others owe their existence to a desire to hold services to a minimum, to serve the cause of suburban pride, or otherwise to further local interests. Nor is it likely, in view of the Supreme Court's recent reapportionment decisions, that state laws will be changed to make such annexations easier for the central city. It is, after all, in most metropolises the suburbs, not the central city, which are grossly underrepresented in the state legislature. In short, given the nature of the present-day metropolis and the laws governing annexation, attacking the problem of fragmentation by extending the jurisdiction of the metropolitan core requires in large measure the geographical consolidation by bilateral action of governmental equals.

Consolidations of two or more municipalities or of two or more counties are beset by legal and political difficulties, and city-county consolidation is both hard to achieve and of limited usefulness. And even where only one county is presently involved, continued metropolitan expansion will render city-county consolidation a temporary and inadequate solution. Moreover, a merger of city and county governments does not necessarily affect the status of other municipalities contained within the county's boundaries; and only two of the seventy-five metropolises have one incorporated municipality while all but seventeen have ten or more. Though mergers of two or more special districts or of special districts with either counties or cities remain realistic possibilities in many cases, it is not surprising that constructive use of geographical consolidation is at present largely confined to school districts.

To be sure, major rationalizations of governmental structure are not impossible. Nashville, Tennessee, has recently adopted a consolidated metropolitan government[1] and Miami, Florida, a federated form of metropolitan government.[2] Nor is annexation a dead letter everywhere, as the record of Phoenix during the 1950s will attest. But such major reorganizations are beset by difficulties and consequently have been so few that they have hardly dented the overall picture of American metropolises.

However one looks at the matter, it is clear that the urban population comprising what are called metropolitan communities typically are dispersed among a number of independent, frequently overlapping, and often conflicting jurisdictions. In this sense at least, governmental fragmentation is a fact of life in the present-day American metropolis.

---

[1] For a discussion of this reorganization, see David A. Booth, *Metropolitics: The Nashville Consolidation* (East Lansing: Institute for Community Development and Services, Michigan State University, 1963). A briefer account is contained in Chapter IX of *Metropolis in Transition: Local Government Adaptation to Changing Urban Needs*, prepared for the Housing and Home Finance Agency under the Urban Studies and Housing Research Program, Sept. 1963.

[2] See Edward Sofen, *The Miami Metropolitan Government* (Bloomington: Indiana University Press, 1963). For a discussion of the difference between the Miami and Nashville approaches, see Daniel R. Grant, "Consolidations Compared," *National Civic Review*, Vol. 52 (Jan. 1963), p. 10.

Furthermore, as the urban complexes continue to expand and the need for a unified response to common problems presumably increases, the governments whose cooperation is required grow, not fewer, but more numerous. It is all very well to say that this situation might have been avoided by careful planning or alleviated even now by the judicious use of various methods of structural adaptation. It was not avoided, and, as Professor Roscoe Martin puts it, "opportunities for the dramatic rationalization of the pattern of metropolitan government are few and far between."

DISPERSAL AND SPLINTERING

Besides the complications resulting from many units of local government in a metropolitan area, two other types of organizational fragmentation—vertical dispersion and splintering—provide complications for mental health programing. Vertical dispersal is the distribution of mental health functions among the federal, state, and local units. Splintering is the division of mental health functions among several departments or agencies within the same governmental level, for example within the state government or within one city.

Mental health agencies in the United States illustrate a variety of organizational patterns for providing mental health services. Washington and Texas are examples of states where these services were divided between state health departments responsible for community mental health programs and departments of institutions with jurisdiction over mental hospitals. New York and Massachusetts were among the first states to create departments of mental hygiene to coordinate all mental health programs. Minnesota is one of the few states locating responsibility for mental health activities, including those of mental hospitals, within a welfare department. Louisiana is unique in that mental health programs there are located in a Department of Hospitals.

Such diversity arises from many factors, such as the historical development of mental health programs, bureaucratic resistance or pressure to change existing organizational structure, and political pressures for or opposed to change. However, several states have recently reorganized (North Carolina and Illinois) or are considering reorganization (Alabama and Pennsylvania) of the agencies responsible for administering mental health programs.

Out of this plethora of organizational variety emerges the question of whether mental health is of sufficient importance to justify full "departmental" status. A number of arguments can be enlisted to support the creation (or maintenance) of state departments of mental health. Perhaps the most convincing case can be made on the generally accepted view that mental illness is the greatest single health problem confronting the nation. Further, establishing a single department would indicate the importance that state political and administrative elites attach to mental health programs and would presumably encourage coordination and consolidation of related activities. A department of mental health could possibly demonstrate its needs more effectively to the state legislature, governor, and the public, and it could be held more directly responsible for the policies pursued. Finally, it might be argued that departmental, as opposed to bureau, status would aid in attracting higher-level professional staff.

Advocates of a separate department often argue that if mental health programs are combined with programs of a department of health or welfare, then mental health interests and claims are often subordinated to those of the older and already established programs. If, for example, mental health programs are merely one component of a public health department, budgetary requests and legislative proposals must first be cleared by an agency head and budget officers who may have limited sympathy with mental health objectives and who must consider the mental health program as only one of a number of competing activities. Moreover, the department head, not the director of a bureau or a division, is often the individual vested with statutory authority to implement a program. This may act as a deterrent to the needed expansion of mental health programs in a subordinate agency. Thus it is not surprising to find professionals responsible for mental health programs urging the creation of a separate department because they believe their program objectives are being hindered by their subordinate position.

While pressures to establish a specialized department exist within the mental health field, state budget bureaus or departments of administration frequently present another point of view. Their objective is often to reduce the total number of departments and independent boards. Excessive specialization, manifested by a large number of departments and boards, creates problems of program coordination and planning, and often leads to the overlapping of services. Moreover, it supposedly weakens gubernatorial control because it becomes extremely difficult for a governor to understand the needs of so many separate departments, each of which generally has direct access to his office. Consolidation of departments with seemingly related program objectives removes to a great extent many of these difficulties.

The resolution of the dispute also depends on other factors such as demography, number and types of facilities, geography, and existing administrative organization. The situation in states where there is only one state hospital and a small population differs radically from states that have an extensive physical plant, a variety of programs, and a large population. The difficulties encountered in coordinating the total program in large states may be substantively different from those found in small states. Thus, a separate department in more populous states is perhaps justifiable, not simply because mental health programs are as important as their advocates argue but because the scope of their operation is so extensive and complex.

Part of the problem of reorganization stems from the ambiguity as to what should be included in mental health programs. Tight professional and agreed-upon definitions are lacking. For example, are the problems of alcoholism or mental retardation or geriatrics most closely related to mental health, public health, education, or welfare? Just as there are pressures to create a distinct department of mental health by combining several functions, there are counter pressures by existing departments to prevent such transfer of functions which they consider integral to their direct professional concerns.

Despite the apparent trend toward unifying mental health activities in a single department, splintering of mental health functions among agencies of a single government seems to be growing. In an earlier governmental period of organization, functional divisions among agencies seemed logical and relatively clean-cut. Thus, at one time welfare, corrections, public health, and education each could be distinguished from the other. But as the public's rising expectation of service and the growth of knowledge about the causes and treatment of social ills have progressed, either of two things has happened: If the old-line agencies did not move progressively toward taking on new responsibilities and adopting new methods, dissatisfied client groups would demand a new agency. To avoid this, aggressive, responsive, or imperialistic department heads moved to broaden the service of their agencies to answer the new demands. In either case, the jurisdictional lines between the agencies become fuzzy. If the welfare department wishes to attack causes of dependency rather than merely provide for dependents, it will move into the mental health, mental retardation, rehabilitation, employment counseling, and job training fields. Education will move toward providing special classes for or integrating into regular classes with special services the emotionally disturbed and retarded. Corrections will identify mental illness or retardation as a cause of social misbehavior and attempt to treat it to avoid mere incarceration.

These splintered services intensify the administrative disputes as their leaders compete for tax money to handle similar problems. Governments have attempted to deal with such dilemmas through several means, particularly coordination.

PROSPECTS OF OVERCOMING FRAGMENTATION

Certain centripetal forces are at work to overcome the effects of fragmented government. The exercise of statewide or regionwide mental health planning is in itself a coordinating enterprise. A major accomplishment of these planning sessions was to bring into contact professionals who had formerly gone their own way. This result of the mental health planning process showed up both horizontally and vertically. That is, contact between state and local leaders was facilitated, and contact among people working in the field in local governments was engendered. Prior to the planning sessions, fellow workers in mental health fields within a metropolitan area often had never before been brought together, had never before worked together, and frequently had not even met each other. Whether this contact can be institutionalized through continuing planning bodies remains to be seen. Once centers become operating units, the staff become so preoccupied with the job at hand that they may tend to drift away from combined efforts.

Universities and their activities are also important in overcoming the isolation accompanying fragmentation. University personnel were generally involved in all phases of the planning process. Typically the local university was the source of training of most of the professionals in the area. Graduates of the university departments of psychiatry, psychology, and social work predominate in the area. Fruit does not fall very far from the tree. Many of the students, while in training, worked part-time in nearby institutions, and most interned locally. What could be more natural than that the institutional and community ties so created would often ripen into job offers? Also, these graduates often maintain contact with the university, either through lecturing or supervising interns in their own shop. A certain prestige attaches to university lectureships, which is necessary especially for those graduates more attuned to community psychiatry than to private practice.

Besides the uncut umbilicals to alma mater, professionals provided a bridge between different community agencies with which they work, because their career ladders often ran from one institution to another rather than upward in their own agency. One director will have worked previously under the director of another institution in the same area. Professional societies are an obvious possible contact, but field studies, perhaps surprisingly, gave small emphasis to this possible source of contact. Several center directors were trying to create or revive a professional society to help them spread the gospel of community mental health. The result of professional ties is a communication channel across jurisdictional and agency boundaries. Thus, admission to a university hospital, supposedly bogged down with endless waiting lists, is surprisingly easy for patients of the professor's star pupils now in the field. And when a job opening comes along, word of mouth provides the most valued recommendations.

The university provides another means of overcoming fragmentation by the community involvement of its professors, as all the field studies reported. Each of these would often be a member of several mental health groups. Thus, the chairman of the psychiatry department may also serve on the board of the community mental health center and be an important member of the state mental health planning task force, a member of the medical advisory committee of the state mental health agency, a consultant to the court, and on the board of a local hospital with a psychiatric wing. It is likely that he wears several hats and that his participation at these various levels will bring some unity of action. It would be comforting to believe that all of these coordinative contacts eventually would result in the care of everyone who needed help by some appropriate agency and that a rational allocation of responsibility throughout the community would result. Such a belief puts too much reliance in an Adam Smith type of "invisible hand" to hope that this would automatically work out. The contacts, being personal, are ad hoc. If a personal contact breaks down, the participants give up the attempt to organize. Certainly, a more formal coordinating system would be necessary if facilities and staff ever became so sufficient as to result in competition for clients. However, that day, for mental health, is not imminent.

The political party, where it is a unified force in government, can be a great coordinator. This is true in Syracuse, where the state is united with local leaders for action, particularly since a key legislative leader is from there. The Minneapolis–St. Paul area has a moderately strong party organization, which has shown some success in coordinating city, county, legislative, and state executive action. But years of split party control between branches and units have not enabled a full demonstration of whatever benefits one party might deliver.

Fundamentally, however, local people are not particularly alarmed about the governmental fragmentation in their areas. They become quite well adapted to the complexities of their local government. This is, after all, all they have known to work with. Government leaders of municipalities typically have a vested interest in the maintenance of their identity. If municipalities were combined into some allegedly more rational system, or if some important service were given up to another unit, their jurisdiction would be less important, or their jobs might not exist. In the face of financial pressures, many local governments might be willing to let go of services so that they would have no further responsibility for them. The likelihood of their whole government's disappearing may seem slight. On the other hand, they may be hesitant to let the single service go for fear this is the harbinger of a trend that will ultimately see a super-government established that will dwarf their own powers.

While the local officials may be familiar with the governmental jigsaw puzzle, it would be erroneous to assume that ordinary citizens are equally well informed. In fact, the people may not be able to master the complexities of their area governments and may fail to enter local government activities because of this. Or, those who truly understand the system may realize the quantity of energy required to mobilize for action and give up before they start. Thus the assumed shortage of interested and dedicated lay people may itself be partially a result of the governmental structure. Still, past experience indicates that for mental health centers to get into action, known community leaders must devote themselves to this field. Thus, the mental health centers program faces the paradoxical fact that its goal of integration into the local community is threatened by the present pattern of community organization.

COORDINATION

Some degree of coordination among fragmented units of government can be achieved merely through informal agreements to cooperate, as is often the case in regard to the reciprocal use of firefighting equipment in case of emergency. Formal compacts under which two or more governments undertake certain mutual obligations can be employed. In many areas, under state "joint powers" legislation, local governments can agree to perform jointly any function which they have the power to undertake individually. The service contract, particularly as developed in Los Angeles county's Lakewood Plan, offers a means for overcoming at least some of the problems resulting from fragmentation. Nor should local officials ignore the usefulness of metropolitan conferences or councils to bring together representatives of the various local governments of the area to discuss common problems. A transfer of functions from one government to another more adequate in jurisdiction or resources, as from a city to a county or from a city or county to the state, involves no structural change yet may be very helpful in meeting changing needs and might even lead eventually to a painless transition to some variety of metropolitan government. In some areas at least a degree of extraterritorial control over zoning and subdivision development has been granted to cities, and this provides a means for avoiding some of the problems accompanying expansion where such power was lacking.

Local units are essentially equals. There is no authoritative body to resolve disputes, allocate responsibilities and ratios of contribution, and decide priorities. Local units, if cooperation is necessary, must bargain, compromise, and contract among equals. This is possible, and in fact would seem well within the typical American skills to handle. Group members and politicians are used to bargaining and compromising. The price of governing this way is the great hunks of time it takes to work out the arrangements, and the leadership required to do it. The costs of this kind of effort are great. The two field studies that ventured to present conclusions on this subject were agreed, perhaps coincidentally, that five years was required in their areas for getting a mental health center in operation. This was, of course, in the days before passage of the federal Act. In the other cities, the mental health interest is yet so new that five years have not elapsed. Perhaps the time period will be shortened with provision of federal planning money, the lure of federal construction money, and staffing money, plus publicity for the subject of mental health.

In short, various forms of intergovernmental cooperation offer at least partial solutions to the problems resulting from the plethora of jurisdictions infesting the modern metropolis. Which approaches can best be employed in a particular metropolitan area will depend on the nature of its needs and the degree to which those needs evoke responsible attention. But the outstanding unavoidable fact is that the governmental fragmentation characteristic of these areas is of such a nature that its elimination by establishing a metropolitan government is ordinarily not even a remote possibility. The division of a metropolitan community into a number of independent jurisdictions may be irrational and undesirable; nevertheless, that is the way American metropolises are and, for the most part at least, that is the way they are likely to remain.

Coordination among fragmented local governments is only part of the problem. Dispersal and splintering also result in conditions requiring coordinative efforts. Various approaches have been tried: coordinating committees, designation of one department as the responsible coordinating agency, interagency task forces, or committees of department heads.

The effectiveness of these techniques is somewhat in doubt since department heads may not have the time or the desire to coordinate their activities. Most interdepartmental committees are strictly *pro forma,* and seldom meet. About the best that can be hoped for is that the officials will come to know each other through contacts in planning meetings and will feel free to pick up the phone and work out problems on an ad hoc basis. Examples of this form of coordination can be seen at the local level in a number of states where local mental health boards are required to include representatives from all agencies concerned with mental health problems.

Where the governor is constitutionally and politically strong, as in New York and Massachusetts, the governor's leadership promotes coordination. Legislative committee chairmen can require coordination by writing it into appropriations language, but legislators are usually prone to champion a single department. In Minnesota, state mental health is pretty much concentrated in activities of the welfare department, yet groups still compete and push separately with differing degrees of success; but the leadership of the several groups have not been opposed to each other, feeling that a gain for one is a gain for all.

At the local level, the community mental health center, if it is directed by people with a broad view of their responsibilities, may serve a coordinating function in a given community. Through joint staff appointments or by placing on its board officials from the court probation office, the public health nurses, the school counseling service, vocational rehabilitation, and employment service, a smoothly working relationship among local agencies might be achieved. Indeed, some state community mental health acts require such appointment practices. The success of this relationship, it should be emphasized, will to a certain extent depend upon the people involved. Institutionalization alone cannot eliminate the personal factor necessary for successful coordination.

It should be noted that before organizational squabbles can be settled some agreement over program objectives and techniques must be reached by those working in the mental health area. Given the extent of mental illness, no one need fear in the near future that agencies will be fighting over a scarce supply of clients. Only legislators and administrators who fear that money is being wasted through "duplication" will strive for administrative neatness to correct the inadequacy. The real fear might better be that some people with needs are not handled at all, but are falling between the stools of specialized agencies or are not responded to because of the absence of a focal point of administrative leadership and power.

XIV: FINANCIAL DILEMMAS AND
MANPOWER LIMITATIONS

UNLIKE OTHER AREAS of health care, the costs of looking after the
mentally ill have traditionally been borne in this country primarily by
the public. Government involvement in providing mental health services is so heavy that caring for the mentally ill, despite the fact that
it involves an area of medicine, is—like education—primarily a socialized
undertaking. While only about 20 per cent of all personal health care
expenditures in this country including the military are publicly financed,
about 70 per cent of the expenditures for mental health services are
publicly financed.[1] Indeed, it has been estimated that between 35 and
40 per cent of all public expenditures for personal health care are
accounted for by mental health services.

There are many reasons why the responsibility for providing mental
health services has been assumed to such a great extent by government.
In the first place, there is the long-term nature of so many types of mental
illness and the inability of individuals, out of their own resources, to bear
the costs of expensive and protracted care. Secondly, and perhaps more
important, the social consequences of serious mental illness are significant and obvious enough to encourage public support. And, of course,
the nature of the illness and the ignorance of society have contributed to
the traditional rejection of the mentally ill with the consequent impulse
toward the creation of public institutions for putting them out of sight
and out of mind.

Whatever the contributing factors, however, the fact is that mental
health services have been for a long time primarily public and the current
level of governmental expenditures in this regard is far from insignificant. President Kennedy spoke of an annual governmental expenditure
of approximately $1.8 billion in his 1963 message. That figure was for

[1] See Robert H. Atwell, "The Financing of Mental Health Services—A National
View," paper prepared for delivery to the Task Force on Planning, National Commission on Community Health Services, Baltimore, Md., Sept. 21, 1964.

1961–1962, when federal expenditures for mental health totaled less than $700 million. Of that figure the great bulk went to specialized clientele groups such as the armed forces, veterans, and federal prisoners. State and local governments, on the other hand, spent almost $1.1 billion, almost all of which went toward the costs of direct patient care. Further, well over 90 per cent of this sum went to public mental hospitals, with only $87 million directed toward community services. Indeed, three states, New York, California, and Illinois, accounted for more than 50 per cent of the community services expenditures.[2]

The sums that will be involved if the program envisioned by the 1963 federal legislation is effectively implemented are staggering. At the estimated construction cost of $1.3 million per center, providing one community mental health center for every two hundred thousand people in a total population of nearly two hundred million would involve expenditures of approximately $1.3 billion. Since, however, the range of population to be served is from 75,000 to 200,000, construction costs will probably be substantially greater. For example, if there were one center for each 100,000 people, costs would be $2.6 billion. Inflation in construction costs over the next several years could easily double this figure.

In computing total costs of the new program it is more important to recognize that annual staffing costs for a center serving 100,000 people were estimated in 1965 at $600,000. This totals $1.2 billion if complete coverage is assumed, and rising professional salaries will steadily push this upward. Where is this money to come from?

FINANCING EXPANDING MENTAL HEALTH SERVICES

It seems highly unlikely that private sector expenditures will rise to anything near the magnitude required by even a relatively modest expansion of mental health efforts, especially if those efforts are to be of the community services variety. Despite the growing affluence of the American population, the same factor which has contributed so much to governmental assumption of responsibility in the past—the cost of private psychiatric care—promises to militate toward continued dependence on publicly supported facilities and services. Nor can one expect very much

---

[2] U.S., Congress, Senate, Subcommittee on Health of the Committee on Labor and Public Welfare, *Hearings on S.755 and 756*, 88th Cong., 1st Sess., 1963, p. 38; and see Atwell, "Financing of Mental Health Services," p. 9.

from private charitable efforts such as United Fund drives unless one assumes either a radical increase in the sums contributed or a very significant decrease in the number of worthy causes clamoring with insistent voices for continued and ever-expanded support.

There remains private insurance. It is estimated that while health insurance covers more than three-fourths of the population, it covers only one-fourth of the medical bills. Restrictions against mental illness in many forms of coverage have meant that insurance pays for a much lower proportion of the mental health bill. Thanks in part to the demands of collective bargaining contracts calling for extended coverage, gradually these restrictions are being removed, but primarily with respect to inpatient services. Presently more than 60 per cent of the room and board charges of general hospitals is paid through insurance against hospitalized illness, and perhaps before many more years a large portion of the hospital room and board for the psychiatric services of these hospitals will also be met through insurance. But what about outpatient and partial hospitalization services, not to mention coverage for the services of psychologists, social workers, and other professionals who are increasingly important in the treatment of the mentally ill? These areas account for a very significant portion of the total costs in the kind of integrated community-based services contemplated by the new program. The obstacles in the way of adequate private insurance coverage for them are formidable indeed. Voluntary health insurance is not a major factor as yet in the payment of outpatient services in the case of physical illness, and mental illnesses pose even more difficult problems in regard to the prediction of incidence, the development of standards of treatment, and the imposition of controls so essential to designing a viable insurance program.

The conclusion seems unavoidable, then, that the bulk of the money for expanded mental health services is going to have to come, as it has in the past, from government. But each level of government in the United States poses its own special problems as a source of adequate funds for this purpose. The legislative history of the 1963 Act and of its 1965 amendments dramatizes the obstacles in the way of financing by the federal government. That history reflects the extent to which the traditional view of the role of the national government in our federal system still prevails. The financial role of the federal government is to be that of providing seed money through the grant-in-aid approach. From one-third to two-thirds of the money for construction is to be raised privately or by public authority at a lower level, and federal contributions toward the costs of staffing the centers will rapidly decline from an initial 75 per cent to zero after only four and a quarter years. Presumably, the entire cost of operation is to be borne at the state or local level thereafter. However realistic or unrealistic this scheme may seem, it is the natural outcome of the continuing political disagreement in our democratic system over which level of government properly should do what, over the advantages and dangers of centralization, over the relative desirability of local control and national standards, and the like.

Even without a great expansion of mental health services such as now envisioned, state expenditures in general have been rising very rapidly during recent years and it is hardly surprising that these increases have been accompanied by a very significant rise in state indebtedness. Moreover, it seems optimistic in the extreme to believe that mental health will be able to do much better than hold its own in relation to other state programs in the near future. If that is the case, it is highly unlikely that state resources will increase anywhere near enough to make future allocations for mental health equal the amounts that will be needed. While it is all very well to argue that in the long run community mental health centers will contribute to a "withering away" of the large mental hospitals with a consequent freeing of funds, the immediate financial irrelevance of this position is evident.

Clearly, the need for currently available services, however unsatisfactory or inadequate, cannot be reduced by community centers until they are built and operating in significant numbers. Thus, at the outset at least, state contributions to new programs are going to require new money, not simply a diverting of presently available funds.

It is also questionable whether, even in the long run, a decline in mental hospital expenditures will result in the diversion of significant amounts to community programs. As already pointed out, mental hospitals have long been the mainstays of the state approach to the problem of mental illness and are currently a billion-dollar-a-year operation. Whatever the attractiveness of the prospect of gradually reducing these expenditures, as the state of California is attempting to do, there are grave doubts whether it can be accomplished. Moreover, other practical political considerations will influence the outcome.

The California experience also suggests there are vested interests that can be expected to feel threatened by any de-emphasis of mental hospital operations and will therefore protest. Administering the present system requires an extensive bureaucracy, and that bureaucracy has long experience in "bunging the barrel" in political competition for funds. Furthermore, the legislative representatives of areas where mental hospitals are located can be expected to resist any cuts in state monies presently flowing into their districts. And it must be remembered that the professional disagreement over the best approach to combat mental illness works to strengthen the hands of those interests working to preserve the present pattern of expenditures.

For these and other reasons, it seems unlikely that the mental hospitals will disappear, even if a network of community centers is successfully brought into existence. They may change significantly; perhaps many will become intensive treatment centers or geriatric installations, providing services beyond the capacity of local centers. But what then? Should such a change occur, would there be a significant reduction in expenditures? Even if the envisioned decline in the mental hospital as the primary facility for treating the mentally ill does in fact occur, it remains to be seen whether that will mean any freeing of presently committed money.

There remain local governments as a potential source of funds for an expanded mental health program. Here the difficulty is perhaps even greater than at the state level. Apart from a very few states, local government efforts directed toward mental health had by the mid-1800s all but disappeared, save for the provision of a limited number of psychiatric beds in public general hospitals and the handling of specific problems such as drug addiction and alcoholism. In recent years, thanks in large part to the stimulus of the National Mental Health Act of 1946, local activity, primarily in the form of support for outpatient clinics, has been on the rise. But how far this can be expanded is highly questionable.

With ever-increasing emphasis on the importance of local action against poverty, the need for increased urban renewal efforts, and the growing demand for better, and more expensive, schools and police protection, local financing capacities are becoming more and more strained. Local government expenditures for hospitals and health in 1962 already totaled $2.2 billion, more than for sanitation, for police protection, or for housing and urban renewal.[3] In view of all this, it is not

---

[3] U.S., Bureau of the Census, *Census of Governments: 1962, Compendium of Government Finances,* pp. 27, 32.

likely that local expenditures on behalf of what has traditionally been a state responsibility will rise significantly in the near future.

LOCAL CONTROL AND FINANCE

As problems in metropolitan areas have become acute, the state has stepped in or has established special units to deal with such activities as water pollution, mass transportation, and even planning. Typically, basic responsibilities are left with local governments, but the state, often with federal assistance, takes on a large share of the cost of new and expanded functions through some sort of aid plan. This has become a universal trend.

In the field of mental health, the 1963 Act proposed a drastic reversal of the trend. An almost exclusively state function is to be transferred largely to the local level. Such a shift poses many problems. Psychiatric professionals are worried about community acceptance of keeping the mentally ill close to home. Local politicians are more likely to think that the attempted transfer of costs to the local government is potentially a greater handicap than the transfer of patients. Both may be true. Attitudes in some localities, as the field studies indicate, suggest that requiring local financial support will simply mean that no community mental health centers will be established. The long tradition of state responsibility for financing mental health activities is everywhere hard to overcome.

It is fair to ask whether local units can reasonably be expected to take on a large, new expense. Local units are reluctant to assume major new responsibilities because they are already seriously underfinanced. The continued growth of younger and older populations, the rising expectations for public services in transportation, housing, renewal, beautification, and fighting poverty result in vastly increased financial needs. At the same time, local governments are hampered in raising money to pay for them by constitutional, statutory, economic, and political impediments.

Local governments throughout the United States are financed in heavy proportion by property taxes. Where there are several layers of local government, each levies on the same property. State statutes typically limit the taxing capacity of local units by specifying the purposes for which tax monies can be spent, and by specifying a millage limit for specific purposes, as well as a total millage limit for all expenses. Local governments in the United States are universally up against these limits. Since property tax receipts are the product of the rate applied to the assessment base, more money can be brought in by raising the base ratio of assessed value to market value if the rate limit cannot be increased. This action is within local powers, but local governments find this politically difficult. To be sure, where there is a will to spend for mental health, a way can be found. Minnesota authorized its counties to levy a special property tax of not over fifty cents per capita for community mental health purposes. So far this revenue authorization has proved sufficient. This is not to say that mental health is adequately supported from the professionals' view, but that the level at which local government officials have wished to support mental health has not exceeded the statutory authorization.

In the Boston area, little opposition to spending by local units for mental health has been evident so far. But apparently this is because local spending for mental health has been very low, less than 1 per cent of local budgets. Syracuse has had a similar experience. In these two cities, however, as vastly increased spending for mental health is contemplated, government budgeting officials are taking a harder look at requests. Houston and Seattle are backed against their statutory tax rates, and, given the low level of public interest in mental health, there is no present prospect of a breakthrough. Local financial response has been virtually nil in the city of New Orleans, although of some significance in adjoining parishes.

It is clear that local spending limits are subject to shifting political winds and that they could be changed by legal or administrative means if the desire were present. But what kind of local political "climate" produces such desire?

The federal community mental health centers program assumes that local financial participation will provide a greater sense of community participation than if the service were wholly funded by the federal or state governments. This is a widespread assumption in all intergovernmental programs. But federal programs differ in the amount of matching funds required. The interstate highway program is financed 90 per cent by federal funds, and many aspects of the poverty program are 100 per cent federal.

Without question, requiring local financing will delay establishment of community mental health centers, and lack of money will be the main reason. The time-honored method of changing local priorities by offering matching money can at least get such a project into competition with other fields of government activity, such as highways or education, which operate with the aid of large grants from higher levels of government. Perhaps the greater the subsidy, the more rapidly the program will be set in motion. If it is true that local involvement varies with the extent of local financing, then the goals of getting the center established rapidly and involving the community are somewhat opposed. If community mental health centers were as large in operation as conceived in the 1963 Act, they would dislocate local budgets so much as to make them politically inconceivable. Present clinics established on a minimal scale continue to be small, token enterprises, and are likely to be thought of as getting about as much support as they deserve. A continuing process of intervention with the political leaders or influential persons and much greater federal aid will be required if community mental health centers are to attain the level of activity envisioned in the Act. If an attempt is to be made to alter present priorities, it is important to understand the relative importance of each governmental activity in the opinion of various segments of the community and especially in the view of the lawmakers who allocate funds among them.

EQUALIZATION OF LEVELS OF SERVICE

Given the fact of local government fragmentation, financing any governmental activity locally carries with it an enduring serious disadvantage—inequality. Local units differ in resources and needs for public services. The location of industry, the quantity of land taken for public use or otherwise exempt from taxation, the quality and number of homes, the rapidity and density of settlement—all of these factors combine to yield vastly different tax resources to counties and cities. As a result, any generalized limitation, such as fifty cents per capita or ten mills per dollar of assessed valuation, means greatly varying revenue available for expanding a service. More usually, it means that wealthier areas are able to afford, with less relative effort, far better services. Thus, the desirability of requiring local support at all for a new government service that should presumably be equally available to all is open to serious question.

Assuming that the aim of the federal act is to provide some minimum level of mental health services to every part of the land, the use of existing units of government is not likely to result in this. Within a single metropolitan area, to say nothing of throughout a state, the various local jurisdictions will differ radically in resources. This means that, unless a drastic equalization factor is built into fund distribution as a part of the policy, some areas will get markedly better services than others. Where the fiscal relationship is one of matching (putting up 50 per cent of the cost), the result is to aggravate existing inequalities. To those that have, more is given. Those who cannot afford the matching get nothing. Thus, in the Minneapolis–St. Paul area, the poorest county, harassed by many demands upon its meager resources, was ten years behind the wealthiest county in starting a mental health center and may not easily catch up in services rendered. The demand for local participation, unless heavily equalized, means a maldistribution of resources.

Early experience under the 1963 Act in allocating initial construction funds indicates, however, that readiness to participate was the prime consideration. In general, those localities that were most ready were those most financially able. Presumably the availability of extra funds was supposed to overcome the political reluctance of local units to spend for mental health. It will have this effect first in governments where a marginal expense can be added without pain. In the longer run the availability of outside funds may well induce new local spending where it causes real sacrifice. This cost, too, raises questions of fairness and equity.

The larger the geographic unit that is the tax base for a service, the less inequity in taxation, because the large unit will encompass more of the industrial, commercial, and residential base of the area. But it is hard to rationalize a stopping point. Ideally the base should be a whole metropolitan region, which is something of an economic system; but, because of migration from outside the area, a whole state or even the nation can better serve as an appropriate tax base. This demographic fact has been the principal justification for the gradual assumption by states and the national government of social costs—the wealth of the country is national, the market is national, and the problems are national. That is why the attempt to require assumption of mental health costs by smaller units will be regarded by some to be a regressive step, especially in the absence of any indication that mental illness is something peculiar to a particular locale or location. To be sure, the use of voluntary hospitals or privately supported centers, sometimes under university auspices as in the case of Tulane University in New Orleans, would solve the financial problem by avoiding the necessity for tax support.

MANPOWER REQUIREMENTS OF AN EXPANDED PROGRAM

During the course of the House hearings on the community mental health bill in 1963, one committee member remarked that he did not "see much point in building centers unless we have adequate staffing, because it seems to me that staffing is more important than going around building buildings." [4] In saying this, the congressman put his finger on a problem of major dimensions that was not necessarily alleviated by the restoration of staffing money by the 1965 amendments. The proposed network of community centers will require a staggering number of pro-

Table 1: Staffing Pattern of a Typical Community Mental Health Center, as Proposed to Congress during Hearings on 1963 Bill and 1965 Amendments

	1963		1965	
Staff Positions	Number	Annual Cost	Number	Annual Cost
Psychiatrists	10	$190,000	6	$135,000
Psychologists	8	93,800	4	60,000
Social workers	8	67,280	6	60,000
Nurses	19	133,570	14	112,000
Health educators	2	19,960	2	20,000
Occupational therapists	4	30,760	2	16,000
Psychiatric aids	32	134,880	24	120,000
Other supporting personnel	25	142,350	14	80,000
Total	108	$812,600	72	$603,000

Source: U.S., Congress, House, Subcommittee of the Committee on Interstate and Foreign Commerce, *Hearings on H.R.3688, H.R.3689, and H.R.2567,* 88th Cong., 1st Sess., 1963, p. 101; and the Committee on Interstate Commerce, *Hearings on H.R.2984, H.R.2985, H.R.2986, and H.R.2987,* 89th Cong., 1st Sess., 1965, p. 48.

fessional personnel. Table 1 summarizes the staffing pattern of a typical mental health center as presented to Congress in 1963 and as revised in

[4] Rep. Paul G. Rogers (Dem., Fla.), U.S., Congress, House, Subcommittee of the Committee on Interstate and Foreign Commerce, *Hearings on H.R.3688, H.R.3689, and H.R.2567,* 88th Cong., 1st Sess., 1963, p. 105.

1965. Even if the lower estimates of 1965 are accepted, then blanketing the country with one center for every 200,000 people would require employing some 72,000 professionals, 30,000 of them from the four basic mental health disciplines of psychiatry, psychology, psychiatric social work, and mental health nursing.[5] Even with money available to pay them, it seems highly questionable whether these professionals will be available in sufficient numbers to make the program a reality.

In an extensive study of manpower needs in mental health for the Joint Commission, Dr. George W. Albee concluded in 1959 that very real shortages existed and that "the prospect for the future . . . is for more shortages." [6] According to Albee, a number of studies indicated that 68 of every 1,000 budgeted positions in nonprivate institutions were unfilled in 1956 and a very high proportion of the vacancies were in the higher professional categories. Of some 3,000 positions available for physicians in state and county hospitals, nearly a quarter were unfilled. While vacancies for psychiatric social workers and registered nurses were slightly less numerous, the extent of unfilled positions for psychologists was much the same. Moreover, even if all the vacancies that existed could have been filled, these public hospitals would still have been far below the minimum standards for mental hospitals set by the American Psychiatric Association. Indeed, Albee reported in 1957 that not a single state even approached these modest minimum standards. Registered nurses were in especially short supply; according to the association's standards, there were less than one-fifth of the registered nurses needed for minimal adequate staffing of the country's mental hospitals. The number of physicians in public mental hospitals was only 40 per cent of what the association considered minimally adequate, and a significant proportion of those employed were foreign interns.

To be sure, the mental health professions have been growing very rapidly. Administration spokesmen pointed out in the 1963 hearings that the estimated 1960 total of 44,200 persons employed in the four core disciplines represented an increase of almost two and one-half times the 1950 figure. But if only half of that increase is assumed to have occurred by 1957, then the pathetic inadequacies reported by Albee

---

[5] And these figures ignore the fact that the staffing pattern as presented apparently assumed a service population of only 100,000, not 200,000.
[6] *Mental Health Manpower Trends,* Joint Commission on Mental Illness and Health Monograph No. 3 (New York: Basic Books, 1959), p. 13.

occurred in spite of the availability of approximately 31,000 of these professionals. During the 1965 hearings it was reported that psychiatrists, psychologists, psychiatric social workers, and mental health nurses had increased to a total of 64,000.[7] Even with this level of increase, however, it is difficult to believe that the shortages in existing institutions reported by Albee have been fully eliminated, and it is worth noting that even the Administration witnesses in 1965 admitted the continued inadequacy of the manpower pool. How then is a program expansion, which when fully implemented will require professional personnel totaling almost half the present supply, to be staffed?

During both the 1963 and 1965 hearings, administration witnesses expressed their confidence that the necessary professional personnel would be found. They and other witnesses favorable to the legislation emphasized the rapid growth in mental health personnel and their confidence that this trend would continue in the future. The staff for the centers would come from a number of sources. It was expected that many psychiatrists in private practice would use the center for their patients or would become full-time staff members. Another source anticipated was the general practitioner or family doctor, who would admit patients to the mental health center just as he would to a general hospital. As the number of admissions to state mental hospitals declined, personnel presently employed there would be freed to work in community centers. But most important of all, increased training efforts, primarily through increased federal training grants, would increase the number of mental health professionals significantly.

Despite the confidence of the program's backers, however, a number of troublesome questions remain unanswered. It has been said that if all the psychiatrists in the United States, plus all the psychiatric social workers, and all the psychologists trained as therapists spent all their working hours with individual patients, they would still be able to treat only one in ten of the patients who need help for emotional ills.[8] The difficulty of remedying this situation rapidly by even drastically increased training efforts is well illustrated by the case of the top level of the professional group, the psychiatrists.

[7] U.S., Congress, House, Committee on Interstate and Foreign Commerce, *Hearings on H.R.2984, H.R.2985, H.R.2986, and H.R.2987,* 89th Cong., 1st Sess., 1965, p. 55.
[8] *Time,* Feb. 8, 1963, quoted in Karl Menninger, *The Vital Balance* (New York: Viking Press, 1963), p. 334.

532 PITFALLS AND PROBLEMS

An NIMH publication in the fall of 1964 indicated that an American Psychiatric Association study had identified 17,809 psychiatrists in the United States.[9] While this figure jibes nicely with the projections made in 1963, almost 1,000 were identified as not practicing, leaving 16,863 who were in active practice devoting at least 50 per cent of their time to the practice of psychiatry. An American Medical Association report, also based on data for the fall of 1964, listed 16,259 physicians (6 per cent of the total) as engaged in the specialty of psychiatry, of whom 3,455, or 21 per cent, were residents.[10] Regardless of which figure is considered more reliable, however, a rapid expansion in the number of psychiatrists is subject to the very real strictures of the training process.

A physician's career begins with his graduation from medical school, which, with few exceptions, requires four academic years of training after three or four years of undergraduate college work. But most doctors continue their education as interns in a hospital the first year after acquiring the M.D. degree. In order to meet the certification standards set by one of the nineteen national specialty boards, an additional two- to five-year period of residency or other formal training is required. According to a recent study of medical school graduates during the period 1948–1961, about two-thirds of the young doctors spent their second year after graduation in residency training and more than half continued their postgraduate training into the third and fourth years.[11] That the great majority of doctors desire to be specialists is borne out by the fact that the proportion of graduates who had made a choice of specialty had increased from two-thirds by the second year after graduation to four-fifths by the fourteenth year. Surgery and related fields were the primary choice; medical fields were next, with psychiatry and neurology claiming 9 per cent of the physicians by their fourteenth year out of medical school. By this fourteenth year half of the graduates held certificates from one of the specialty boards and two-thirds of the specialists were diplomates. About 60 per cent of those practicing psychiatry and neurology had been certified by the American Board of Psychiatry and Neurology.

[9] U.S., Public Health Service, *Mental Health Manpower: Current Statistical and Activities Report* (Washington: U.S. Government Printing Office, 1964), p. 1.
[10] "Medical Education in the United States, 1964–1965," *Journal of the American Medical Association,* Vol. 194 (Nov. 15, 1965), p. 779.
[11] See Maryland Y. Pennell, "Career Patterns in Medicine," *Public Health Reports,* Vol. 80 (Feb. 1965), pp. 155–62. This article has been drawn on freely throughout this paragraph.

The period of formal training required for certification as a specialist in psychiatry is long and expensive, and the number of psychiatrists who can be trained under these conditions is limited. Specializing is, of course, a matter of personal choice and a doctor may specialize without certification by a national board. Indeed, of the physicians reporting themselves as engaged in full-time psychiatric specialization in 1961, only 42 per cent were diplomates; and even excluding those who were still in training programs the proportion certified was only 51 per cent.[12] But surely the community centers program assumes that "psychiatrists" means specialists who have taken some or all their residency in psychiatry, and the American Psychiatric Association spokesman at the 1965 hearings cited 800 as the number of new psychiatrists being turned out each year.[13] The question is whether the realities of the training process will allow an increase sufficient to meet the need within the four-year period during which staffing grants remain available. It seems highly unlikely.

UNEQUAL DISTRIBUTION OF PROFESSIONAL MANPOWER

The availability of professional personnel in sufficient numbers is not the only manpower problem, however. Given the community focus of the new program, the geographic location of available personnel becomes as important as their numbers. Again, the psychiatrists will serve to illustrate the problem. These medical specialists are not spread across the country in accordance with population distribution. As of late 1964, five states—New York, California, Pennsylvania, Massachusetts, and Illinois—with approximately a third of the nation's population, accounted for over half the psychiatrists in active practice. As can be seen in Table 2, the proportion of the nation's active psychiatrists practicing in three of these states was considerably greater than the percentage of the American population residing there. It seems highly likely that a similar imbalance in the availability of psychiatrists exists within each state. As the nature of the five states with the largest numbers suggests, mental health professionals are presently clustered in the large metropolitan areas. Given a persistent shortage that puts them in an advantageous

[12] U.S., Public Health Service, *Health Manpower Source Book: Section 14, Medical Specialists* (Washington: U.S. Government Printing Office, 1962), p. 164.
[13] House, *Hearings* (1965), p. 204.

Table 2: Proportion of Practicing Psychiatrists and Proportion
of United States Population in Selected States

	Psychiatrists		Population	
State	Number	Per Cent of U.S. Total	Number (Millions)	Per Cent of U.S. Total
New York	3,690	21.9	16.8	9.4
California	2,100	12.5	15.7	8.8
Pennsylvania	1,079	6.4	11.3	6.3
Massachusetts	943	5.6	5.1	2.8
Illinois	801	4.8	10.1	5.6
Total	8,613	51.1	59.0	32.9

Source: Data on psychiatrists from U.S., Public Health Service, *Mental Health Manpower: Current Statistical and Activities Report* (Washington: U.S. Government Printing Office, 1964); population data from U.S., Bureau of the Census, *Census of Population, 1960* (Washington: U.S. Government Printing Office, 1961).

market position, they have settled in areas that provide an unlimited supply of potential patients, professional contacts, and other facilities and opportunities. How are the needed professional personnel, even if available in sufficient numbers, to be induced to spread themselves as needed as the new centers are built? It is all very well to say that physicians will be attracted to the locations where facilities are made available, but this assumes a diminution of the attractiveness of the big cities, an assumption which has yet to be demonstrated.

It also has yet to be demonstrated that psychiatrists in sufficient numbers will be willing to accept salaried positions in community centers. Private practice, especially psychoanalysis, is highly lucrative, and the training process is lengthy and very expensive. Commenting on the reports of the Joint Commission on Mental Illness and Health, Elaine Cumming observed in 1962, "There is a seepage of manpower out of the core field of the treatment of the seriously mentally ill into private practice where the least seriously ill are treated." [14] Without casting aspersions on the motivations of medical professionals, one wonders what assurance there is that even a greatly expanded training program would not work primarily to increase the availability of treatment for middle-class neurotics, rather than to staff adequately the proposed network of

[14] "A Review Article—The Reports of the Joint Commission on Mental Illness and Health," *Social Problems*, Vol. 9 (Spring 1962), p. 397

centers. At the very least, it remains to be seen whether further adjustments in the direction of higher salaries for the centers' staff such as that reflected in the 1965 projections will not prove necessary.

Some centers may allow doctors to conduct private practice in the center after hours, which would provide greater opportunities for supplementing income than have been available in state mental hospitals. Joint appointments and consultantships could be arranged in a flexible system. This combination of possibilities may indicate that decentralization of psychiatric and related services may be the way to make public practice more attractive and, in turn, attract more top quality people into the field.

On the other hand, economies of scale must be maintained to get maximum use from staff, and to justify higher pay. Small units may not be able to afford an adequate recruiting campaign. Within a single metropolitan area, competitive differentials among mental health centers will arise. Some counties or cities are more prestigious than others; some may have generally better reputations in the operation of community mental health facilities or other community facilities than others. Some will certainly be more remote from a university, medical center, or private practice location, which could make it harder to get professional staff.

Finally, the supposed effect on the manpower problem of the decline in mental hospital admissions deserves comment. In the first place, the need for personnel in the hospitals can be reduced only after the centers are built, staffed, and assuming part of the patient load. Consequently, this expected decline in the future provides no relief from the problem of initial staffing for new centers. But more importantly, the program assumes that, with greater emphasis on the treatment of mental illness and availability of service in the community, a greater percentage of the mentally ill will seek and obtain care than before. If this proves to be the case, then it does not follow that the centers will necessarily take over part of the mental hospitals' present load in the near future; they may well be occupied primarily with meeting new demands for service created by their presence. Given the present short supply of professional personnel, there is a very real danger that the creation of new facilities will produce a competition for staff between them and presently existing, still direly needed, institutions. It remains to be seen whether an initial "robbing Peter to pay Paul" situation can be avoided.

All of these manpower difficulties finally come down to the same basic problem: the present shortage of professional personnel and the need for drastic increases in the number available in the very near future if the new program is to have any chance of success. But this will be expensive, and, as indicated above, the launching of the new program is itself likely to increase the expense. The conclusion cannot be avoided that present manpower realities serve to increase the complexity of what is already a problem of major proportions—finding the money to finance the community centers program.

SUPERVISION OF FEDERAL GRANTS

If the policy of the new Act is to change radically the direction of present mental health activity, not only must a very large dose of outside money be offered, but there must be a good deal of supervision and encouragement (not to say friendly harassment) to bring about any substantial change. Most participants and directors are likely to believe that what they are doing is the right thing, but that they are not adequately financed to do it as well as they would like. When the opportunity arises for them to get more money, therefore, they will try to get it without changing their current orientation and *modus operandi*.

Where much of the money is local, the local administrators will be reluctant to change the thrust of their present programs. The more money that is made available on specified conditions, the more likely is change in the desired direction to transpire. No change is automatic, however, if the outside money is minimal or is a single grant for construction. The influence will be much less than that of a firm continued support that becomes a vital part of the budget.

The relationship between grantor and grantee is two-way. Money alone will not accomplish the change. Experience strongly suggests that most communities would use the new federal money available to do more of what they are already doing. Where the state community mental health program is under the same agency that operates other institutions, the state is content to start small centers and let them grow somewhat toward comprehensive care. State agencies operating state hospitals do not wish to suffer displacement.

Where large mental hospitals have long been accepted, as in New York state, the community mental health center is likely to be merely a smaller version of the standard hospital located downtown rather than in a remote rural area. In Houston, the likelihood is that many of the mental health services will merely be brought together under an administrative umbrella and be called a community mental health center with no really different direction of operation. In Seattle, community mental health centers, depending upon which state agency ultimately winds up in control of them, could be extensions of the state mental hospitals or supervised by the Department of Institutions, provided the recent move by the governor designating that agency as the mental health authority is upheld legally. In Boston, since the state already controls community clinics, and local government units are forbidden to treat mental health, state control seems most likely to be great. In New Orleans, however, new community centers are developing, although it is also true that the 1950 vintage clinics have been turned into "centers" by change of nomenclature.

This variety among community mental health centers may or may not be desirable. It may be that the field of community psychiatry is still so new as to require this experimental approach. Surely the time will come, however, when a better device than trial and error will have to be applied in the provision of mental care. If central professionals, as in the National Institute of Mental Health, have a doctrine in mind for public policy, this doctrine may be drastically changed, even subverted, in practice across the country. Leadership, defined as instruction combined with persuasion, with an ultimate coercive power to close the tap, must be rendered by the grantor if he is to accomplish change. But preserving the apparent initiative and control of the local directors will be necessary—that is, allowing them to change their programs gradually and seemingly under their own ideas and desires.

In Minneapolis, the county mental health center was once oriented to in-house treatment of the acutely mentally ill. Under encouragement from state officials, its local staff attended planning meetings where the intent of the new program was explained and demonstrated. The center has since moved in the direction of greater comprehensiveness and of handling mental illness at stages other than acute. It has done this in the face of unpublicized professional criticism on the one side and prodding from community agencies on the other.

Perhaps this community-by-community administrative leadership job is the ideal way to build a long-lasting, broadly conceived mental health program in every community across the land. That is, rather than imposing a national professional agency's preconceived ideas of a center with federal funds, the centers should be allowed to grow cooperatively toward an emerging goal. Whatever is done, by whomever financed, will have to be done by the seriously limited pool of professional people now involved. More of the newly trained professionals will be oriented toward community mental health than in the past. Under no circumstances can a sudden transformation in the care of the great numbers of mentally ill persons be expected. But the speed and direction of change can be profoundly affected by the quantities of outside money injected into the operating level, depending upon the degree and competence of the influence sought to be extended along with the money.

XV: DECISION MAKERS AND INFLUENTIALS

BOTH THE EXISTING PATTERNS of mental health services and the prospects for the federal Act depends upon the structure of influence and decision making in mental health in the various state and local communities. Who wields effective power over mental health services? What is the role of public officials? How influential are the various voluntary organizations in shaping mental health policy? What do the field studies contribute in answering these questions about decision making at the state and local level?

Two analytical approaches frequently employed by political and social scientists have been used in the field studies: interest groups have been examined and the community power structure outlined. Used with discretion both methods can add greatly to available knowledge about the decision-making process in mental health programs.

Influence is as deceptive as it is important. If influence is conceived as the capacity to control operations and shape program and policy decisions, then there are numerous gradations associated with the various groups and individuals involved in the policy field, and the influence of any one of them will vary with time and circumstance. Yet, while no attempts were made to develop formal quantitative criteria for measuring the roles of particular groups and individuals in mental health, their activities were readily apparent and can be described in sufficient detail to serve analytical needs. By focusing particularly on those who by function (e.g., mental health professionals, state hospital administrators, etc.) seem logically to belong in the policy process, as well as on those who are identified as direct or indirect participants in actual decisions, the principal elements in the influence structure can be outlined. The task was simplified by the fact that state mental health programs are low-pressure, low-priority affairs, with only those groups and individuals immediately and professionally concerned likely to care much about it. They tend as well to be dedicated, outspoken, and often conspicuous.

This situation operates both to limit the number of persons and groups in the influence network at the state and local level, and to give considerable visibility to those who are in it.

PUBLIC OFFICIALS IN THE DECISION PROCESS

The group theory of politics, formulated by Bentley and elaborated by Truman, has often been accused—rightly or wrongly—of failing to take into account the role and influence of public officials.[1] According to some critics, the group theorists have portrayed the nongovernmental interest groups as the sole agents of influence, and the course of public policy as a vector of those forces, with official policy makers cast as essentially passive or helpless bystanders. What light do the field studies shed on the actual roles of public officials?

Since state legislatures are formally designated as official policy makers for those within their jurisdictions, it might be well to begin by considering the role of their members in general and with particular reference to mental health programing. Viewed in general terms, and with a few exceptions, the fifty state legislatures have a low estate that contrasts sharply with their position atop the formal policy structure. To some extent this is a matter of personnel. Particularly in the lower houses there is a staggering rate of turnover among members, due partially to the tendency to view the state legislature as the first step toward higher office. This general political inexperience, coupled with rawness in the legislative process, low pay, lack of office space, and the like, exacts a heavy toll in the lawmakers' performance.

There are also institutional forces at work to downgrade the state legislators. Often they are handicapped by state constitutional limitations. Biennial sessions, though declining in use, are still the prevailing pattern, so that many matters demanding careful attention can never get it. In some states the political context leaves legislators highly vulnerable

---

[1] Arthur F. Bentley, *The Process of Government* (Bloomington, Ind.: The Principia Press, 1949); David B. Truman, *The Governmental Process* (New York: Alfred A. Knopf, 1951). For critical assessments of the group theory of politics see Peter Odegard, "A Group Basis of Politics: A New Name for an Old Myth," *Western Political Quarterly*, Vol. 11 (Sept. 1958), p. 689; Stanley Rothman, "Systematic Political Theory: Observations on the Group Approach," *American Political Science Review*, Vol. 54 (March 1960), p. 15; and R. E. Dowling, "Pressure Group Theory: Its Methodological Range," *American Political Science Review*, Vol. 54 (Dec. 1960), p. 944.

to pressure group influence. The assemblies themselves seem determined to compound their difficulties by clinging to archaic or obsolete practices.

It does not necessarily follow, however, that state legislatures are therefore of no significance in the state policy process. In some states the legislative branch remains the dominant one; in others, it has been overshadowed by the executive. Probably the greater part of the legislatures fall in the intermediate position, neither dominating state policy nor relegated to an insignificant role.

The tendency for state legislators to play primarily a ratifying role is confirmed by the findings in all six states covered in this study, for in no case was the state assembly found to be in the forefront of the policy process. Legislative action regarding mental health was often nothing more than a *pro forma* gesture to ratify leadership decisions, but even when a vital choice was made in committee or on the floor the basic alternatives were developed elsewhere, for instance by the governor's office as in Minnesota, or by the bureaucracy as in Massachusetts. The principal and sometimes quite important exceptions involved individual legislators who took an interest in mental health problems and even influenced policy details for one of two reasons. Some were strongly motivated to act on behalf of mental health because of mental illness or retardation among their relatives and friends. Others were simply in quest of public installations such as hospitals and clinics for their particular districts. Hospitals mean jobs and dollars for constituents. The location of state mental hospitals always has been a matter of primary concern to members of the legislatures. Increased local activity in mental health in New York state apparently expanded the role of legislators from the Syracuse area, and there would seem to be a high potential for such in the Minneapolis area, where the legislative delegation has a long tradition of serving as a super city council.

While legislatures have not played a significant innovative role in general mental health policy making, neither have they emerged as active obstructionists. None of the field studies reported any notable blocking or delaying by the legislative branch where the policy innovators were reasonably unified and where they had provided the necessary leadership. The Massachusetts legislature usually goes along with the governor's mental health budget proposals and on occasion even increases the funds recommended. In Louisiana, executive budget proposals are sometimes cut, but not viciously. In Minnesota and New York, where mental health programs have relatively high priority among state programs, the legislatures have allowed that status to prevail, even if they did not bring it about. In the low-priority states of Washington and Texas, the legislatures have been willing to take favorable action whenever sufficient leadership was available to give saliency to the issue. Thus, with the possible exception of New York, which has actively promoted the improvement of mental health services, most state legislatures often are content to reflect the views of the majority of their constituents.

The greatest impact of these bodies may very well be found in the tendency of leadership elements to limit their proposals in anticipation of legislative disapproval. Particularly in the states where mental health programs are low in priority, there is some scattered indication of the emergence of a "self-fulfilling prophecy" in this respect, for an estimate of legislative coolness to mental health policy proposals may very well result in lack of proper effort to cultivate the lawmakers. While the field data do not bear directly on this question, there is reason to believe that the basic difficulty in getting increased legislative support for mental health is not so much hostility as indifference and ignorance. It is less a problem of changing legislative opinion than a matter of getting opinions formed at all. The function of "educating" the state's legislators on the needs and problems of mental health has not always been properly performed.

While state legislatures have been declining in status and power, the governors of the various states have been slowly improving their overall position. The governor's position as political leader has been strengthened, with the inevitable result that he has become more and more responsible for legislative and policy leadership. This has been reinforced in some states as in New York by varying degrees of administrative reform designed to make him chief of the executive branch in fact as well as by title. When fully armed with administrative authority, budgetary powers, and such constitutional powers as the legislative veto, a governor who is also a skilled and popular political leader is often able to dominate policy making in state affairs. Even those who lack the administrative and constitutional weapons of influence, as in Texas and Minnesota, may be able to utilize their political power for policy purposes. Thus, while the presence or absence of formal powers constitutes an important variable, the governor's role is also greatly affected by the kinds of priorities he sets in the field of public policy and by the political skills that he brings to the office.

In Minnesota every governor since Youngdahl (1948–1951) has recognized the political popularity of the subject by making the further development of mental health services a major objective, and they must be credited with contributing importantly to the development of services in that state. In other states studied, however, a common thread runs through the reports. The governors have on occasion been influential in molding or in speeding up policies and programs in the mental health field, as did Governor Volpe in the fall of 1966 when he called the Massachusetts legislature back into special session and forced through a reorganization of the community mental health centers. Similarly the governors of New York, on occasion, have strongly supported particular mental health programs. But few of them have cared to make it a major campaign or legislative issue. Although the governors are the apex of formal political leadership in the states, their support for new mental health programs has been tacit and the rationale primarily political. Except for Minnesota, effective communications between proponents of local mental health programs and state chief executives had hardly been adequate until the passage of federal legislation filled the horizon with pots of federal gold. If there is, outside of Minnesota, any capital in mental health as a political issue, a host of governors have generally overlooked it.

Although overshadowed both in constitutional theory and in political activity by the governor and the legislature, officials in state agencies are able to influence greatly the course of public policy. By pressing for legislative enactments, by winning budgetary support, and by implementing patterns, they give policy their distinctive imprint. Whether this potential is realized depends partly on the political context in which it functions, and partly on the drive and capabilities of the agency's leaders.

In considering the role and influence of state mental health administrative agencies it is helpful to note that their opportunities really begin with utilization of their expertise to identify policy needs and alternatives in the care of mentally ill persons. While there were naturally variations in the degree of accomplishment, in all six states studied, with the exception of Texas, there was a real concern with this function. The outstanding examples are the Department of Mental Health in

Massachusetts and the Department of Public Welfare in Minnesota, both of which have contributed importantly to national as well as state policy development. The relevant departments in New York and in Washington were also actively engaged in confronting mental health problems. In Louisiana the whole state and local programs owe much to the efforts of "Blue" Walters, a long-time state hospital official. Only in Texas did the agencies seem to be lagging badly in this first stage of policy influence, and even there the administrators in the mental retardation area were moving with some alacrity.

But such is the influence of the political environment that success in the next stage of influence, "educating" other participants, varied tremendously. In what is undoubtedly a cause and effect relationship, the Department of Public Welfare in Minnesota both contributes to and benefits from a climate of public and political opinion that is well disposed toward mental health programs. The Department of Mental Hygiene in New York, the Department of Mental Health in Massachusetts, and the Department of Hospitals in Louisiana also appear to be properly attentive to their "educational" responsibilities. In Washington the conditions operate to limit sharply the efforts of the Department of Institutions. In Texas, again with the exception of those dealing with the mentally retarded, the state agencies were not proceeding with any apparent vigor to press the case for better services with either the public or with state political leaders.

The final stage of the influence process for these agencies is the mobilization of public and governmental support for their proposals, and here one finds the widest range of accomplishment. In Minnesota, Louisiana, and New York, it would appear, the agencies have with other elements been especially successful in winning support. In Massachusetts strong agency efforts have produced considerable gains within the limitations imposed by broader state fiscal considerations. In Washington the mobilization of support by agencies has been hampered by rivalry and conflict between the Department of Institutions and the Health Department, as well as by general budgetary problems. One finds in Texas perhaps the least effective performance by agencies in attempting to mobilize for purposes of influencing state policy, although it is worth noting that they played an important role in organizing the mental health planning committee that did eventually weld together a structure of influence.

Thus, although conditions did not always enable these officials to have a great deal of impact, individual leaders of state agencies, such as Jack Ewalt in Massachusetts, did have considerable effect in all states except Texas. Deserving to be called professionals by virtue of their approach to administration as well as by their medical training, these administrators have undoubtedly contributed importantly to an atmosphere of administrative sophistication in the total state picture. Their approach was often described as expansive, but it is difficult to label innovative and pioneering thrusts as empire building or aggrandizement when existing levels of service are so low and the needs so shockingly evident.

On the local level, the influence of public officials is most evident in Minneapolis–St. Paul, New Orleans, and Syracuse. In each case an unusually effective county official played a very important role in furthering the development of local mental health programs, and other local officials have taken supportive positions. In Massachusetts the constitutional arrangements leave little room for local public mental health services, and hence it is not surprising that there has been virtually no influence exercised by local officials. In Seattle local officials have generally shown little interest in or concern with mental health problems, but they are clearly a key element in the decisional process, since their unwillingness to provide funds for mental health services are felt, and felt heavily, in that community. The same generalization holds for Houston, although there are conspicuous exceptions. Thus the county judge has labored consistently if not always effectively for expanded services, and administrators in the Galena Park school district have gone far beyond most other districts in their mental health program. Still, it is generally true that local officialdom has given ungrudging support to mental health services only when they put no strain on the budget.

One can say, then, that local officials are acquiescent in a field that is dominated by state officialdom on the one hand and by private organizations on the other. Operating in an atomized, fragmented, often chaotic atmosphere, local officials are not apt themselves to produce a unified approach to the handling of problems in a field so broadly defined. The studies of the six communities reveal occasional instances of vigorous effort by political leaders seeking to realize mental health goals, but on the whole one cannot detect widespread involvement.

However, if there is a further growth of local public mental health programs, then local officials, particularly county officials, may emerge as brokers between state, federal, local, and private interests in mental health.

Another vital part of the total context of mental health policy making is the existence of several major professional groups with an important stake in existing and proposed programs. These include such directly involved groups as psychiatrists, psychologists, psychiatric nurses, psychiatric social workers, therapists, and the like, and also such secondarily involved groups as the entire medical profession. Professionals in any complex industrial society such as our own are highly functional, and one of the questions to be considered is whether they play equally important roles in the policy process.

Certainly the most important organized medical group is the American Medical Association. It is a federation of 54 state, commonwealth, and territorial associations, which in turn are composed of more than 1,900 component medical societies. Authority moves up from the component societies through the state and territorial associations to the national body, through the process of electing delegates. With a membership of some 202,000, the AMA includes approximately 70 per cent of the nation's physicians.

The extent of AMA activities is reflected in the total cost of operating the association. In 1965 expenses totaled almost $28 million. Among its many educational activities are the sponsoring of more than a thousand scientific meetings a year, postgraduate programs for physicians, several programs of educational and research grants and fellowships, the maintenance of an extensive medical library, a comprehensive information service providing guidance for physicians on drugs, and cooperation with other organizations in fostering health education. The AMA also serves the public as well as the medical profession through its activities on behalf of medical standards.

The activities that have the most direct bearing, both actual and potential, on the success of a particular public program are the AMA's legislative and publications programs. The association or the state medical societies analyze pending legislation of medical interest at both the national and state levels. It is an active pressure organization, supporting, opposing, even initiating various types of governmental activity.

Psychiatrists are, of course, physicians, and as such most are members of the AMA. And among the thirteen association councils set up to deal with professional or technical areas is the Council on Mental Health. The fundamental role of the council is to recommend policies and develop programs in mental health. In this role, the Council on Mental Health has played an important part in furthering mental health programs. Yet it must be remembered that while the AMA supported that part of the 1963 legislation authorizing construction grants, the House of Delegates overrode the Council on Mental Health to oppose successfully the initial staffing grants and that, when the 1965 amendments reinstated the staffing money, they were passed over the AMA's opposition.

The American Psychiatric Association is the oldest national medical society in the United States. Founded in Philadelphia in 1844 by thirteen distinguished physicians who administered mental hospitals, the association gradually broadened in scope from its origin as an organization of superintendents. Operating under its present name since 1921, the APA's membership has roughly doubled each decade since the 1930s. The membership now totals about 15,000, which is 80 per cent of the association's estimate of the total number of psychiatrists and psychiatric residents in the United States.

There is a district branch of the association in nearly every state, and some states have more than one. Requirements for membership in a branch are the same as for membership in the association, and since 1963 new members must belong to a district branch provided there is one in the area where they reside.

While lacking the resources and political muscle of the AMA, the APA has long been an active proponent of extensive governmental activity on behalf of mental health. It has been a consistent supporter of ever-higher appropriations for the National Institute of Mental Health and has vigorously urged the adoption of a new approach to the mentally ill through the community mental health center model. The association's role in bringing about the Joint Commission's study and its active support of the 1963 legislation were discussed in a preceding chapter. The association exerted every effort on behalf of the staffing provisions in 1963 and redoubled its efforts after the initial failure. Only a little over a month after President Johnson's 1965 health message, for instance, the APA convened a conference for leaders in state mental health planning from all over the country; it was clearly designed to stimulate grassroots support for the staffing amendments, which it hoped would be translated effectively to key congressmen.

There is a surprising similarity in the findings of the field studies regarding the role and influence of the various professional organizations at the state and local level. In Seattle individual psychiatrists were found to be of critical importance in the making of community mental health decisions—their support is essential and their veto nearly absolute. However, as a formally constituted group, the Seattle psychiatrists have not been particularly active, and most of them give little attention to community problems. The meetings of the Northwest Chapter of the American Psychiatric Association tend to be poorly attended, and it has taken no positive action regarding community mental health. The situation regarding the psychologists and the medical society is no better. Psychologists are still a small group and thus far have failed to organize themselves for effective public action. The medical society in Seattle is well organized, and it is no stranger to the public arena. Nevertheless, far from providing positive leadership, it has been content to play a passive if not vaguely hostile role in the establishment of community mental health centers.

Essentially the same conclusions were drawn from the study of Houston. The state medical society and its mental health committee are clearly the most significant of all organized groups concerned with mental health, but their greatest influence is negative. The state society was found to have been involved along with others in the decision to seek a planning grant for a community mental health program, and its officials were deeply involved in some of the infighting that took place during the life of the Planning Committee and during the legislative consideration of reorganization of the state mental health administrative system. There was nothing, however, to indicate any long-term concern with mental health programing, or to warrant assigning the society credit for progress made. Much the same can be said of Houston's medical society.

So far as psychiatrists in Texas are concerned, their state society was found to be relatively weak. It was rather generally agreed that the Houston Psychiatric Society is similarly impotent. The psychologists and social workers appear to be even less significant as groups. Both have organizations at the local and state level, but in no case is there a paid staff, and their influence is minimal.

The investigation of influence in mental health programing in Minnesota and in the Minneapolis–St. Paul area revealed approximately the same pattern. The state medical association has been on the whole a passive force, acquiescing in public mental health programs in exchange for rules (backed by a means test) limiting such services to indigent persons. A Minnesota Association of Psychiatry has only recently been organized, and the private practitioners among its members are not particularly interested in public policy.

Professional organizations in Massachusetts and in Boston are found to be somewhat more involved in policy issues. For example, such a highly specialized group as the Associated General Hospital Psychiatrists has worked assiduously to promote the incorporation of comprehensive mental health centers into private general hospitals. The state medical societies keep a close eye on public policy but, while they are certainly respected, they may not have much political power. Certainly there is nothing approaching large-scale organizational involvement, for only a small fraction of the members of the mental health community were found actually to exert much influence on the shaping of public policy regarding mental health.

In Syracuse the medical society, and the area chapters of the American Psychiatric Association, the American Psychological Association, and the National Association of Social Workers are seen as part of the influence structure, but the investigation there cast serious doubt on the assumption that these groups as organizations wield effective power. Although the findings are not without ambiguity, there is some reason to believe that it is a case of influentials wielding power not derived from their organizational offices.

What overall conclusions are to be drawn from these sketches? While the situation reported varies from one area to another, there are certain elements of similarity that need to be noted. As a general rule professional groups tend to function most effectively in the political system as "veto" groups, and the field of mental health provides no exception to that rule. The hostility of any of the major professional groups would in most instances suffice to force accommodative modifications, and certain of them, most notably the psychiatrists and the medical societies, can probably block all efforts at policy innovation if sufficiently aroused.

On the whole the professional groups were more or less won over to the idea of a new departure in mental health services. None chose or was forced to exercise its veto power. That is not to say that there was uncritical acceptance, or that they did not seek modifications in the mental health centers plan. The AMA opposed staffing grants. There was some professional opposition in Massachusetts to separating the centers from general hospitals, and the medical profession in Texas was apparently ready to block the administrative reorganization of services unless the statute specified that the commissioner of mental health services had to be a psychiatrist. But despite these qualifications it is generally true that the various professional groups have acquiesced in the decision to develop community mental health centers.

Third, this acquiescent role should not be confused with an innovative one. While professionals in either public or private practice were invariably involved in the decisions to seek state and local implementation of the federal statutes, their organizations played minor parts. It appears that the organized professional groups were not in the policy vanguard.

It is worth considering why the professional groups failed to play a more significant role. There are at least three factors that seem to be important in that failure. One is the division of professional opinion regarding public mental health programs, and particularly those with the potential impact of community mental health centers. One confronts in almost every case the doubts and reservations of physicians about public psychiatry, sometimes expressed openly as in Massachusetts, sometimes implicitly as in Texas. The psychiatrists themselves are divided on a host of professional issues, ranging from the question of the wisdom of varying from the traditional one-to-one relationship of doctor and patient to the merits and demerits of the psychoanalytic approach. The proposals for community mental health centers added new issues, such as the advantages of a community-centered approach versus the state hospital tradition, or the proper location of community centers (general hospitals or physically separate facilities). Psychologists and social workers, and some psychiatrists, tend to prefer more emphasis on the preventive aspects of mental health services rather than relying on treatment after the onset of mental illness. With these and other professional differences so much in evidence, it is hardly surprising that the organized groups fail to stand out as policy innovators and leaders.

A second factor militating against a group role is the well-known conservatism of the professional groups involved. While this term can be applied in a political sense particularly to the medical profession in general and to some but certainly not all psychiatrists, it is used here in a broader sense to refer to the cautiousness, resistance to change, and lack of innovative spirit that are so often found among the professionals involved, social workers no less than physicians.

A third explanatory factor is that the organized groups, with the conspicuous exception of the American Medical Association, are not geared for involvement in the policy process. In some instances the organizations exist locally only on paper, and even when there is a functioning structure and a dues-paying membership the orientation is apt to be narrowly professional and/or social in nature. Rarely, if ever, is there a paid staff or office facilities. The means for propagandizing members and the general public, for research and analysis of substantive policy issues, for mobilization of group resources—all these prerequisites for successful entry into the policy sphere are largely absent. The preoccupation of the professionals with their private practices or with their own agencies and programs undoubtedly contributes heavily to this pattern, but whatever its causes the consequence is a marginal involvement in policy affairs.

It cannot be stressed too heavily that the foregoing has dealt only with the role of organized professional groups. These generalizations, however, are applicable as well to the vast majority of professional personnel, for the field studies are unanimous in reporting that most of them were not involved in policy affairs even in individual, unorganized ways. However, in each case it was found that a few professionals were deeply concerned with public policy matters, often playing leading roles. Thus one should not conclude that there is no professional influence on decisions, but rather that it is the product of individual motivation and effort, rather than being group-inspired and directed.

There is still another category of groups involved in mental health programing, which for want of a better term will be labeled "voluntary." It includes basically two types of organizations: the local, private, nonprofit agencies providing mental health services; and the lay associations organized at the state and local levels essentially as pressure groups, typically without providing any direct services. The former includes a variety of agencies dispensing a wide range of services; often they are at least partially supported by United Fund or Community Chest programs. These will for purposes of this discussion be designated as "private" agencies. The second category has several components, but the most prominent ones are the various state and local mental health and mental retardation associations.

For many years the private agencies have been the backbone of community mental health operations. They have often been the instruments if not the innovators of such successes as have been achieved, but on occasion they have represented stumbling blocks to successful program development. Typically each has its own niche carved out in the local spectrum of programs. As a general rule each is an independent agency, locally based and supported in most part. Normally a governing board operating under a charter serves as the official policy maker for the agency, but with day-to-day affairs in the hands of a professional staff. Depending on the size of the agency and the nature of its operations, the executive director who heads the staff may be either a psychiatrist or a social worker. Membership in the organization is open to all, but in practice it is apt to be limited to a relatively few interested persons.

The field studies suggest three perennial concerns of the private agencies. The first is originating, developing, and overseeing specific programs. Administrative structures must be organized, clientele accepted, administrative and professional personnel recruited, governing boards constituted. In some cases the agency must fit its efforts and ambitions into some sort of planning by a community council or its equivalent; in other cases each agency is on its own in developing and managing programs. It becomes literally a program instigator, implementer, and protector.

A second type of concern is financing. A certain element of uncertainty and insecurity is introduced by the lack of fixed and foreseeable sources of funds. Although it is true that few agencies ever suffer complete economic collapse, many do find it necessary from time to time to reorient their program to adapt to the financial realities of the situation. Usually a great variety of sources is tapped: membership dues and contributions, fees from clients, United Fund support, and grants from foundations and governments.

Finally, private agencies are concerned with a number of what might be broadly termed communication needs and problems. Each must somehow fit into the total pattern of voluntary and public agency programs in a functional way. While this is always troublesome, it is particularly so when there is no effective coordinating or planning body to facilitate such integration.

There is great variation in the relative importance of the services provided by these agencies. The mental health services available in Houston and Seattle were mostly provided by them. Their relative share of the service load fell in Minneapolis–St. Paul and New Orleans but still represented a sizable contribution to the total effort. In Syracuse and even more in Boston the efforts of such agencies were pretty well overshadowed by the programs of state and/or local governments.

Although their professionals were often involved in state mental health planning activities, there is no evidence that the agencies as such played important roles. At the local level the private agencies would seem to have considerable potential for influencing the shape and structure of local mental health because of their linkages through their boards of directors with social and economic dominants or their lieutenants. Unfortunately, in this respect the agencies tend to be undone by their parochialism. Where unchecked, each agency functions more or less independently, expanding or reorienting its own activities largely as it can and as it pleases. In thus retaining freedom to chart its own course, each agency at the same time tacitly surrenders any claim to influence over similar decisions by other agencies. Justifying and protecting against encroachment their individual spheres of action become the major preoccupations of the private agencies.

Effective coordination to overcome these centrifugal tendencies is thus an important prerequisite to agency influence. The inability of private agencies to do much to mold mental health policy in Seattle and Houston despite their predominance in the provision of services is undoubtedly due in substantial measure to weakness of the coordinating body in each case (the Community Council in Houston, the United Fund organization in Seattle). By contrast, the finding of a more important role for the private agencies in Minneapolis and in Syracuse is paralleled by a report of a stronger structure of coordination in those cities.

While the unchecked parochialism of private agencies hinders their effectiveness in the development of broader programs, there is another factor at work that should not be neglected. The private agencies loom particularly large in Seattle and Houston mostly because of the paucity of publicly provided services, but that very paucity is testimony to a lack of community interest and involvement that relentlessly saps the private sector as well.

In concluding this discussion of the private agencies it might be well to recall the questions raised in the Syracuse study concerning their long-range future, for in greater or lesser degrees the same questions apply to other cities as well. Reduced to their starkest form, these questions ultimately concern the capacity of private agencies to retain their distinctive character and roles. They are apt to decline in relative importance as more comprehensive public mental health programs are increasingly extended to the various communities. Survival will demand increased bureaucratization and professionalization, bringing them closer and closer to resembling their public counterparts. Their uniqueness may then consist essentially of the element of private financing. This fate is hardly inevitable, but to escape it will require more concern with the nature and functions of private agencies than has been in evidence so far.

The second type of voluntary organization to be considered here concentrates not on the provision of services but on the many activities involved in mobilizing support for mental health programs. It is best exemplified by the mental health associations and associations for the mentally retarded operating at all three levels of government.

By far the most important supportive group is the National Association for Mental Health (NAMH) and its state and local affiliates. Indeed, in a directory of national, state, and local agencies "to which individuals can turn for psychiatric help and mental health services" included in the *Encyclopedia of Mental Health,* the only "State Sources" listed other than public authorities were state divisions of NAMH.

Supported entirely by voluntary contributions from individuals, business firms, and foundations, the NAMH includes well over 800 state and local affiliates and has member organizations in 48 states and the District of Columbia. These local associations vary considerably from one area to another in size and strength, but through its affiliates the association has over a half million members. In addition, more than a half million nonmember volunteers serve in the work of the NAMH during the year. The state and local programs are carried on with assistance, guidance, and materials from the national headquarters.

Among the numerous local activities of the mental health associations are the sponsoring and supporting of research; consultation, fund raising, and public information programs for the improvement of mental hospital conditions; recruitment, training, and placement of volunteer workers in mental hospitals; assistance of various types to the families of the mentally ill; and social, vocational, and medical rehabilitation programs. But from the standpoint of generating public support or opposition to any particular public program, by far the most important functions of the National Association for Mental Health are its widespread informational and educational activities.

Among the state mental health associations, those in Minnesota, Louisiana, and New York appear to exercise the most positive influence. With centralized organizations which set out to enroll community influentials as members, they diligently promote the development of local chapters, sponsor numerous projects, and above all attempt to inform their own members so that they can better educate their communities about mental health. A rather elaborate procedure has been worked out by the Minnesota association for the development of a legislative program, and it is typically active in the legislative arena, with at least a modicum of effect. Yet the difficulties that emerged after the death of the association's long-time director suggest that at least some of its influence was peculiar to the man rather than the organization. In New York and Louisiana the associations have been effective in dealing with the state legislature.

But in the other field studies the state mental health associations were found lacking in effectiveness. Although their representatives often participated in policy conferences, planning committees, and legislative arenas, these associations were seldom perceived as key elements in the policy process. This assessment may reflect in part a tendency to see the state associations as essentially auxiliaries or fronts for the dominant state agency involved in mental health (e.g., the Department of Mental Health in Massachusetts or the former Department of State Hospitals and Special Schools in Texas). It may also be that the state associations lack the capacity to attract the dedicated and devoted laborers necessary to give a voluntary group the means for exerting influence. Finally, it may well be that the state groups simply lack knowledge of the ways in which influence is gained and exerted, both in public and private arenas.

At the local level the spectrum of effectiveness for mental health associations is somewhat more extended. At one extreme are the local units in Massachusetts, which have been very influential is establishing and supporting community mental health programs. It may be that their outstanding record in that state reflects the administrative structure which enables them to tie into service-providing programs. At the opposite end of the spectrum are the mental health associations in Seattle and in Houston, both of which have a history of weakness and ineffectiveness. These failures at the local level are far more damaging to mental health program development than those of the state associations because there they were expected to carry the principal burdens of education and mobilization of the general public and of special sub-publics. Their inability to discharge those functions was thus of critical importance. Often areas of greatest need have poor organizations, or none at all.

In the scrutiny of mental health associations it was inevitable that comparisons would be made with the National Association for Retarded Children and its state and local affiliates. Although the field studies did not explore in depth the activities of the association, the prevailing impressions are that its chapters function much more successfully than their mental health counterparts, showing both more initiative and more capacity to follow through with program developments. While their aggressive tactics unquestionably antagonized some, most observers nevertheless felt compelled to recognize their industry and determination, and to acknowledge their right to be seen as influential within the areas of concern to them.

One cannot escape the question, "Why?" No doubt the mental retardation groups benefit from the clearer and narrower focus of their concern, for the areas covered are much more sharply defined than those involving mental health. It may be too that public opinion regarding the mentally retarded is somehow less a problem than opinion pertaining to mental illness. While these are logical possibilities, the speculation most encountered in the field studies stressed the differences in commitment of participants. Those active in mental health associations participated for all sorts of reasons, but those active in associations for the mentally retarded typically were involved because that misfortune had struck their own families. Seemingly, there is no substitute for the concern that arises from personal and familial circumstances.

COMMUNITY POWER STRUCTURE

No less significant for an understanding of mental health programing is that aspect involving informal and/or unorganized groupings of influentials in a community, summed up in the phrase "community power and decision making." The way in which influence is exerted in a community in general has obvious relevance for a consideration of mental health policy making, and each of the field studies deals with the issue of how the community under scrutiny generally goes about making decisions before examining the process with specific reference to mental health. Explicitly or implicitly, each field investigator in his analysis of community power in general tended to do so within the framework of two polar models: the elitist model and the pluralist model. The elitist model, associated with such figures as Floyd Hunter and Robert Presthus, is pretty well summed up in the following statement by Presthus: "Elitism connotes domination of the decisional process by a single group or a few men, limited rank-and-file access, little or no opposition and a failure on the part of most of the adult community to use their political resources to influence important decisions." [2]

In sharp contrast is the pluralist model, associated with such scholars as Robert Dahl and Nelson Polsby.[3] Its essential features are the absence of any ruling elite, with power and influence effectively dispersed among various strata, and with significant opportunities for many people to participate in decisions.

Which model seems to be more useful in describing power and influence in the six metropolitan centers?

Community power in Syracuse has been studied in depth by others, and the conclusions reached do not support Hunter's hypothesis of monolithic power. Instead of one there were many leadership groups. According to some respondents in the field study, general decision making in the community is a process involving both compromise and power—the former recognizing the legitimacy of other interests and

[2] Robert Presthus, *Men at the Top* (New York: Oxford University Press, 1964), p. 25.
[3] Robert Dahl, *Who Governs: Democracy and Power in an American City* (New Haven: Yale University Press, 1961); Nelson Polsby, *Community Power and Political Theory* (New Haven: Yale University Press, 1963).

then proceeding in a mediational or brokerage capacity, the latter exploiting weaknesses to override opposition.

This general pattern of influence and decision making in Syracuse is roughly paralleled by that found in the field of social services, including mental health. There is a somewhat more clearly identifiable set of influentials, perhaps because of the greater role of private and nonprofit organizations, and their strategic position continues undiminished. However, this is a very elastic and definitely nonmonolithic structure, appearing to be more a loose coalition of various influentials than a tightly knit oligarchy, with admission rather easily attainable by those of recent eligibility.

Superficially this appears to be a stable and continuing system, but considerable evidence indicates that its key elements are increasingly doubtful of their capacity to function successfully. This doubt, seemingly, is a consequence of the emergence of government and the professions into prominent places in policy making in the field of social services. The pattern of community influence is now being shaped by the local-state or local-federal relationship, and the community influential is one who is able to affect these intergovernmental relationships. In such a situation, more formal and more institutionalized processes of decision making are to be expected. To be influential, community leaders must master the legal and bureaucratic skills respected in governmental circles, and must as well develop contacts in this governmental system and the persuasive powers needed to take advantage of them, along with an instinct for strategy. The specialized skills needed are such as to imply that an inner-core influential may be forced to work full time at mobilizing and wielding influence.

Although these tendencies in Syracuse are still in an early state, they are operative. In addition to its implications for the future role of existing influentials, this development raises questions about the brokerage function. The need may be for brokers with a new set of skills more appropriate for mediating conflicts between governmental agencies, or between administrators and professionals, or between influentials in public and private sectors.

Although it has not been exhaustively analyzed, the situation in Seattle has some elements of the elitist as well as the pluralist model. One view of Seattle leans toward the notion of an elite "establishment" composed of a rather large number of civic, professional, and business leaders. There tends to be considerable dispersion of activities and interests, resulting in several fairly well-defined spheres of influence (education, transportation, etc.). A second view finds less overall unity and coordination, and hence stresses what is termed a "multi-nucleated" decisional process, the essence of which is decentralization of control among numerous, formally independent jurisdictions in the metropolitan area.

The value and relevance of this view are apparent when one turns from the general picture of decision making to the more specialized one of mental health. Decisions on mental health programs are dispersed among several agencies (mostly private), each distinguished by its autonomy and jurisdiction. The vital linkage of these agencies to the community is provided by their governing boards, composed of the most strongly motivated lay and professional people. Most of the mental health programs were brought about as a result of the expenditure of considerable energy by this relatively small number of people.

Yet, because there is no overall guidance or direction, the result is an atomized and fragmented system of decision making, one that in the terms of an economist would be judged as approximating that of "laissez faire." Because public services are so limited, governmental involvement in mental health decision making at the local level has been negligible. Significantly, the principal force attempting to impose order and direction in the local system has been state inspired—the Planning Committee and its work.

The Boston field study suggests that policy decisions there involve members of three groups. One is composed of officials in the local governmental structure, such as the mayor, city council, school committee, and director of the Urban Redevelopment Authority. Leaders from the private economic sector such as those in banking, business, and industry make up the second group. Because it is the main source of mental health activities, state government—meaning the governor, legislature, and agencies—constitutes the third group. Newspapers are not seen as particularly effective or influential, and labor primarily figures in "bread and butter" issues. Both of these may be increasing in general importance, however.

Although there have been no definitive studies of the patterns of influence in Boston, informed observers are of the opinion that the situation there bears little resemblance to the "elite" model of community power. The business community of Boston can be mobilized sometimes for support for specific programs, especially those of benefit to it, but the leaders in that sector seldom initiate and probably cannot veto policy proposals. Anything of major importance has so many ramifications that the business community is apt to be badly divided, so much so in some cases that no effort is made to mobilize its support.

The overshadowing role of the state in providing mental health services at the local level makes any discussion of community decision making in that area somewhat academic. Certain financial figures may be involved in the voluntary agencies that abound in Boston, but this reflects personal interests and commitments rather than any group or class behavior. Seemingly, mental health is a peripheral concern for the "multi-centered" power structure of Boston.

To the extent that one can speak of community influence in mental health decisions, the process seems to center around the formally constituted policy makers, particularly the governor and legislature. Behind them, however, looms the Department of Mental Health, subject both to internal and external pressures for policy proposals and actions from the local level. Internally, the chief forces are the professionals in the Division of Mental Hygiene, spokesmen for the local mental health centers, and the state hospitals and special schools, representatives of the institutional and medical outlook. Externally, there are several groups that attempt to influence the department's course of action, most notably the professional groups and the local mental health associations.

It appears from the comments on community power in the Minneapolis–St. Paul area that, while there is considerable influence exerted by business groups, the roles of other private elements and of public officials and party leaders are sufficiently significant to cast doubt on the validity of any "elitist" explanation of the pattern of influence and power there. A study of opinion leadership in local and metropolitan affairs found public officials to be foremost. Economic groups, broadly classed as business, commercial, and labor groups, are important. Civic groups figure in the process, as do the political parties. There is little evidence of monolithic power in Minneapolis–St. Paul.

The pattern of decision making there in the field of mental health can be deduced from several examples. The general picture that emerges is of a relatively decentralized decisional process. Thus a mental health center was finally established in Dakota county only after some five years of preparation that involved garnering support from every conceivable source: professionals, public officials, Chamber of Commerce leaders, union officers, administrative agencies, and so on. However, the Minneapolis–St. Paul field study also makes a number of references to key structures of influence and to knowledge or lack of knowledge of them, suggesting that there are several centers of influence that provide some degree of centralization in the process of decision making. Still, the leading roles played by public officials and by spokesmen for groups and organizations with broad constituencies leads once again to the conclusion that nothing approaching a monolithlic power structure is involved in mental health programing.

Although community power has not been systematically investigated in Houston, there are limited indications of a pluralistic structure. Among the relevant evidence is the existence of several competing centers and bases of power, such as business and industry, organized labor, Negroes, the professions (especially law and medicine), and the political activists; the porosity of the political system, which offers rapid penetration and elevation; the opportunity for significant participation in many organizations and activities; and the tendency to refer issues, including specific ones, to the electorate. Clearly, Houston does not seem to conform to the "elitist" model of community decision making.

All indications are that this general pattern of decision making also applies to the specific area of mental health policy making. There have been so few significant mental health decisions in Houston that one is tempted to describe it as not merely a pluralist but even an anarchical situation. There has been very little leadership within the mental health community, and such as there is has not been able to tap effectively the leadership of the larger community. In part the difficulty is that power and influence tend to be so greatly dispersed that mobilization for mental health programs becomes a formidable undertaking.

For the New Orleans area, the pattern of influence is highly variegated. The historical decision that mental health as a public function should be a state function puts first premium on the roles of state officials, particularly the commissioner of mental health, the governor, and, to a lesser extent, the legislature. Local officials on the whole take little or no part in mental health decision making. This is particularly true of the city of New Orleans, but less true in Jefferson and St. Tammany parishes. Community groups such as the Mental Health Association, the Retardation Association, and the Committee on Alcoholism have been active. Their political efforts have focused on Baton Rouge, and they also are concerned with the operation of the United Fund and the Social Welfare Planning Council. These community groups were heavily involved in the New Orleans regional planning under the Community Mental Health Centers Act. The leadership of the community groups is not drawn from the cream of New Orleans society and business elites, although it is fair to say a few top community people were instrumental in getting the more significant mental health groups founded. The leadership of the groups is heavily sprinkled with professionals: the doctor, the psychiatrist, the social work professor, the lawyer, the educator, the nurse. The topmost New Orleans society and business leader seems to feel it is necessary for him to belong to the Boston Club and "best" Mardi Gras krewe, and that it is nice to work with the United Fund or the Cultural Attractions Fund. But he and the local politician stay out of mental health. There results a vacuum, not so much of power but of no-power, and the second and third ranks of the community elite structure hasten to fill it up. It should also be noted that organized labor has taken an interest in mental health, both in New Orleans and statewide.

What overall significance is there in the data just summarized for the six field studies? One of the most obvious points is the diversity of the patterns of general community influence. On the whole the areas discussed are characterized by somewhat pluralistic tendencies in the decision-making process, with little indication of a monolithlic power structure in any of the communities. However, there are almost infinite varieties and degrees of pluralism, and each community is to some extent unique.

A second noteworthy point is that there appears in each case to be a reasonably close resemblance between the general pattern of influence and the pattern for mental health policy making. One does not find examples of highly centralized decision making in mental health; the pluralism of the general community carries over into that specific field.

A third and closely related point is the absolute necessity of understanding the community's influence system and of knowing how to function effectively within it. Given the degree of pluralism present, this is not an easy undertaking. There are few manuals available for the beginner, and in any case it is necessary to temper general rules to particular situations. In each of the field studies there are examples of failures or inadequacies in mental health programing that can be traced to poor comprehension of the policy-making process. Those in the mental health field are not necessarily any more lacking in this respect than others, for this appears to be a fairly common problem. But it may be that the training and the folkways of the mental health professionals make the acquisition of such knowledge more difficult for them. It would be interesting to compare their political and community involvement with that of other professions.

It follows from these observations that the task of mobilizing community support for mental health programs calls for certain highly developed skills. The point is made most emphatically in the Syracuse study, where a sketch of the desirable characteristics of mediators pointed to a full-time job for them. The same report also brought out the possibility that there may be long-term trends toward change in the nature of the skills involved in community influence. It also follows from the pluralistic context of mental health programing that policy proposals must be designed with clear understanding of the various influences that must be brought into supportive roles.

But perhaps the most important conclusion to be drawn from the summaries touching the influence structure and the decision-making process is that the time span from program conception to adoption is apt to be far longer than is commonly anticipated. The five years of careful work that was behind the adoption of a mental health center for Dakota county, as noted in the Minneapolis–St. Paul study, may be far more typical than one would like to believe. The amount of time required undoubtedly varies greatly from one city or state to another and from one type of program to another, but it is to be expected that mobilization of community support will be a slow, sometimes glacial, process. It is true that shortcuts sometimes can be found, but such good fortune is not common and may carry with it unfortunate consequences of the tendency to use the budgetary process, with its one- or two-year cycle, as an instrument of policy development.

But even in the states where there is more leadership in evidence, there are often conspicuous gaps and failures. Without in any way denigrating the leaders who have performed ably, it appears that there have been countless opportunities for even more effective leadership. It seems likely that the failure of adequate leadership to emerge under even relatively more favorable conditions, as well as under the less favorable ones, is related to several factors. Among them is the existence of considerable fragmentation at all levels, for governmental and program fragmentation impedes leadership by discouraging attempts and by exacting a heavy toll in time, effort, and failures. Another factor appears to be the lack of sufficient knowledge of the system of community influence and decision making. One cannot play the game well if the rules and players are not sufficiently familiar, and there is evidence that among mental health personnel there is a decided unfamiliarity with the rules and players of the power and influence games.

XVI: ACTION ALTERNATIVES

THE POLITICS of mental health involves two interacting processes: policy adoption and policy implementation. Federal action beginning with the Mental Health Act of 1946 and culminating in the community mental health program initiated in 1963 represents the end product of the process of adoption. In pushing through the legislation of 1963 and 1965, the mental health enthusiasts implicitly argued that there should soon be a center serving every community. But if it required two decades to complete the process of adoption, this study suggests that it is likely to require as much time for implementation. Even this time estimate may prove overly optimistic, however, unless further energizing action is taken.

In the enthusiasm of adoption, the federal legislation of 1963 was heralded as a "bold, new program" designed to transform mental health operations in the United States. In the more sober light of practical problems of implementation a much different image emerges. What emerges is a "brave program," since it was the brainchild of a small group of professional people and not a grassroots movement. The program endorses a concept of mental illness and treatment challenged even by some mental health groups. It is not a program that readily fits into established administrative and political patterns at either the state or local levels. Instead, it threatens many of these established patterns. Further, it faces fierce competition from other governmental programs for scarce resources of men and money. Above all, it presumes the existence of viable communities at the local level, when oftentimes viable communities do not exist at all.

Action to prevent and combat mental illness generally has not been at the forefront of pressing social issues. Until recently it has been a low-pressure, low-priority business compared to the other concerns of politicians and civil servants. The stigma attached to mental illness has clouded its public visibility. Under pressure from the national government, the status of mental health as a public concern has been raised. The leadership of a low-pressure public policy is likely to be limited in numbers and vitality. Those whose dependents have been afflicted by mental illness, and those fortunates who have been helped, are the immediate interested public. The mentally ill themselves are not organized for political action despite their sizable stake in public policy; public officials and surrogate organizations have to act in their behalf. In this situation government officials have greater freedom in the decision-making process than in the usual pattern of interest group–government relations. They may be less arbiters of interest group claims and more free agents whose chief problem is to decide what to decide. As a consequence, a program is likely to be adopted which is attuned to professional views of desirability without being subjected to the practical compromises that normally are assured by the realities of interest group politics.

The proponents of community mental health legislation have accomplished a great deal in the last few years. They have seized the attention of Congress and the President with sufficient force to pass a major piece of enabling legislation and funding, and to secure additions which they could not attain initially. They have launched mental health planning projects in many states where these projects never would have occurred without federal stimulation and financial support, or would have been of far lower quality without federal guidelines and minimum standards. This planning has involved state and local political leaders and influential citizens who probably would never have otherwise become familiar with the issues involved. Thus the mental health surrogates have had great success in initiating the community mental health program.

At the same time, there are serious obstacles to the realization of their dreams. Some of these are a result of the nature of the proposals themselves, while others evidently reflect the lack of knowledge by the plan's sponsors and administrators of the political realities of the federal system and of state and local governments and related private social service organizations. The nature of these misconceptions and practical obstacles suggests certain policy accommodations and strategies of action which may be essential to further progress.

What further action is needed? Where should it be taken? The dimensions of the national mental health program provide some clues. The federal program envisages four distinct action inputs resulting in a single output: comprehensive mental health services.

The first and most significant input is the federal legislation itself, coupled with federal funds to support it. The basic act of 1963 assumes an implementing path following the traditional federal-state pattern of action: through NIMH to the mental health agency in each state and thence to the local community.

A second input envisaged is positive action of the local community itself toward achieving community mental health services. It is presumed that local public opinion will give support to the goal of community mental health and that local public officials will move to endorse this goal by providing funds and other necessary legal and administrative arrangements. The local action contemplated by the federal program does not exclude local private mental health agencies from participation in implementation. On the contrary, the Act endorses a bringing together of public and private services into a comprehensive community program.

A third input comes from the mental health profession itself. The federal program enunciated in 1963 embraces a new concept of mental health, one not completely accepted within the profession, and one not fully tested by practice and time. Only the profession can provide the continuing appraisal of the new program and the needed professional skills demanded now and in the future.

A fourth input consists of the administrative skills and know-how necessary to build a mental health organization comprising the local community, the state, and the federal government, and, equally important, the skills to make a complicated federal-state-local organization function effectively.

When the action envisaged by the federal program is analyzed against the various existing political environments—national, state, and local— in which implementation is to take place, critical friction areas appear. These critical areas develop in part from the nature of the new federal program itself and in part from the nature of the particular environment in which action is required. In each friction area experience indicates that additional inputs are required to produce a successful community mental health program. Furthermore, the pattern of future action must be flexible enough to allow selection among several alternatives, for what may work well in one state or metropolitan area may only lead to frustration in another.

THE PROFESSIONAL INPUT

The burden of innovation and execution falls upon the professionals. The role that they played in conceiving the 1963 program has been set forth in some detail. Clearly without the leadership of professionals in NIMH, supported by professionals at the state level and by professional societies, there would have been no new program. It hardly needs to be said that the professionals have an equally important role in carrying out the program by providing services and by directing the operations of the community centers. However, the great sums of money involved and the substantial participation of the federal government mean that the professionals will be engaged in a much more complex administrative relationship than previously.

Federal control inevitably follows the federal dollar. Even with small grants to mental health clinics during the last two decades the federal government has to some extent set accounting and personnel standards which had to be followed. These will be refined, but—more important —as governments develop program budgets they will demand better ways of measuring the kind and extent of treatment as a means for determining the effectiveness of one program compared with another.

Operating at public expense imposes the obligation of developing criteria that can be used for management purposes, including planning and control. Some sort of therapy standards similar to those used by the medical profession in regard to surgery must be developed. They may not be as specific but they should show the seriousness of the illness, the kind of treatment, and the results achieved. They must provide some sort of yardstick relating treatment to dollars spent. They must do more than simply indicate the number of hours the professionals are on duty and the number of patients seen.

Auditing the level of services in the mental health field poses a real problem. How is this to be done? One alternative is to leave it to the individual professional consciences of those working in the field. This is not a very satisfactory solution because the criteria must be translated into the language of governmental administration, and it must be consistent and generally applicable. On the other hand, there are real dangers in having standards imposed on the professionals from the outside. It is imperative, then, that professional groups in the mental health field work actively to establish precise criteria for professional performance, as is done in other professional practices.

More than a mere auditing exercise is involved in the question of therapy standards. Mental health programs will compete with governmental programs of long-standing priority whose accomplishments are by and large readily translated into material, quantitative terms. Superficial as these terms may be when used as justifications for funds, realistically, proponents of public expenditures for community mental health centers must be prepared to present a strong case before tough-minded, quantitatively oriented officials. Whether the formal requirements of contemporary management be program and performance budgets, cost-benefit calculations, or input-output analyses, those responsible for mental health programs must be prepared to provide the best possible justification in the technical medium demanded.

NIMH has interests of its own in the development of standards of this kind. One objection that is frequently raised against the community mental health program is that nothing really will be changed, and that professionals in community centers will go on doing just what they have done in the past. Given the judgment of professionals who were responsible for the new program, it is evident that it represents a commitment to a different type of professional activity. To ensure that their goal is reached, NIMH will need to develop professional standards for the activities it is sponsoring and for the therapy which is used.

Finally, if health insurance programs are expanded to cover outpatient treatment, more exact standards will be needed. In the past, Blue Cross and Blue Shield have been reluctant to insure for outpatient services because of the difficulty of defining mental illness and evaluating the treatment. Inpatient mental services, especially in general hospitals, are theoretically subject to greater control and consequently they are viewed in a more favorable light by insurance companies. As more precise knowledge of the costs and effectiveness of diagnosis and therapy permits a more reliable degree of predictability, insurance companies can be expected more easily to incorporate mental illness in their coverage schemes. In a broad sense, then, mental illness and the evaluation of effective treatment should be conceptualized in such a way as to provide an adequate rationalization for public support.

Another area about which professionals should be concerned is how manpower resources can be regrouped in the interest of more effective utilization. The field studies confirm earlier national surveys in pointing out that the number of professionals is far smaller than what is needed even today. The new program will increase the need. The various mental health professions have an obligation to examine and devise solutions to this problem. The problem has two aspects: First, how can psychiatrists and clinical psychologists, now engaged in private practice, be induced to participate in the community center program; and how can their duties be assigned according to the kind and degree of skill needed? Second, how can greater use be made of trained administrators as in the hospital field and of other professional groups such as psychologists, adjunctive therapists, social workers, and psychiatric nurses?

The years immediately ahead should be a time for experimentation, for trying out differing staffing and administrative patterns and arrangements. Contract relations between professionals and public agencies might be more fully exploited. Community mental health services must be made professionally attractive so that the best possible talent will be attracted. Among the professions themselves, then, there must be awareness of the need to find ways and means to regroup and greatly expand professional resources to provide for their most efficient utilization.

The figures established for the manning of new community mental health centers are, according to the findings of the field studies, unrealistic. Even in areas such as Boston and Syracuse, where the professional skills exist in sufficient numbers, there is no indication that professional persons are willing to switch to community mental health activities in large numbers. In most other areas demands of current programs cannot be met because of existing shortages. Securing competent manpower for community mental health centers in the immediate future is beyond hope without the sort of crash program that would require treating mental illness as a national emergency.

In view of the impossibility of providing adequate staffing, it is necessary to devise measures to cope with the problems of mental illness that require fewer, and less professionally skilled, persons. The mental health professions must define the skills and design the systems necessary for training such persons. Great emphasis should be placed on providing imaginative, effective, and realistic staffing alternatives for the near future. New concepts of skills required to care for the mentally ill should be developed, especially in semiprofessional and nonprofessional areas.

THE COMMUNITY INPUT

Most metropolitan areas and the units contained within them, particularly the city governments, are short of funds and are fighting hard for a greater share of state income. Shifting part of the responsibility for mental health programs from the state to localities will necessitate moving traditionally state-financed programs to local units. Yet, most local governments cannot afford to shoulder even part of the burden. Nor have they much financial flexibility in contemporary state-local relations. Constitutionally creatures of the state, units of local government generally are restricted in their financial freedom, to say nothing of their resources.

At this juncture, it is difficult to predict just what impact the federal program will have on the division of financial responsibility between state and local governments. However, a few things are clear. Local governments' heavy reliance upon the relatively inflexible property tax will pose a major barrier to their assumption of major financial responsibility for mental health services. Moreover, even where the tax base can be expanded to produce adequate revenues, there will be a natural reluctance on the part of local officials to finance what has traditionally been a state responsibility. And this reluctance will be accentuated in poorer areas because placing the financial burden on a higher level of government offers obvious equalization advantages.

No doubt one reason why communities and states with the best existing services have been successful in obtaining federal money is the fact that they had manpower with expertise in grantsmanship. They had sufficient personnel who talked the same language as the Washington professionals. This is not true in the poorer states. Indeed, an economically depressed state often cannot obtain such personnel until a grant is assured. If this is not corrected it will mean that those "with the mostest will get more." Moreover, the scarcity of manpower in poor states and local communities is made more acute because of new federal grant programs in education and poverty, as well as mental health. People who have expertise in drafting proposals and answering federal questionnaires are often equally useful in any one of these programs at the local level. To be sure, areas which now have the least resources in mental health will obtain some grants. But the most lucrative grants, those which can provide the most significant breakthroughs, require a level of imagination and skill in drafting proposals that is readily available only in the wealthier states.

Moreover, the federal grants-in-aid as well as the administrative stipulations placed a premium on state plans and planning rather than community plans and planning. Community planning efforts were encouraged at best as contributions to regional reports and to the state plans. In no substantial manner were the localities assisted in bringing forth a comprehensive mental health plan of their own. The state plan occupied the center of the stage, and it was to this plan that local initiative was expected to defer.

Secondly, in most instances, the planning staffs of state departments of mental hygiene, health, or institutions were strengthened. And with additional resources at their disposal, they often demonstrated monopolistic and autocratic tendencies in their relations with local groups. This was justified by claims of professional superiority, statutory requirements, statewide coordination, uniformity, and lack of time. Staffs of local governments and voluntary agencies, and even other state departments, proved to be no match for the recipients of the federal grants.

This relationship between state and community planning may have been all but inevitable. The state's heavy involvement in the care of the mentally ill gave it a great stake in providing leadership for statewide planning. Another explanation could be found in the desultory record of localities in earlier attempts at community planning. Mental health agencies at the local level were largely operational in outlook, under great pressure to solve day-to-day problems, and sensitive to the posture and interests of particular constituencies. Moreover, planning agencies in local government structures tended to be dominated by physical planners rather than social engineers, while the planning undertaken by such voluntary bodies as Community Chest tended to be "soft," largely directed at determining needs or inventorying resources and overly responsive to fund-raising situations and existing patterns of influence. In addition, there was the problem of jurisdiction. Members of health committees of boards of supervisors, mental health boards, and so forth showed considerable jealousy when even technical tasks were taken out of their hands and assigned to professional staffs not directly subject to their authority. It is little wonder that effective planning had not developed at the local level.

There is no doubt about the NIMH commitment to planning as a critical facet of community mental health development, but it seems certain that NIMH anticipated valuable secondary consequences of a political nature. The guidelines for mental health planning stressed participation of all segments of the community in a calculated attempt to broaden the base of support for mental health. This implied the desirability of airing interagency and intersector disputes with the expectation that in this way the disputes would be resolved. In most cases neither of these goals was reached. Political leaders outside the mental health fields for the most part did not participate in the planning, and interagency disputes were rarely resolved.

There can be no doubt that the NIMH grants did encourage "plans for planning" and "comprehensive state plans." But plans of these kinds are one thing and "construction plans" for community health centers are quite another. And the very emphasis on state responsibility, crucial in the comprehensive planning endeavor, ignores some of the hard realities of construction planning and bodes ill for the program's goals of community acceptance and local involvement.

Construction planning is inevitably more political than comprehensive planning. It involves the expenditure of public funds, the allocation of largesse, the acquisition of real estate, and the downgrading or upgrading of adjacent property. Moreover, since centers once built must be staffed, it involves employment. Construction decisions are still the stuff politics is made of: they grease the wheels of the state and also the local political machinery. Planning in this connection invades the preserve that the politicians consider naturally their own, and over which they are constantly striving for control. It seems highly unlikely that there is much hope of success for construction planning that emphasizes participation of the mental health community as opposed to the general political apparatus to the extent that characterized comprehensive planning.

Moreover, construction planning is also location planning and is of direct and vital concern to local communities. Where centers should be situated, given the size of the population to be served and the function to be performed, are technical challenges, problems which could well be solved at the state level. But such decisions are not merely technical ones; there are always political priorities to be recognized and accommodated. Each locality has its own decision-making patterns, and if local resistance is to be avoided and community responsibility encouraged, then these patterns must be taken into account far more decidedly than has been the case in most mental health planning activities thus far.

Planning experience to date has pointed up other problems. In jurisdictions with more people than the prescribed maximum service population, insistence that a center serve only residents of a smaller district will make local governmental support difficult to obtain, unless enough centers to serve the whole area are begun simultaneously. Few citizens wish to pay taxes to support a service for which they are ineligible because they live in the wrong neighborhood. In jurisdictions with populations too small for a center, on the other hand, local governmental support will be complicated by the necessity of first obtaining intergovernmental agreements, which in many cases will require legislative authorization.

The field studies show a diverse complex of mental health services of varying size, nature, and effectiveness operated by county, municipal, special district, and semipublic agencies. Even within a particular metropolitan area, there is great difference in how effectively the same level of government operates in the mental health field. Thus, even the most cursory study of the conditions in an urban area—even one with such limited mental health services as are found in Houston—shows that there would not be a clear and unchallenged field of operations for a new community mental health center. There would have to be an accommodation with a number of other mental health institutions, activities, and services which could not be expected to give up the institutional ghost merely to create a neat organization chart. Further, political structure and political power are so fragmented among independent or substantially autonomous governmental entities and agencies, especially at the local level, that there could not be an enforced consolidation even if the will to attain such a goal existed. Those areas where speedy action on planning and establishing community centers is likely because of their long tradition of providing well for mental health are also those which will require the greatest degree of coordination with existing agencies.

Evident in the early discussion of the idea of community mental health services was a belief that the community as a whole must be convinced of the validity and need for this new public service and should express this approval in an appropriate manner. A vast array of studies of decision making in urban areas, however, has shown that such broad-based interest and participation ordinarily cannot be expected. The ideal of popular decisions popularly arrived at is infrequently realized in metropolitan areas; at most, that segment of the citizenry who choose to cast a ballot express their general approval or disapproval of the conduct of the city's business. In certain cases a particular decision will be referred to the voters; this is especially common in respect to levels of taxation. Yet, even here, there is usually a relatively low level of citizen participation.

The field studies indicate mental health is a fairly technical function, and most of the significant decisions concerning it are taken within a limited arena of private and bureaucratic politics. In metropolitan areas the significant decisions about mental health are usually taken by mayors and councils, community service organizations, groupings of mental health professionals, hospital trustees, or other local and state officials. The decisions so taken are crucial and commit the community (and especially the relevant agencies and institutions within it) just as completely, and with far less effort, as would a major public debate and popular vote. Indeed, this type of decision making may be preferable because it does not offer an occasion for the mobilization of the often virulent opponents of mental health activities, whether such opposition springs from ideological sources, from hostility to rival institutions, or from a desire to hold the public purse strings tight.

The extent to which there will be effective local control of community mental health centers when such are established is still to be determined as local treaties between the existing parties at interest are worked out. A federal program of locally controlled centers may well be foredoomed in many cases. Struggles which have already occurred between state agencies on the one hand and the advocates of substantial power for local boards of directors on the other are indicative of the conflict which can be expected when centers are dependent upon large subventions from state and federal funds.

Moreover, given the realities of local decision making, it is not at all clear that support for local control will be forthcoming from the communities themselves. In many parts of the country, mental health has long been viewed as primarily a *state* responsibility. In fact, Massachusetts has a Constitutional provision to this effect, although a monopoly is hardly evident in practice. However, this feeling persists among hardpressed municipal leaders, as evidenced in Houston by the mayor's attempt to disengage the city from any responsibility for health services. In view of the tremendous fiscal, organizational, and coordinative problems faced by urban governments (and especially central cities in metropolitan areas), it is hardly surprising that there is a marked lack of enthusiasm among many local officials about accepting responsibility for a potentially vast new function. They have all they can do to keep up with the mushrooming of what have traditionally been local functions.

The notion that mental health centers can be independent units each serving a restricted population and still integrated into the pattern of related social and medical services defies the realities of modern metropolitan living. Existing central city and suburban facilities and services are frequently intertwined, with specialized facilities in either place serving the entire area. It may well be argued that truly comprehensive mental health services can be provided most efficiently by a network of varied facilities dispersed across the whole of the metropolitan area. In that case it also could be argued that the cost should be borne by the entire area.

Since there are few cases in which a single municipal jurisdiction encompasses an entire metropolitan area, this suggests that the county, or counties, included in the metropolitan area should be the fiscal goat, or else that there should be a special district established for such services. However, suburbanites are reluctant to take any action which might appear to "bail out" a central city, even though the proposed activity would benefit them as well. Consequently, responsibility for community centers may shift to the state level, since state taxes, if adequately devised and collected, may approximate a fair taxing of a metropolitan area without requiring a political solution of central city–suburban hostilities or suspicions. However, to the extent that financing of community mental health services and centers is provided by larger units such as states and counties, the geographic area served will probably have less and less to do with existing communities and will move toward the service-area type.

Thus, while the original concept of community mental health services was based upon a substantial concern for the relation of such activities to the social and political construct of a specific community, the implementation of the program may well increasingly diverge from this ideal. A community mental health center is likely to serve a number of distinct communities and other areas as well which have no particular sense of being communities themselves or of belonging to the larger community in which the CMHC is located. Once such a center is established, it presumably will develop a "community of interest" insofar as mental health services and related activities are concerned. While this may be as much of a community as is possible in our fragmented and spatially extended conurbations, and while such enterprises may be locally controlled to varying degrees, what is likely to emerge seems a far cry from the somewhat romantic views of the originators of the idea. Still, the advantages of community involvement—acceptance of the notion of treating the mentally ill at home, enlisting the cooperation of related professionals, etc.—may well be achieved without requiring that mental health centers be established in some sociologically integrated and well-defined local political unit. These can seldom be found in any large metropolitan setting today.

In view of the difficulties of mobilizing local communities for action, it is perhaps not surprising that, so far as establishment of community mental health facilities has gone, the accomplishments have been much less than expected. By mid-1967 federal grants to the extent of some $77 million had been approved, of which approximately one-fourth went to projects located in four states—California, New York, Massachusetts, and Illinois—which already had the most mental health facilities. No grants had been made in Idaho, Mississippi, Montana, Nebraska, or Nevada, although grants were pending in several of these states. Moreover, publicly supported centers shared about equally with privately supported projects. The extent to which publicly supported projects drew their funds from local governments as opposed to state governments varied so much from state to state that no clear pattern emerged. But construction and staffing grants were made to a wide variety of public and private agencies including general hospitals, county and city mental health centers, and universities. Thus, one might conclude that, while some new community facilities were in the pipeline, probably few were in operation by mid-1967. Grants had been made to projects in five of the six metropolitan areas covered by field studies.

The five years' experience with the mental health program so far has been sufficient to lead to a series of conclusions regarding desirable courses of action for the future. In those states in which the planning process has brought together (often for the first time) disparate groups and individuals to develop a plan for publicly supported mental health programs, the process should not cease once the plan is devised and submitted. A planning body, broadly based, can serve in an advisory or even a policy-setting capacity. It can provide the most effective linkage between the professionally oriented agencies at the state and metropolitan levels and the communities they serve. It can also provide communications between professionals and lay leaders. The broad spectrum of community groups, organized for planning purposes, should be encouraged to remain organized for policy leadership and public support.

The field studies revealed, in some instances, a failure or inability to bring in politicians and community leaders at all stages in the development of mental health programs. In those regions dominated by voluntary programs the tendency has been to shy away from obtaining assistance from outside the mental health complex. Yet, community influentials, including business and professional leaders, mass media managers, and politicians in and out of office are vital to the successful support of a program. Since they are busy persons, a strenuous effort must be made personally and informally to secure their active participation. One must, for example, go far beyond the issuance of formal invitations to meetings. An active campaign of recruitment should be aimed at maximizing the involvement and contributions of nonprofessional leaders. At all levels, then, community leaders should be more directly involved in mental health planning and support.

Above all, however, a specific type of nonprofessional who is needed in the establishment and maintenance of community mental health centers is the lay community organizer. These persons are not those engaged in treating patients, but those who have an interest in organizing community support. They may be identified with one program or agency, or with the support of mental health activities generally. These activists, strongly committed to doing something for mental health, ought to receive special training and recognition for their labor. They can be particularly helpful in preparing the way for a new center.

Even more so than at the state level, coordination of mental health and related services is crucial at the local level. If the community mental health program is to be an integral part of the total social service complex, then coordination with related services is imperative. Coordination can take the form of joint referral services: coordinating boards to oversee cooperative services; regionwide coordinating councils, including representatives of public, professional, and citizen groups; and intergovernmental interdepartmental coordinating committees with action responsibilities. Such a system should be patient oriented, and its design should not lose sight of the need to assist the mentally ill. If the assumptions of the proponents of community mental health centers are correct, it follows that the community's resources must be developed and harnessed to provide a therapeutic environment for the mentally ill, and to identify those who are in need of assistance.

Some forms and manifestations of mental illness may be symptomatic of cultural deprivation. Mental health centers in poverty pockets will pose special problems, not only in therapy but in coordinating the functions of the center with the services directed toward alleviating conditions contributing to deprivation. The design of centers in poverty stricken sections of the community should take into account the special role imposed upon them by location.

Community leadership should encourage the expansion of insurance programs to cover mental health services along the lines of existing labor and industrial contracts. Labor and industrial contracts are usually restricted to inpatient services for a period of from sixty to ninety days, though firms such as General Electric and International Business Machines do provide for limited outpatient services. Close cooperation with officials of local insurance associations, particularly Blue Cross and Blue Shield, in developing broad insurance coverage should be maximized.

The practice in most communities has been to restrict services to persons with low incomes and, to be sure, no claim can be made that adequate facilities and services exist for the poor. But where this practice prevails, middle-class people pay the largest proportion of their income for mental health services. The wealthy patient can pay for private services, the poor may have services provided at public expense, or for minimal fees, but the middle class enjoys neither of these advantages. Income cut-off levels for services have not kept pace with inflation. In the new community mental health centers, fees should be minimal and services made available on a fee basis to the entire community, and fees should vary in proportion to income.

Patients and their families are less likely to object to inpatient services at general hospitals than to centers specifically designated as facilities for the treatment of mental illness. An additional advantage of close association is the availability of medical facilities. Community plans should recognize that the physical connection of community mental health centers to general hospitals offers realistic advantages. It may not be possible, however, to offer the array of services required of a mental health center within the physical confines of a hospital. Therefore, some treatment centers, even diagnostic centers, may have to be kept separate from the hospital. Administratively, however, such facilities might remain associated with the hospital; certainly such an association would facilitate acceptance by insurance companies of coverage for mental illness.

THE ORGANIZATIONAL INPUT

In the states and localities, mental health programs are administratively atomized. Unevenness in resources and achievements results from this condition. Atomization in the midst of governmental fragmentation may sound horrendous to the uninitiated; consequently they are prone to seek simple and rational organizations for programs. However, anyone familiar with American state and local government knows that simplistic solutions will never work, and that ingenious planning and sagacious administration will be required to bring about an acceptable level of mental health services throughout the land.

In states with weak mental health agencies, communities have had to rely on local, voluntary programs. The inevitable consequence has been inconsistent coverage and service and, most important, program isolation. Programs and organizations were set up as autonomously governed structures with little or no relation to other programs. A typical pattern is something like this: a psychiatric clinic here, a child guidance center there, each independently run, supported by private and community contributions with perhaps a direct grant from a federal or state agency for research, training, or, as in welfare cases, to cover services rendered. Such organizations generally owe their being to a board of lay and professional governors very likely led by a vigorous individual whose removal could lead to chaos and disaster.

Where public services are dominated by private, voluntary organizations, effective integration—if it comes at all—follows the establishment of individual units. Cooperation and coordination are usually limited to the needs of those who run the autonomous units. Integration is based largely on informal ad hoc arrangements and the establishment of communications networks, sometimes taking the form of referral services.

Integration of a sort may also be provided through the financial activities of Community Chests and United Funds. But such agencies do not concern themselves with the development of the broad spectrum of mental health services. Their interests are limited largely to funding what exists, to providing a balanced array of voluntary, community-supported social service programs of which mental health is but a part. They must maintain a realistic view of anticipated revenues and weigh these against the increased costs of services to which they are already committed. Community funding agencies are in no position to promote the massive increment of mental health facilities and services thought necessary by federal and state agencies.

Referral services, Community Chests, informal communications among professionals do not knit together mental health activities. Even in Boston, where local mental health associations have formed the backbone of existing programs, or in Minneapolis and Syracuse, where county programs are developing vigorously, the services are piecemeal. The splintering of mental health services and responsibilities at the local level indicates the need for a strong agency. If it is impossible to accomplish this locally, as seems likely, a strong state mental health agency would appear desirable.

A vigorous state agency to carry out mental health programs need not have separate departmental status. What is really important is the capacity to lead in the mental health field. Where such an agency should be placed in the pecking order of state governmental organization will vary from state to state. In some states it will be important for the agency to have independent status; in other states, combination with public health or welfare units will have significant advantages. Each state has its own governmental and political subculture and therefore it is difficult to prescribe a single organizational framework applicable to every state. A good state agency is one that has mastered the political culture of its state and provides program leadership and support, regardless of its location in the administrative structure.

Federal and state mental health officials should make more effective use of the governor's office and executive budget agencies. The growing importance of the chief executive in program development is one of the facts of life of American government. In those states with central budget agencies, usually attached to the governor's office, the instruments for initiative and support are such that the executive enjoys certain advantages over state legislatures. Battles are won or lost in the governor's office and, once lost, are difficult to retrieve through the legislature. But the governor's office, in view of the low priority usually attached to mental health, is not likely on its own to seek out the needs of a mental health program. The state mental health agency, therefore, must develop a procedure for making more effective use of the governor's office and executive budget agencies.

Typically, a number of state agencies provide services related to mental health other than the unit whose primary function is mental health. These include departments of education, of health, social welfare, and perhaps the department of institutions, corrections, or hospitals. In view of the universal existence of splintering in mental health, broad program coordination among agencies concerned becomes essential. One approach to solving this problem would be to create a social services coordinating council.

To be effective such a council should possess power, both political and administrative, and expertise. Thus, a two-tiered structure is suggested. One tier, composed of agency heads and a representative of the governor's office, might assign priorities to problems and adopt recommendations for solutions. A second tier composed of experts from the agencies might identify problems and prepare recommendations for resolutions of problems as assigned by the first tier.

Closely related to the problem of coordination is the planning process. The state mental health agency should develop a continuing planning mechanism that would collect essential data and draw up realistic short- and long-term projections. Planning for construction of centers and the development of programs should be a continuing process. Since planning to date has been primarily a state effort, it would appear most practical to continue at that level. However, larger metropolitan areas or cities should be given greater encouragement to plan for their areas.

The initial emphasis generally should be on policy planning, involving discussions among large groups of professional and lay leaders. From the continuing interaction of this process a clear pattern of professional and lay leadership should emerge. A necessary adjunct to policy planning, of course, is program planning executed by professional and administrative personnel who organize, collect, and process data and provide suggestions and alternatives to the policy groups. In the long run the costs of effective planning ought to be more than compensated for by more imaginative programs and better organizational arrangements. Moreover, the demands that a good planning program makes for the articulation of goals and for specificity in implementation help avoid shoddiness in operations.

One evident area of organizational improvement that deserves close attention is the utilization of the professional administrator. A psychiatrist who must spend all of his time in administration is depriving the community of a vitally needed resource. On the other hand, a professionally skilled administrator can provide mastery of the formal instruments and techniques of management, as well as serve as an effective link between professional personnel, other public agencies, and the community. Management, particularly public administration, is increasingly demanding and professionally oriented. A career professional administrator is probably better qualified to translate the needs of a public agency into effective legislation and budgetary requests than a person who regards himself as a psychiatrist first and administrator second. This is not to disparage those psychiatrists who have become brilliant administrators, but, given the anticipated increase in mental health facilities, full utilization of the growing profession of management may be crucial. Following the lead of hospital administration and the best practice in public and business administration, greater use ought to be made of professional administrators in the management of community mental health centers and other public psychiatric facilities.

One advantage of a professional administrator may be that he is trained to deal with the complexities of record keeping and communications. The establishment of community mental health centers means the involvement of many agencies. The problem of records communication becomes acute when many people in numerous professions are concerned with a patient's well-being. Systems of access to various kinds of psychiatric and medical information must be set up without jeopardizing the individual's status and dignity. An imaginative system of record keeping and records transfer is needed, designed to recognize both the patient's needs and his right of privacy. Adequate systems should therefore be devised for maintaining patient records, particularly within the network of community health and welfare services.

The Federal Input

The various practices of American federalism have modified relations within it, but do not alter the constitutional fact that the nation is a federal union of states. Action at the national level sparked the recent movement toward planning and programing in mental health throughout the country. The national impetus was twofold: program design and money. The outline of the program of community mental health centers was presented to the states. Money was made available for state planning, for the construction of centers, and, more recently, to aid in staffing the centers. As with any federal grant-in-aid program the theory holds that the option to accept the money and attendant obligations rests with the states. But the bait of money is not easy to resist and, even if rejected, can stimulate action.

The federal government had the option of dealing with the states or, alternatively, developing a system of direct relations with local communities and organizations within communities. By the mid-1960s ample precedent and rationale could be provided for either alternative, or a combination of the two. Even though state departments concerned with mental health varied from vigorous and successful to virtually nonexistent, it would have been a strategic error to have by-passed the states in program development and implementation. The state planning process has not always gone smoothly, but it has been especially important for the states with modest programs.

Working through state agencies also provides the most efficient means of helping the communities. Dealing with the fifty states is easier than dealing with thousands of local units of varying size, purpose, and capacity. Quite apart from the fact that local governments are legally creatures of the state, there were compelling, practical reasons for retaining strong state-federal relations.

Against the single standard and position of the federal government, states are disparate in their development and resources, in capacity and achievement, and in their manner of dealing with mental illness. Nevertheless, the state governments in the field studies, regardless of their level of achievement, have been the major contributors to mental health activities. The traditional state responsibility for the care of the mentally ill placed the states in a central position. If comparatively little state-sponsored or -supported local activity has taken place in Washington and Texas, it was not because of any absence of authority, but rather the lack of priority and direction. Four of the states studied had vigorous agencies and programs.

Whatever the level of state involvement in mental health, states still are the crucial building blocks of the federal system. Not only do they currently provide the bulk of the public expenditures for the care of the mentally ill, but they also exercise broad powers over what their local subdivisions can do. In many cases state-enabling legislation is necessary to allow local communities to provide the matching funds required by federal grants. Thus, states can exercise effective vetoes and state support may often be a prerequisite for local governmental involvement.

But state administrations across the board face increased program commitments, increased costs of current operations, and proportionately decreasing revenues. The states view the fiscal future with uncertainty. The fact that the fault may lie with inadequate revenue systems which skittish legislators are reluctant to reform does not remove the unfortunate reality. To compete effectively with time-honored high-priority programs, mental health advocates must move their programs closer to the front rank of pressing need. But in those states in which this has yet to be done, officials and others eager to champion the cause of mental health do not wield nearly enough influence to reorder priorities. The federal requirement that a state commit itself to long-range development of mental health services may prove to be one of several illusions held by federal mental health officials in their expectations of state and community support.

In light of this situation, it is not surprising that some states have not provided and may not be able to provide the vigorous leadership necessary to carry through implementation of the mental health program. Where this is the case the federal government should assist in strengthening the state mental health agency. This may appear deceptively easy. But if a state mental health agency is less than adequate, NIMH must be willing to bargain with the governor's office and be prepared to use its discretionary power over awarding grants and approving plans to ensure the development of a strong agency. This will have advantages for both the states and the federal government. The states will retain their role as full partner in the implementation of the program and the federal program will benefit from the state agencies' detailed knowledge of local problems.

If attempts to work through state agencies prove unsuccessful, NIMH should cooperate with local governmental units and voluntary agencies in arranging for demonstration and pilot projects. The primary purpose of demonstration units should not be to by-pass the state, but rather to foster local interest, which in turn might result in pressure on the state to become active. A few well-placed demonstration projects might spark action at the state level so that the traditional pattern thereafter could be utilized.

Even where vigorous state agencies exist, financial problems pose stumbling blocks. One major stumbling block is that federal grants-in-aid offer short-term grants for long-range problems. The federal program asks the states and local governments to make a long-range commitment to support each community mental health center constructed without a similar commitment on the part of the federal government, even though mental health is declared to be a national problem. In this situation, the political power structures in the states are understandably loath to place a long-term lien on their financial resources in the interests of a low-priority program. The action necessary here is clear. The federal government should recognize the problem of longe-range funding and take steps to ensure that the grant-in-aid program will provide long-term federal funds to match the long-range commitments of state and local finances to the mental health program.

Another major stumbling block is the cost-sharing formula established under the federal acts of 1963 and 1965. To assume that a substantial portion of the cost of construction and of annual operating expenses could be borne by the local community is, in most places, unrealistic. Local government revenue sources, severely tried, are the least flexible among the three levels of government. At the local level, competition for available money for government services is increasingly fierce. As a relative newcomer and at this juncture not powerfully organized in most places, mental health cannot be expected to compete successfully. Moreover, the fragmented governmental structure in metropolitan areas often means that large blocs of the potential financial resources are politically isolated from needy areas. And even in well-to-do areas the atomization of funds earmarked for special purposes often precludes diversion to new programs, however worthy. If the goal of a network of centers in communities across the country is to be realized within a reasonable time, the federal government should revise its grant program, not only to commit more money, but also to operate on a long-term basis so as to assure continuing support. Moreover, the cost-sharing formula should be revised to provide a much greater proportionate contribution by the federal government. This is particularly crucial in the poorer states, and not simply because their resources are limited. States differ not only in resources but also in the professional status that comes from participation in their program. Unless one assumes a missionary zeal on the part of mental health professionals far greater than has yet been demonstrated, one should expect that as the more prestigious states obtain federal grants to expand services they will siphon off manpower from those states where it is already scarcest. To avoid this effect and to reverse the present concentration of mental health professionals in the prosperous urban areas, it may be necessary to include a manpower bonus and incentive plan in the cost-sharing formula.

Moreover, the field studies have indicated that, with the possible exception of Boston, the development of community mental health programs depends upon the provision of manpower not presently available. Training programs should be intensified, even modified, to produce needed professional and nonprofessional personnel at an increasing rate. The federal government should make every effort to encourage state agencies and universities to expand their training services and facilities. Expanded grants for training programs and for fellowships and residencies are needed to fill the yawning gap. Further, NIMH should consider requiring persons trained under government auspices to render some sort of public service, with due compensation, of course, after receiving such training. Given the acute shortage of psychiatrists, for example, it makes little sense to use public funds to train a psychiatrist who goes into a private practice largely limited to the upper middle class. In short, the training efforts of federal and state agencies are basic to the accomplishment of community mental health programs and need great expansion.

The community mental health program demonstrates clearly the extent to which the traditional pattern of intergovernmental relations in the United States has been altered. The mix is indeed changing: in this and other programs federal initiative and financial capacity are directed at stimulating community action programs, and federal leadership is directly applied to what has traditionally been a state preserve. But, to paraphrase Mark Twain, reports of the demise of the federal system are greatly exaggerated. There have been, and will continue to be, important alterations in the roles of the national and state governments. But the changes have come about through a continuing process of bargaining, pressuring, inducing, bribing, supervising, demonstrating, harassing, encouraging, and publicizing. This has been a two-way relationship, with both levels learning, teaching, and adjusting.

Even during the period of the field studies, considerable improvement in mental health services could be observed. State and local mental health leaders want to be thought well of professionally by the federal bureaucracy so they constantly change and grow under the incentives that come from the bargaining process. They do not always admit that they change, perhaps because they do not want to admit that what they have done in the past was not adequate. Yet change they do, and similar flexibility is also necessary on the part of federal officials.

Indeed, it is this two-way relationship of adjustment that suggests the critical elements of the action necessary for the successful unfolding of the community mental health program. Organizational and governmental realities together with experience to date clearly indicate that, whatever the importance of other inputs, the *sine qua non* of the community centers program is the continued catalytic and structuring role of the federal government. It is at this level only that the conflict between programmatic ideals and practical problems of implementation can be readily reconciled. But even at this level, such reconciliation can occur only when professional zeal is adequately tempered by political adaptability and administrative flexibility. Thus, while successful implementation of the mental health centers program as envisioned by the legislation of 1963 does not call for abandoning the basic concepts inspiring the program's adoption, it will require a franker recognition of how dependent upon federal initiative and support those concepts are. A continued federal input of massive proportions is the crucial support that the professional, community, and organizational segments need and is therefore the keystone of the national community mental health effort.

INDEX

Action for Mental Health (Report of the Joint Commission on Mental Illness and Health), 42, 45–46
Administration, psychiatrists in, 152–53, 251; professional management, 583; *see also* Authority, mental health
Adrian, Charles R., quoted, 493
Adult Clinic (Syracuse), 290, 304, 320, 324, 325
Aftercare: New Orleans, 243; Syracuse, 301–2; Boston, 352; Minneapolis–St. Paul, 419, 425, 447
Aged, care of: Texas, 96; Houston, 104–5; New Orleans, 246; Massachusetts, 351, 353, 398
Agencies, mental health
——county: Houston, 108, 115, 129
——local: role in community care, 488–89; coordination of, 519
——private: Houston, 111–12, 115–17, 129; functions, 552; local importance, 553; potential for policy making, 554
——federal: Texas, 113–14; Boston, 347
——state: Texas, 102–3; Washington, 175–78, 182–83, 184–85, 187; Massachusetts, 352–55; Minnesota, 418–19
Albee, George W., 530
Alcoholism, treatment for: Houston, 100, 130; Washington, 172, 176, 198–99; Louisiana, 200, 239; New Orleans, 241, 244; Massachusetts, 352–53; Minneapolis–St. Paul, 416; Minnesota, 418
Amendment of 1965, 58–61
American Medical Association (AMA), 50, 52, 58–59, 546–47
American Mental Health Foundation, 53
American Neurological Society, 145
American Psychiatric Association, 61, 470, 547–48

Anti-Aid Amendment (Mass.), 349–50
Appel, Kenneth, 38
Associated General Hospital Psychiatrists (Boston), 367, 386, 392
Associations, mental health: Houston, 122; Washington, 186; Louisiana, 247, 261; New York, 307, 313, 319; Massachusetts, 368, 369; Minnesota, 438, 439; functions, 555; influence, 555–56; on mental retardation, 556
Asylums, 3, 12, 236–37
Authority, mental health: state variations of, 6; state tradition of, 584; *Texas:* early history, 98–99; Texas Department of Mental Health and Mental Retardation (*q.v.*); Texas Education Agency, 99–100; Texas Youth Council, 100; Commission on Alcoholism, 100; Child Welfare Clinic, 100; *Washington:* Department of Health (*q.v.*); Washington Department of Institutions (*q.v.*); rivalry, 179, 182–84; *Louisiana:* administration, 238; psychiatrists in, 251; Louisiana Department of Institutions (*q.v.*); *Syracuse:* and state policy, 289–90; county, 290–91; federal, 292; state monopoly, 303–4; county coordination, 317–18; dispute on, 324–26; *Massachusetts:* state monopoly, 347; multiple agencies, 354–55; federal-state-local relations, 347–51; Massachusetts Department of Mental Health (*q.v.*); *Minnesota:* state agencies, 418–19; Minnesota Department of Welfare (*q.v.*); vertical dispersal of, 447–48; and community centers act, 448–49

Baylor University, 106, 130
Beck, T. R., 13
Bellak, Leopold, quoted, 473